This book will be of great interest to all stakeholders in the HIV and AIDS response community. The authors and editors of this timely collection provide a much-needed interrogation of policy discourses that frame the "end" of HIV and AIDS in the near-term as a desirable and reachable goal. No one can argue with the objective of ameliorating the HIV pandemic, but language matters. Constructs, such as a "post-AIDS" era, an "AIDS-free generation," and "ending AIDS," do violence to people with HIV, who will continue to live with the disease for decades, even if new HIV transmissions are halted by 2030 as many campaigns aspire. The experience of people living with HIV and AIDS, which includes stigma, discrimination, marginalization, and criminalization, is not sufficiently captured by discursive structures that persistently reduce the pandemic to a biomedical, rather than a relational and social, phenomenon. The engaging historical, theoretical, and empirical analyses in this book interrogate the meanings that circulate around biological science claims – that virological suppression (resulting from use of antiretroviral drugs) leads to zero new HIV transmissions, which equals the "end of AIDS." They document the ways in which the persistent biomedicalizing of the HIV pandemic and its response shifts attention away from social and cultural processes that are as central to the story of AIDS – and to its ending – as is the virus itself.

Judith D. Auerbach, Sociologist and Professor of Medicine, University of California, Berkeley

Phrases such as "disease control," "elimination," and "eradication" are core concepts in public health; so central, in fact, that they deserve much greater exploration. This is true in general and in efforts to "End the Epidemic" of HIV in the US and around the world. Initiatives to end the HIV epidemic (ETE) tend to focus on epidemiological, clinical, and health disparities aspects of the epidemic. Often given less attention are examinations of critical sociological, psychological, anthropologic, and social justice factors in ETE efforts. For instance, what does it mean, symbolize, and experientially feel like to be a person living with HIV in a time when the epidemic is said to be ending? Will ending the epidemic be achieved in a way that addresses long-term comprehensive health and well-being for persons living with HIV? Will these efforts serve to address societal factors in a way that actually builds HIV-related health equity? These are just a few of the types of questions explored in "Post-AIDS." This volume is highly synergistic across a variety of disciplines and examines in a wide-reaching and nuanced manner the definition of a "post-AIDS" world and the societal characteristics of that future time. "Post-AIDS" is meant to challenge our traditional notions of what it means to end an epidemic, and to greatly expand our thinking about the core public health concepts of disease elimination and eradication.

David R. Holtgrave, Dean, SUNY Empire Innovation Professor, & Distinguished Professor, School of Public Health

Post-AIDS provides a necessary and scathing critique of the "end of AIDS" discourse. It is simultaneously an examination and an indictment of the ways that "end of AIDS" rhetoric is already driving trends, policy, funding, and programmatic priorities in the U.S. and globally – at unspeakable cost to people living with HIV, especially those who are Black, Indigenous, and people of color. The biomedicalization of the HIV response has left unanswered calls for basic dignity and humanity of those who are most vulnerable, for housing and food security, healthcare access, and compassion; our lives are measured not by joy or safety but in viral loads. A "post-AIDS" vision is quite frankly, impractical, when we understand AIDS as a syndrome of interlocking oppressive syndemics – racism, homophobia, transphobia, and criminalization of pleasure – which are far from over.

In the United States alone, there are over a million people currently living with HIV. There is no "post-AIDS" for us until we are cured or dead; in an era beyond AIDS we perhaps become relegated to an inconvenience to be overlooked, rather than a danger to be policed, surveilled, and controlled.

This book is required reading for anyone who considers themselves a human rights HIV activist in the 21st century.

Naina Khanna, Co-Executive Director of Positive Women's Network, USA

Post-AIDS Discourse in Health Communication

This book examines the discourse of a "post-AIDS" culture, and the medical-discursive shift from crisis and death to survival and living. Contributions from a diverse group of international scholars interrogate and engage with the cultural, social, political, scientific, historical, global, and local consumptions of the term "post-AIDS" from the perspective of meaning-making on health, illness, and well-being.

The chapters critique and connect meanings of "post-AIDS" to topics such as neoliberalism; race, gender, and advocacy; disclosure; relationships and intimacy; stigma and structural violence; family and community; migration; work; survival; normativity; NGOs, transnational organizations; aging and end-of-life care; the politics of ART and PrEP; mental illness; campaigns; social media; and religion. Using a range of methodological tools, the scholarship herein asks how "post-AIDS" or the "End of the Epidemic" is communicated and made sense of in everyday discourse, what current meanings are circulated and consumed on and around HIV and AIDS, and provides thorough commentary and critique of a "post-AIDS" time.

This book will be an essential read for scholars and students of health communication, sociology of health and illness, medical humanities, political science, and medical anthropology, as well as for policy makers and activists.

Ambar Basu is Professor in the Department of Communication at the University of South Florida.

Andrew R. Spieldenner is Executive Director of MPact: Global Action for Gay Men's Health & Rights and Associate Professor in the Departments of Communication and Women, Gender & Sexuality Studies at California State University-San Marcos.

Patrick J. Dillon is Associate Professor in the School of Communication Studies at Kent State University at Stark.

Routledge Research in Health Communication

1 Communicating Women's Health
Social and Cultural Norms that Influence Health Decisions
Edited by Annette Madlock Gatison

2 Culture, Migration, and Health Communication in a Global Context
Edited by Yuping Mao and Rukhsana Ahmed

3 Immigration and Strategic Public Health Communication
Lessons from the Transnational Seguro Popular Project
Edited by Robert C. Smith, Don J. Waisanen, and Guillermo Yrizar Barbosa

4 Post-AIDS Discourse in Health Communication
Sociocultural Interpretations
Edited by Ambar Basu, Andrew R. Spieldenner and Patrick J. Dillon

Post-AIDS Discourse in Health Communication

Sociocultural Interpretations

Edited by
Ambar Basu, Andrew R. Spieldenner
and Patrick J. Dillon

Routledge
Taylor & Francis Group
NEW YORK AND LONDON

First published 2022
by Routledge
605 Third Avenue, New York, NY 10158

and by Routledge
2 Park Square, Milton Park, Abingdon, Oxon, OX14 4RN

Routledge is an imprint of the Taylor & Francis Group, an informa business

Library of Congress Cataloging-in-Publication Data
A catalog record for this title has been requested

ISBN: 978-0-367-43048-1 (hbk)
ISBN: 978-1-032-07752-9 (pbk)
ISBN: 978-1-003-00094-5 (ebk)

DOI: 10.4324/9781003000945

Typeset in Galliard
by codeMantra

Ambar: This book is dedicated to my parents, *Baba, Kakima, Ma, Kaku.*
Andrew: This book is dedicated to all people living with HIV, including those who have transitioned.
Patrick: To Mom and Dad – thank you for your continued love and support.

Additionally, we, Patrick, Andrew, Ambar, also dedicate this book to Dan Brouwer's spirit, warmth, and ally-ship.

Contents

Figures and Tables

Figures

Picture

Tables

Contributors

Peter Aggleton is a social scientist with a background in sociology, policy studies, international development, and health. He is an Emeritus Scientia Professor in the Centre for Social Research in Health at UNSW Sydney, Australia, and holds honorary professorial positions in the School of Sociology at the Australian National University in Canberra, and in the Centre for Gender and Global Health at UCL in London. He is an Adjunct Professor in the Australian Research Centre in Sex, Health and Society at La Trobe University, Melbourne. Peter is well known internationally for his analytic work on the social aspects of HIV; youth, gender, and sexuality; and sexual and reproductive health and rights. His research interests concern equity, equality and citizenship and the ways in which gender and sexuality sit within the broader field of politics, national and international development, education and health.

Ambar Basu is Professor in the Department of Communications at the University of South Florida, USA. His research explores how individuals and communities living at the margins of society communicate about health, illness, and well-being. With particular emphasis on theorizing culture as a site of social change, his scholarship is committed to locating health inequities in the context of cultural, political, economic, geopolitical, and development agendas in marginalized spaces. Ambar has served as Senior Editor for *Health Communication* and co-edits a Routledge book series titled *Critical Cultural Studies in Global Health Communication.*

Nicola Bulled is a public health anthropologist and independent contractor based in the United States. Her scholarship interrogates health inequalities, using mixed methods to examine the intersection of biology with the social to offer multi-level perspectives on public health programming, service delivery, and policy. Her specific fields of interest include HIV, infectious diseases, disease prevention technologies, health communication, and community collaboration.

Roberta Chevrette is Assistant Professor in the Department of Communication Studies and Women's and Gender Studies Faculty at Middle Tennessee

State University, USA. Her critical rhetorical and qualitative research employs queer, feminist, and postcolonial frameworks to interrogate gendered and racialized formations of identity, belonging, and difference. She is co-author of the book, *Dangerous Dames: Representing Female-Bodied Empowerment in Postfeminist Media.*

Brianna R. Cusanno is a doctoral student in the Department of Communications at University of South Florida, USA. She uses qualitative and mixed methods research to examine the ways in which power, politics, culture, and identity influence and shape communication between patients and clinicians. Ms. Cusanno's work also explores how social justice organizing and narrative pedagogies can be incorporated into medical education. She has been awarded competitive grants at local and national levels, including a National Science Foundation Graduate Research Fellowship.

Patrick J. Dillon is Associate Professor in the School of Communication Studies at Kent State University in Stark, USA. Dr. Dillon's scholarship explores health inequality in contemporary society. He focuses, in particular, on advancing health communication scholarship in three primary areas: (1) end-of-life care, (2) HIV/AIDS, and (3) substance abuse. Dr. Dillon has served as a primary or co-investigator on funded research projects totaling over $1.6 million; his published scholarship appears in leading journals such as *Communication Theory, Health Communication, Psycho-Oncology,* and the *Journal of Substance Abuse Treatment.*

Gary W. Dowsett is Emeritus Professor and former Deputy Director (1997–2019) at the Australian Research Centre in Sex, Health and Society, La Trobe University, Melbourne, Australia. A sociologist, he has long been interested in sexuality research and the rise of modern gay communities. Since 1986, he has been researching HIV/AIDS in Australia and has undertaken many international HIV/AIDS and sexual health projects. He was Associate Professor in Sociomedical Sciences (2002–2005) and in Clinical Sociomedical Sciences (2005–2009) in the Mailman School of Public Health, Columbia University, New York, USA. In 2003, he was elected to the International Academy of Sex Research. In 2006, he was appointed to a Personal Chair in Sex, Health and Society at La Trobe University. In 2008, he was admitted as a Fellow of the Academy of the Social Sciences in Australia. In 2014, he was appointed Adjunct Professorial Fellow at the Centre for Social Research in Health, UNSW, Australia. His research focuses on sexuality; sexual health; HIV/AIDS; gay communities and cultures; men's health; and LGBTIQ+ experiences of cancer.

Mohan Jyoti Dutta is Dean's Chair in Communication in the School of Communication, Journalism, and Marketing at Massey University, New Zealand. He is the Director for Centre for Culture-Centered Approach to Research and Evaluation (CARE), developing culturally-centered, community-based projects of social change, advocacy, and activism that articulate health as a human right. Dutta's research examines the role of advocacy and activism in challenging marginalizing structures, the relationship between poverty and health, political economy of global health policies, the mobilization of cultural tropes for the justification of neo-colonial health development projects, and the ways in which participatory culture-centered processes and strategies of radical democracy serve as axes of global social change.

Scott A. Eldredge is Associate Professor in the Department of Communication at Western Carolina University in Cullowhee, North Carolina, USA. His scholarship explores family communication and health, as well as patient–provider interaction. Specifically, his research agenda is built around issues involving intimacy, uncertainty, trust, and relational development and maintenance. Using qualitative research methods, he examines how social and relational dynamics shape the management of health and health care.

Somrita Ganchoudhuri is Associate Faculty in the Centre for Communication Skills at the Singapore Institute of Technology, Singapore. Her scholarship explores communication inequalities in the health landscape. She uses research methods to examine various communication processes, strategies, and tactics to explore access to communicative spaces that leads to effective and equitable communication solutions.

Joy V. Goldsmith is Professor in the Department of Communications and Film, and Founder of the Center for Health Literacy and Health Communication at the University of Memphis, USA. Joy conducts research about communication and illness, specifically in the context of chronic illness. Joy co-authors a program of research named COMFORT, a communication-driven model and training system for improving healthcare communication and health literacy. Her numerous books and articles in clinical as well as communications journals address health literacy, communication training, oncology nurse training, interprofessional communication in healthcare, and family caregiver communication.

Satish K. Kedia is Professor in the Division of Social and Behavioral Sciences, School of Public Health at the University at Memphis, USA. He also has a certificate in Medical Behavioral Sciences from the Medical School at the University of Kentucky. His research interests include alcohol and drug abuse treatment and prevention, sexuality and HIV/AIDS, cancer, caregiving and adherence, and program evaluation and impact assessment. Dr. Kedia has received upward of $12 million in research grants as principal or co-investigator. He has published more than 90 research articles, book chapters, and edited volumes on various public health topics.

Nivethitha Ketheeswaran is a doctoral student in the Department of Communications at the University of South Florida, USA. Her research uses qualitative methods to understand health organizing as situated in colonialism. Nivethitha also explores decolonizing as a method of narrative healing through art, dance, and creative writing.

Bernice McCoy is a PhD Candidate in Applied Anthropology at the College of Arts and Sciences at The University of South Florida, USA. Her dissertation research uses a life-course approach to assess how the wider social, economic, and cultural context shape the lived-experience of aging with HIV and being diagnosed with HIV as an older adult. She focuses, in particular, on highlighting the experiences of African American men living with and aging with HIV in Hillsborough County, Florida, USA. In addition to capturing life experiences, she also assesses the quality of current services for these aging, minority adults and identifies strategies to maximize the effectiveness of these programs to best serve this population. Other research interests include the areas of medical anthropology, health equity, sexuality and sexual risk-taking, HIV/AIDS stigma, substance use and abuse, and women's health.

Richard Parker is a social scientist with a background in social anthropology, sociology, and the social and political dimensions of health. He is currently Senior Visiting Professor in the Institute for the Study of Collective Health at the Federal University of Rio de Janeiro, Brazil, and Professor Emeritus of Sociomedical Sciences and Anthropology at Columbia University, USA. For the past three decades, Richard has directed the Brazilian Interdisciplinary AIDS Association (ABIA), based in Rio de Janeiro, and for nearly two decades has served as Co-Chair of Sexuality Policy Watch, a global forum of researchers and activists from a wide range of countries and regions engaged in the critical mapping of conditions prevailing in sexual politics landscapes globally and locally. For more than fifteen years he has also served as the Editor-in-Chief for the journal, *Global Public Health*. His research has focused on the social and cultural construction of gender and sexuality, the social aspects of HIV and AIDS, the relationships between stigma, discrimination and social inequality, and the politics of global health.

Bre Rivera is the Founder and Program Officer of the Black Trans Fund (incubated by the Groundswell Fund), the first in the United States to center joy and liberation for Black trans communities. Having over 10 years of experience funding and resourcing communities, Bre serves as a board member of the Positive Woman's Network-USA, Transgender Resource Center of New Mexico, and Grantmakers for Girls of Color.

Jaime Shamado Robb is Assistant Professor at the Diederich School of Communication at Marquette University, USA. His scholarship explores health inequality in contemporary society. He uses qualitative research methods to examine how the day-to-day health experiences of marginalized populations are impacted by macro-level social forces, such as health policy, economic inequality, and racism. He focuses, in particular, on advancing health communication scholarship that engages critically with the experiences of individuals living at the margins of the dominant health system.

Nancy Romero-Daza is Professor in the Department of Anthropology at the University of South Florida, USA. As a medical anthropologist, her main areas of interest are HIV/AIDS, substance use and abuse, health of minority groups, sexual and reproductive health, food insecurity, and the political economy of health. She has conducted research in Florida, Connecticut, Puerto Rico, Costa Rica, Haiti, and Lesotho.

Ariel Sabillon is a first-generation Honduran-American on a mission to build bridges across space, time, and culture. Through years of experience in spiritual and emotional healing and self-directed study of the quantum universe, Ariel has been able to heal himself from trauma and forge a path for himself as a trailblazer. Ariel is a shamanic practitioner, healer, and seeker who, with the guidance and wisdom of his ancestors, is bringing forth the medicine required to maintain and build the vision of a unified prosperous Earth.

Andrew Spieldenner is Executive Director of MPact: Global Action for Gay Men's Health & Rights, and Associate Professor in the Departments of Communications and Women, Gender & Sexuality Studies at California State University-San Marcos, USA. Dr. Spieldenner's writing is at the intersection of health and culture, particularly looking at HIV and the LGBTQ+ community. A longtime HIV activist, Dr. Spieldenner currently serves as Vice-Chair of the United States People living with HIV Caucus.

Laurel Sprague is Chief, Community Engagement Division, at the Joint United Nations Programme on HIV/AIDS (UNAIDS). She came to UNAIDS from the Global Network of People Living with HIV (GNP+) where she served as Executive Director. Dr. Sprague has worked with, for, and as part of communities living with HIV since 1992, focused primarily on monitoring and challenging HIV-related stigma, discrimination, and criminalization. Since 2009, she has supported networks of people living with HIV in multiple countries and regions to implement the PLHIV Stigma Index. Previously, she worked with the HIV Justice Network and the Sero Project, both organizations focused on ending criminalization of people living with HIV, where she led their social science research activities and monitoring and evaluation efforts. From 2005 to 2015, she taught political science at Wayne State University in Detroit, USA.

B. Liahnna Stanley is a doctoral student in the Hugh Downs School of Human Communication at Arizona State University, USA. Her research accounts for health inequities for individuals and communities living at the margins, specifically Indigenous communities. She braids a mix of methods including critical qualitative research, creative writing, and poetry to study health experiences of Indigenous communities in the context of colonial structural forces. Her work centers interwoven Indigenous knowledges and ecologies to reimagine radical forms of Indigenous health and healing that are beyond Western perspectives of health.

Robert Suttle is a scholar-practitioner and activist. His professional interests and efforts have focused on movement-building, issues of social justice and inclusion, student affairs, and higher education. Robert is recognized as a leading consultant, speaker, and activist in the global HIV movement, advocating for meaningful involvement of communities most impacted, centering Black communities and communities of color, connecting his advocacy to decriminalize HIV to other movements around prisons, policing, and criminalization. He currently serves as a global advisor to the HIV Justice Network.

Sachiko Terui is Assistant Professor in the Department of Communications and Film and Co-Director of the Center for Health Literacy and Health Communication at the University of Memphis, USA. Her research interests include health disparities and intercultural aspects of communication. She uses both qualitative and quantitative research methods to address communicative challenges pertaining to linguistic and cultural aspects of health and health management, communication interventions, health literacy, and health disparities experienced among marginalized and underserved populations. Her recent projects center in interdisciplinary collaborations, including communities and healthcare organizations.

Acknowledgments

Ambar Basu: Patrick and Andy, thank you for your friendship and intellectual camaraderie. It has been such a joy working with you two! At Routledge, Suzanne (Richardson), thank you for your patience and continued guidance in these difficult times; my gratitude to Tanushree (Baijal) as well for your care and attention to detail in the last leg of this project. And an immense THANK YOU to our colleagues who contributed to this book!

My gratitude to my colleagues (staff, student, and faculty) in the Department of Communication at the University of South Florida. Thank you for the shared spaces and imaginaries! Steve Wilson and Patrice Buzzanell, thank you!

My dearest friends, Subhro, Munu, Mohan (Dutta), PD (Patrick Dillon), Ryan (D'Souza), Shaunak (Sastry), Iccha (Basnyat), Ratul (Anustup Basu), Monu (Manisha Basu), Rahul (Chakraborty) – thank you for indulging me!

Nanu (Viola), Bunu (Angsumala Tamang), Sellars (Dillon), thank you for being the warmth and comfort of family.

Muni (Ankur Pal), I am grateful for your unconditional diligence in taking care of our parents in the most onerous of times.

Babijaan (Kohana) and Munai (Mahuya Pal), thank you for your love, care, patience, and unblemished support, always, but especially over the past few months when we have had to negotiate grief and separation.

Andrew Spieldenner: I am lucky enough to be part of a large network of support, friendship, and family. Thanks to my co-editors Ambar Basu and Patrick Dillon for their constant grace and dedication. This book emerged from conversations over the years with Jeffrey Escoffier, Robert Vazquez-Pacheco, Daniel Brouwer, George Ayala, Martin French, Shinsuke Eguchi, Tomeka Robinson, Gust Yep, Debanuj Dasgupta, Heather Harris, Kimberly Moffitt, Ronald Johnson, Ariel Sabillon, Barb Cardell, Naina Khanna, Charles Stephens, Vanessa Johnson, Laurel Sprague, Vince Crisostomo, Sean Strub, Marco Castro-Bojorquez, Miriam Vega, Phill Wilson, Julian Carter, Stephanie Hsu, Julia Johnson, Cecilia Chung, Kali Lindsey, Satoshi Toyosaki, Alex Garner, Deion Hawkins, Gary Dowsett, Christopher Turnbull, Sean Sasser, Wilson Ong, Douglas Yaranon, Reggie Williams, Deloris Dockrey, and Ron Simmons. While some have passed, their imprint remains on my thinking and writing. I have been nurtured through the editing process by meals, texts, and long calls with Phillip Baskerville, Kimberly White-Smith, Chloe White-Smith, Cary Robertson, Elijah Robertson, Cecilia "Lia" Uy-Tioco, Roddrick Colvin, Carlos Ramirez, Michael Pearl, Josiah Jennings, Aaron Foster, Lore/tta LeMaster, Gloria Pindi, Katherine Brown, Ranjeeta Basu, Claudia Calhoon, Jules Kim, Jonathan Gunthorp, Alexander Pastoors, Ruth Morgan Thomas, Judy Chang, Amistad St. Arromand, Judi Tidwell, and the Spieldenners: Lien, Bob, Francis, Patrick, and Mai Lien. Thanks to the Golden Girls – Kevin Williams, Bolivar Nieto, and Christian Castro – for surprise adventures and always being there. Finally, my dog Ace died while editing this book after 15 years together. I miss you, Ace.

Patrick Dillon: This project has been a significant undertaking, and I am immensely proud of the way that it has come together. I am also incredibly thankful for all the people who made it possible.

Thank you to my co-editors, Ambar and Andy, I could not have asked for better collaborators; you are both wonderful scholars and even better friends. To our contributors, thank you for putting your faith in us to showcase your work as part of this volume; I appreciate your collective dedication and enthusiasm for this project and can't wait for others to read the wonderful chapters you have written. A special thank you to my chapter co-author, Satish; it's been a great honor to partner with you over the past several years. Thanks as well to Suzanne, Tanushree, and the rest of the team at Routledge for believing in this project and guiding us through the publication process.

Thank you to my wife, Maggie, for being a constant source of love and encouragement; I am continually grateful for the chance to build a life with you. To my two boys, Liam and Graham, thank you for making my life so much fun and always reminding me to make time for what's most important. Thanks as well to my parents, Tim and Trish, and my brother, Mike; I appreciate you pushing me to be my best but always having my back even when I am not. Thank you to my extended family members, friends, and neighbors for supporting my work – and for humoring me when I spend too much talking about it.

Thank you to everyone in my hometown of Flint, MI – especially my teachers, coaches, and other mentors – for positively impacting my life in more ways that I can name. Thank you also to all my professors and fellow students at Central Michigan University and the University of South Florida; I appreciate you believing in me and helping me realize my dreams. Finally, thanks to all my current and former colleagues from the University of Memphis and Kent State University; your commitment to being great educators and producing meaningful scholarship inspires me every day.

Dreaming a Post-AIDS

An Introduction to the Discourse

Ambar Basu, Andrew Spieldenner and
Patrick J. Dillon

In 2014, the Joint United Nations Programme on HIV/AIDS (UNAIDS) proclaimed a fast-track to ending AIDS by 2030 (see UNAIDS, 2014). In March 2021, UNAIDS reiterated this lofty goal (UNAIDS, 2021). National governments and international public health organizations appear to have a plan to end the HIV epidemic by 2030. In the United States of America (U.S.), the federal Centers for Disease Control & Prevention (CDC) has funded End the HIV Epidemic (EHE) plans in every state (https://www.cdc.gov/endhiv/index.html). On February 5, 2019, former U.S. President Donald Trump announced that the fight against AIDS was almost won and that HIV transmission would be eliminated in America and the rest of the world by 2030. Soon after Trump's declaration came widespread media attention to an article published in *Nature*, which reported that a previously HIV-positive man living in London may have been "cured" following a bone marrow transplant (Gupta et al., 2020). These stories and declarations dovetail with the recent public health discourse on worldwide HIV and AIDS initiatives, namely, the "90 – 90 – 90" (i.e., 90% diagnosed, 90% receiving treatment, 90% virally suppressed; UNAIDS 2014) rhetoric, which is similar to the World Health Organization's 2015 promise of ending the AIDS epidemic (WHO, June 2015).

During and following the XI International AIDS Conference (1996) in Vancouver, the term "post-AIDS" began to circulate in mainstream medical and public health discourse. In 2013, O'Brien wrote that the watershed success of the HAART (Highly Active Antiretroviral Therapy) cocktail in allowing people to continue living with HIV "as opposed to dying from AIDS" led to "what commentators term a 'post-AIDS' culture, whereby a discourse of crisis and death has evolved into one of survival and living" (p. 74). Close to three decades into this medical-discursive shift, questions are being – and need to be – raised on what "post-AIDS" signifies and how the idea is communicated. Are we really in a "post-AIDS" culture where U(undetectable)=U(untransmittable)[1] is a moniker for "living well[2]" with HIV and AIDS? This edited volume will present essays that interrogate and engage with the sociocultural interpretations of the "post-AIDS" discourse.

Sontag (1989) wrote about the early days of AIDS, and the pathogenic and moral/cultural decay associated with it. Living with HIV and/or AIDS was

DOI: 10.4324/9781003000945-1

certainly not a "living-well" condition. Sontag successfully highlighted the unpleasant metaphors/meanings associated with AIDS. Walker (2020) and Mazanderani and Paparini (2015) note that there is a shift in the meanings associated with AIDS, and, as always, these meanings matter. In other words, the communication (i.e., meaning making) of and about HIV and AIDS matters, more so now than ever before. Walker questions the prevailing attributions to AIDS, chiefly those that allude to being in a "post-AIDS" time, because, she says, the sociocultural and geopolitical entrenchment of HIV and AIDS prevention and cure continue to (un)balance medical-technocratic progress towards a "normal" life with AIDS. Walker explains:

> In the context of HIV and AIDS, language has always been a crucial tool used to generate and perpetuate attitudes and approaches...the language of AIDS matters and, in this context, the language of 'post-AIDS', in particular, has its own semantic and linguistic resonance ... to be a citizen with HIV in the 'post-AIDS' era, means...embodying a quite new HIV identity...'Post-AIDS' is premised not just on the political and economic commitment to treatment and prevention but, fundamentally, on the 'normalisation' of HIV.
>
> (p. 9437)

Comprehensive scholarship on "post-AIDS" complexities is, however, rare. Most articles and books on this topic focus on particular communities, more specifically the gay community (in the West) and their experiences (Butler, 2004; Rofes, 1998). While the gay community in the West has been a torchbearer of modern AIDS social movements, this singular focus on a particular group of individuals (at the risk of homogenizing gay individuals and their communities) risks erasing the enormity of the local and global efforts required to reach the HIV-free-world target. After all, there are large pockets of global spaces that do not have access to HIV medical therapies; the stigma of living with HIV and AIDS still overshadows activists' efforts even in the "developed" Western world; gender and work-related structural violence, as well as neoliberal agendas of the security–health–commerce nexus, are still pertinent to HIV prevention and cure (Basu, 2017, Dillon, Basu, & Romero-Daza, 2016; King, 2002).

What then are the current meanings circulated and consumed on and around HIV and AIDS? What are the commentaries and critiques of a "post-AIDS" time? Are we really living in such a time? The turn of the US federal website "aids.gov" to "HIV.gov" supports this symbolism. The current use of the term "HIV" and the reduction in the use of the term "AIDS" ostensibly reflects scientific and medical understanding of the disease, but it also demands a change in personal, organizational, and discursive identities. Where once "person living with AIDS" and "person living with HIV" were considered different in terms of both identity (AIDS was considered closer to dying) and access to certain governmental benefits (such as housing and food vouchers) and treatments (including medications against pneumocystis pneumonia), they are now collapsed and utilize other biological and social markers to determine access to these treatments and benefits. What, then, are the multiple intersections of meanings and materiality (Mazanderani & Paparini, 2015) associated with a "post-AIDS" temporality, a context that is marked by public health experts discussing functional cures of HIV and claiming that HIV virologic suppression reduces the possibility of disease transmission to zero? While the science behind virologic suppression is not being challenged, the meanings that circulate around the science claims must be interrogated.

The essays in this book connect with the cultural, social, political, scientific, historical, global, and local consumptions of the terms "post-AIDS" from the perspective of meaning-making on health, illness, and well-being. They typically respond to a primary research idea that guides this book project, which is: How is "post-AIDS" or the "End of the Epidemic" communicated/made sense of in everyday global–local discourse? The essays map meanings of "post-AIDS" to topics such as neoliberalism, race and gender, advocacy, indigeneity, disclosure, relationships, stigma, family and community, survival, transnational organizations, aging and end-of-life care, HAART and PrEP (Pre-exposure Prophylaxis), campaigns, and social media.

Structure of the Book

The book's essays are presented in two interconnected sections. The first, called, "Debate, Discourse, Politics," offers first, a historiography of the "post-AIDS" discourse, and then, several debates on global–local politics that nuance this discourse. The second section, titled, "Rhetoric and Relations," teases out linkages between relational (interpersonal, family, and community) networks and the "post-AIDS" phenomenon.

Section I: Debate, Discourse, Politics

The first essay, "Revisiting "Post-AIDS:" Understanding Gay Community Responses to HIV Then and Now," **by** Gary W. Dowsett, Richard Parker, and Peter Aggleton, is a seminal piece that lays the foundation for our deliberations on the "post-AIDS" concept(s). This essay is a historiography of "post-AIDS," a term first coined and put on the world stage in 1996 by Gary W. Dowsett, the essay's first author. This is a must-read for anyone interested in our book and for any and all interested in the global history and politics of HIV and AIDS. Dowsett, Parker, and Aggleton trace the trajectories, politics, and fissures that have characterized the discourses on HIV and AIDS in the past 50-odd years. They note that the term "post-AIDS" — as it was initially framed — is distinct from its contemporary "end of AIDS" usage(s). The "end of AIDS" story is a mirage; as they note, it is "a fantasy world that almost completely ignored the grim reality on the ground, largely disconnected from grassroots experience and invented in conferences and board rooms." Dowsett and co-authors argue that the narrative that we are almost into the "post-AIDS" era is spearheaded by a global initiative to re-biomedicalize HIV and AIDS – a move away from the community-centered socio-cultural movements to address living contexts of those affected or likely to be affected by HIV and AIDS – that gained prominence in the early 2000s.

We find a similar logic put forth in the essay "Biocommunicability and the Biopolitics of 'post-AIDS'" by Nicola Bulled. According to Bulled, AIDS remains the "epidemic of the poor," "rarely mentioned in public discourse beyond grand announcements of an 'end to AIDS.'" This public silence, however, Bulled states, does not reflect the lived realities of people living with HIV (PLHIV). Bulled's essay presents a content analysis of "recent reporting on three diverse responses to PrEP for HIV prevention: public media campaigns to promote consumer demand in the U.S., public activism to obtain access to PrEP in the U.K., and highly restricted PrEP distribution in South Africa." Bulled uses concepts of "biocommunicability" to conclude that current health reporting continues to "operate as a form of governmentality, reducing agency, increasing risk, and perpetuating disease." Bulled defines "biocommunicability" as a "set of normative assumptions regarding the production, circulation, reception, and valuing of biomedical information – and biomediatization – the co-production of biomedical knowledge." In South Africa, for example, Bulled explains, media portrayals of successful treatment programs belie the continued existence of "gender-based socio-economic disparities, gender power dynamics, and a lack of female-controlled HIV prevention options." Bulled concludes that critical attention must be afforded to how media as "biopolitical agents" that largely frame "post-AIDS" discourse manufactures consent about "who is deserving of access to PrEP and … justifying restrictive and discriminatory access policies."

The next essay by Andrew Spieldenner, Laurel Sprague, Robert Suttle, Ariel Sabillon, and Bre Rivera, entitled, "Last people Standing: People Living with HIV after the 'End of the Epidemic,'" is a scathing critique of the "end of the epidemic" narrative by a "community of people living with HIV." Written as a conversation between the authors and presented seemingly as a rejoinder to those in charge of framing and eulogizing a nearly-there "post-AIDS" condition, this essay is a vindication of the violence(s) inflicted on PLHIV through an "end of epidemic" discourse. The authors write:

> You promised this would be over, but it's only over for you. You wanted us to be compliant patients, taking our pills. But some of us do not have healthcare, some of us are dealing with jobs and housing and mental health and discrimination.
>
> Your vision of the "End of the HIV Epidemic" is not the same as ours.

Spieldenner and co-authors present their bodies as evidence of continuing AIDS-related violations; they demand an end to the narrative about the end of AIDS: "What is – exactly – ending? We hold the disease in our bodies, and barring a cure, this will not change. Many of us are marginalized across identities and these produce particular vulnerabilities. How do these end?" Spieldenner and co-authors agree that neither treatment access nor a drop in transmission can be a marker of the "end of AIDS." An end to HIV and AIDS should mean a suitable addressal of structural violations that "facilitate risk – stigma, mental health, lack of healthcare, racism, sexism, transphobia, homophobia, prisons, religion (the church in the US), homelessness, and people-first treatments," they add.

The connections between structural violence and the "post-AIDS" utopia are carved out further in the next essay, "A Dramatization of post-AIDS stigma: A Pentadic Analysis of the CDC's 'Let's Stop HIV Together' campaign." The author, Jaime S. Robb, dissects the CDC's "Let's Stop HIV Together" campaign, noting that it promotes a clear "post-AIDS" framework without accounting for the social and structural realities of people who are either living with or are most vulnerable to HIV and/or AIDS. Inspired by Kenneth Burke, Robb's analysis notes that the CDC campaign "celebrates the medical advancements for treating and managing HIV/AIDS" but "utilizes various rhetorical moves ... to flatten the multiple economic and political constraints that accompany surviving with HIV/AIDS in the 'post-AIDS' world." Robb explains that the CDC campaign begins as a message of de-stigmatization but quickly pivots to focusing on PrEP as a sort of panacea towards an "AIDS-free society." The author surmises that any attempt to move towards a "post-AIDS" utopia should, at the very least, make efforts to "recognize the linkages between structure and culture, agency and voice, the notion of multiple and shifting contexts, and spaces of resistance" for individuals and communities vulnerable to HIV and AIDS. Hence, there is a need for a shift away from PrEP and towards "highlighting the array of lived experiences that show the complexities involved in living with HIV/AIDS from various class and cultural perspectives." This focus on PrEP, and the corresponding possibilities of governmentality and surveillance that such a focus creates, is revisited in Roberta Chevrette's essay in Section II of this book.

The linkages between structural violence, HIV and AIDS, and strategies of resistance and survival are presented in the next chapter, titled, "Indigenous HIV/AIDS in the Context of 'Post-AIDS' Discourse: A Meta-synthesis of Qualitative Research." Authors B. Liahnna Stanley, Nivethitha Ketheeswaran, and Brianna R. Cusanno synthesize 14 published qualitative research articles that engage with how "Indigenous Peoples of the Americas living with HIV and/or AIDS ... discuss the health implications ... in the context of contemporary 'post-AIDS' discourse." Stanley and co-authors present three broad themes: "(a) Structural and Symbolic Violence, (b) (Silently) Making Sense of HIV/AIDS and Identity, and (c) Resilience, Agency, and Resistance." The authors argue that Indigenous Peoples' health and HIV/AIDS experiences must be located in the context of the historical colonization they have faced and continue to face. "Post-AIDS" is part of a colonial project, they add, one that works to "further marginalize Indigenous health." Drawing from Syndemics Theory to story an integrated and holistic ideation of health and healing, Stanley, Ketheeswaran, and Cusanno critique the biomedical mechanization of health evident in the "post-AIDS" narrative and point to the resulting erasure of local Indigenous realities that actually inhere health meanings, rituals, and strategies. They explain,

"The notion of 'post-AIDS' promotes colonial ideals that carve deep, cognitive and cultural erasures of health and healing while simultaneously superimposing modalities of health that reduce health to an isolated biomedical issue."

The final essay in Section I is titled, "Neoliberal Hegemony and National HIV/AIDS Policy in India." Authors Somrita Ganchoudhuri and Mohan Jyoti Dutta argue that dominant discourses on HIV and AIDS in India, created and sustained by the National AIDS Control Organization (NACO) and its affiliated state units, perpetuates a neoliberal logic of "individualist intervention" promoted by the NGO–pharma–Global North[3] axis. "Diseased bodies become sites of intervention and markets for pharmaceutical companies keeping 'humanitarian reasons' and greater 'self-protection' in mind while facilitating the neoliberal agenda of free enterprise and private property," they note. This neoliberal agenda, Ganchoudhuri and Dutta claim, frames the "the risk agenda of national control around the high-risk individual, decontextualized from the structural contexts of HIV/AIDS." The authors point to a paradox in this neoliberal ideology and its claim to ending AIDS in that the Indian state's campaign to end AIDS "constitutes impossibilities of eliminating HIV/AIDS" because NACO's "end of AIDS" rhetoric is essentially directed towards re-structuring health as a "private commodity" for transnational profit, and for "dismantling the existing public health systems, and introducing large-scale precarities" that cause *(more)* violence to the margins.

Section II: Rhetorics and Relations

Section II of our book includes essays that plot the debates, histories, and discourses on "post-AIDS" to the domain of relations, thus making obvious the networks between macro-, meso-, and micro-communicative structures. Policies, campaigns, and debates constitute discursive structures at the macro and meso levels, they prop up other meso-level and micro-level communicative and material structures such as stigma, lack of access to health, and lack of social support, which in turn tune the notes that influence micro-level interpersonal relations, and meso-level family and community communicative rules, rituals, habits, and relations. The essays in this section highlight lived experiences that coalesce around exigencies related to living with or being vulnerable to HIV and AIDS.

The first essay connects "post-AIDS" to the concept of social death. In their essay titled "'I might as well be dead': Aging with HIV in the 'Post-AIDS' Era," authors Bernice McCoy and Nancy Romero-Daza explain that for older PLHIV, "post-AIDS" era medical benefits that help to prolong life obfuscate the "challenges of the aging process while living with a heavily stigmatized disease." Isolation, invisibility, and rejection in social networks characterize their social death, even as these older PLHIV continue to be poster-exemplars of a "post-AIDS" medicalization that keeps them biologically alive. This essay "presents the life stories of six African American men – three diagnosed in the pre-HAART era and three after the advent of HAART – and their personal philosophies on life and death in the 'Post-AIDS' era." As we witness the "greying of the epidemic,"

McCoy and Romero-Daza explain that the biomedical industry's predilection towards prevention often absents PLHIV from the prevailing AIDS discourses. As an instance, they quote one of their research participants:

> HIV is so mainstreamed now...so much is focused on prevention and so that those of us who've been living with it for so long are sort of being forgotten. Which don't get me wrong, [prevention] is good, but, don't forget about us! A lot of programs that were once available back in the day have kind of fallen to the wayside. We [individuals living with HIV] are all lumped together now, but we aren't all the same.

McCoy and Romero-Daza conclude that "social death adds an additional layer of exclusion to a population already plagued by multiple social inequalities" based on, among other things, HIV status, sexual identity/orientation ageism, and homophobia.

Patrick J. Dillon and Satish K. Kedia elaborate on similar exclusions, particularly (those brought forth by) the stigma that African American women living with HIV encounter in their daily lives. In their essay, "The Continued Impact of HIV-related Stigma on African American women: A Meta-ethnographic Synthesis of Qualitative Research," Dillon and Kedia, like other authors in this book, argue that "post-AIDS" discourses "overlook the daily challenges of living with HIV," which is a particularly salient omission when it involves "groups who encounter intersectional vulnerabilities" such as "African American mothers living with HIV." The authors use the socioecological framework to identify important structural/social, interpersonal, and individual-level factors that impact these women's lives. They note that these factors "offer insight" into the disconnect between "post-AIDS" discourse and the realities of living with HIV. "The success of biotechnical innovations such as antiretroviral therapies (and, more recently, pre-exposure prophylaxis) have undoubtedly transformed the experience of living with HIV and emboldened policy makers to cast an optimistic vision of a 'post-AIDS' world. However, suggesting that the proliferation of these technologies signal that society has moved beyond HIV is a misplaced notion," Dillon and Kedia argue. They add that, for African American mothers, living with HIV brings with it stigmatized conditions that affect "every area of their lives – contributing to negative health outcomes, limiting their ability/willingness to seek needed social support, and compromising their ability to care for themselves and their children."

The next essay in this section, "'YOU FUCKING DESERVE HIV:' Seeking PrEP Information, Disciplinary Power, and Queer Technologies of the Self on /r/AskGayBros," by Roberta Chevrette, identifies how disciplinary technologies are reproduced in conversations between members on the subreddit AskGayBros. Through a critical analysis of these conversations using Foucault's technologies as a theoretical framework, Chevrette points to how these conversations challenge PrEP as biomedical technology purported to end AIDS. The technologies of production, technologies of power, technologies of signs, and technologies of the self allows Chevrette to "examine how contemporary gay subjects navigate contradictions inherent in 'post-AIDS' discourses." "Among these contradictions," the author asserts, "is the fact that, through successful treatments, it has now become possible to live a healthy life as a person who is HIV positive, and yet HIV stigma remains pervasive .... Livable lives needs to be looked at vis-à-vis the call to end AIDS, for till lives with AIDS become livable, there can be no end to AIDS."

"It is against this backdrop of stigmatization, an ever-present disease threat, a myriad of relationship choices, and a 'post-AIDS' discourse dismissing the disease as any real threat that HIV negative men attempt to form close, romantic partnerships," notes Scott Eldredge, the author of the next essay, "Intimacy Uncertainty and post-AIDS Discourse: HIV and the Role it Plays as an Uninvited Third Party in Serodiscordant Relationships." Eldredge, like authors of several other essays in this book, punctures the feel-good claims about an AIDS-free world through mere adoption of appropriate medical technologies. The author sheds light on how uncertainties (via living with HIV/AIDS) play out in intimate relationships between serodiscordant partners. Drawing on in-depth interview data, this essay presents the "experience of nine HIV negative partners of gay men living with HIV." Eldredge explains that HIV and AIDS still sit "at the center of issues salient to conceptualizations of intimacy within these relationships, causing these men to both reflect on their past experiences and understandings of the illness, as well as contemplate both their personal future, and future of their relationships." The prevailing "post-AIDS" discourse, the author maintains, has successfully subsumed the relational realties associated with living with HIV and/or AIDS, the reality that, "20 years after that 'end-of-AIDS' moment Rofes (1998) writes about, gay men are still struggling to manage uncertainties related to HIV and intimacy, both physical and emotional, as they attempt to form and maintain committed, romantic partnerships."

It is quite evident in the essays discussed above that the "end of AIDS" vocabulary needs to pay substantive attention, among other issues (some discussed in our essays), to the lived realties of those most affected, or likely to be affected, by HIV and/or AIDS. The next essay in this book offers us a glimpse into how one might begin to do so. Sachiko Terui and Joy V. Goldsmith report on the processes of delivering a visual health literacy resource, focused on HIV, for undergraduate students in a large U.S. city. In their essay, "The Experience of Building and Testing a Visual Health Literacy Resource for HIV Prophylaxis," Terui and Goldsmith write that "undergraduate students received training and delivered communication-centered HIV interventions to their peers using the Social Network Strategy in Memphis, TN – a city with high HIV transmission rates." Analysis of the intervention data revealed that "the use of visual aid produced stronger assessments of HIV as non-deadly disease" and HIV-related stigma emerged as a critical component of the prevailing narratives on HIV among students who participated in the project. A vital part of similar interventions could, thus, be a focus on socio-cultural contexts of HIV and/or AIDS, including persistent stigma, instead of one on the medical technology–surveillance axis promoted by the CDC and comprised of diagnosis, prevention, treatment, and response.

Concluding Remarks

The authors of the essays in our book have marked "post-AIDS" variably. As editors, we tried our best to stay true to the authors' interpretation(s) and usage of the concept. Our goal was to curate for our readers a broad canvas that documents these unique dispersions vis-à-vis any attempt to design any order or singularity. We believe that the formulation and sustained diffusion of the term "post-AIDS" runs a remarkable danger of medicalizing and homogenizing the multiple and ongoing struggles related to HIV and AIDS. In a way then, our goal in presenting this collection of essays is political, in that we attempt to counter the dominant monolithic discourse that the global society as a whole, and the Global North (which has dictated most HIV and AIDS policies and practices) in particular, purports, which is that we are poised to enter an HIV-free era. Each essay in this book challenges this dominant "post-AIDS" discourse.

This edited collection also marks a pivotal moment in our research careers. All three of us – i.e., the book's editors – have been invested in scholarship on HIV and AIDS for multiple years. In our research with communities at the margins, such as poor female sex workers, transgender women in sex work, African American mothers living with HIV, and minority men who have sex with men, we increasingly stumbled upon a fragmented discourse on HIV/AIDS and health. While some of our research participants made sense of HIV/AIDS as a manageable condition, several others emphasized the intricately localized urgencies that condition how they make sense of HIV/AIDS. These localized problem–solution determinations appeared to contradict the monolithic sanitized picture that a "post-AIDS" narrative put forward. Several groups of our research participants did not have access to HAART and other urgent health services; they were subjected to debilitating socio-cultural sanctions that adversely affected their health and lives. HIV and AIDS was critical to how they made sense of and performed health, quite unlike the projected "post-AIDS" scenario of living comfortably with HIV and/or AIDS. As government and multilateral agencies become oriented around "post-AIDS" and look towards an ending in resourcing and political capital around HIV, those people marginalized in society and vulnerable in the HIV epidemic will remain in danger. An interrogation of this "post-AIDS" phenomenon was, thus, apt and politically pressing.

We also view this work as a starting point for the broader engagement of "post-AIDS" discourse(s) among health communication scholars. While health communication researchers publish their work broadly, we find it noteworthy (and a bit disheartening) that there is a dearth of "post-AIDS" scholarship featured in the discipline's two most prominent journals: *Health Communication* and the *Journal of Health Communication*. A quick search of these publications reveals that there are only two explicit references to "post-AIDS," which can both be found in recent issues of *Health Communication* (Hajek, 2019; Kedia, Dillon, & Basu, 2020); there are similarly limited references to the "end of AIDS" (de Souza, 2007) and efforts to "end the epidemic" (Khan, 2020; Wilson, Bleasdale, & Przybyla, 2020). A closer examination of these manuscripts reveals that the authors primarily mention these issues in passing – e.g., when positioning their study within the broader HIV-related discourses (de Souza, 2007) or considering the implications of their findings (Kedia et al., 2020) – rather than making them the focus of their analysis. As evidenced by the essays included in this volume, we believe that health communication researchers (and those from related disciplines) have much to contribute to the burgeoning "post-AIDS" literature; hence, we further position this work as an invitation for our disciplinary colleagues to join the book's contributors in further examining/interrogating the various meaning and implications of "post-AIDS" discourse(s). As Gary W. Dowsett, Richard Parker, and Peter Aggleton, co-authors of the first essay in this book, note: "Put quite simply, the 'end of AIDS' is nowhere in sight."

Notes

1 *U=U – a contemporary framing of the undetectable=untransmittable notion with regard to HIV viral suppression.
2 On its website, the U.S. Centers for Disease Control and Prevention (CDC) presents narratives of people living well with HIV. Aaron notes, "*HIV, taking my meds makes you undetectable. And that makes me unstoppable.*"
3 We use the term "Global North" to signify those geopolitical cultures and networks across the globe (and beyond human-mapped boundaries) that continue to control global resources, wealth, and power. This means that there indeed are pockets of the "Global North" in "developed" countries and vice-versa.

References

Basu, A. (2017). Reba and her insurgent prose: Sex work, HIV/AIDS and subaltern narratives. *Qualitative Health Research, 27*(10), 1507–1517. doi: 10.1177/1049732316675589

Basu, A., Dillon P. J., & Romero-Daza, N. (2016). Understanding culture and its influence on HIV/AIDS-related communication among minority men who have sex with men. *Health Communication, 31*(11), 1367–1374. doi: 10.1080/10410236.2015.1072884

Butler, P. (2004). Embracing AIDS: History, identity, and post-AIDS discourse. *JAC, 24*, 93–11.

de Souza, R. (2007). The construction of HIV/AIDS in Indian newspapers: A frame analysis. *Health Communication, 21*, 257–266. https://doi.org/10.1080/10410230701307733

Gupta, R. K., Peppa, D., Hill, A. L., Gálvez, C., Salgado, M., Pace, M., … Olavarria, E. (2020). Evidence for HIV-1 cure after CCR5Δ32/Δ32 allogeneic haemopoietic stem-cell transplantation 30 months post analytical treatment interruption: A case report. *The Lancet. HIV, 7*, e340–e347. https://doi.org/10.1016/S2352-3018(20)30069-2

Hajek, C. (2019). Gay midlife men's intergenerational and interpersonal (non) accommodation in the negotiation of HIV infection risk: Implications for sexual vitality, generational distinctiveness, and self-preservation. *Health Communication, 34*, 1731–1740. https://doi.org/10.1080/10410236.2018.1517710

Kedia, S. K., Dillon, P. J., & Basu, A. (2020). A qualitative exploration of "mother first" identity and antiretroviral adherence among African American women living with HIV in the Mid-South region of the United States. *Health Communication, 35*, 1190–1199. https://doi.org/10.1080/10410236.2019.1623641

Khan, S. (2020). Examining HIV/AIDS-related stigma at play: Power, structure, and implications for HIV interventions. *Health Communication, 35*, 1509–1519. https://doi.org/10.1080/10410236.2019.1652386

King, N. B. (2002). Security, disease, commerce: ideologies of postcolonial global health. *Social Studies of Science, 32*(5–6), 763–789. https://doi-org.ezproxy.lib.usf.edu/10.1177/030631270203200507

Mazanderani, F. & Paparini, S. (2015). The stories we tell: Qualitative research interviews, talking technologies and the 'normalisation' of life with HIV. *Social Science & Medicine, 131*, 66–73.

O'Brien, C. (2013). Performing POZ: Irish theatre, HIV stigma, and "post-AIDS" identities. *Irish University Review, 43*(1), 74–85.

Rofes, E. (1998). *Dry bones breathe: Gay men creating post-AIDS identities and cultures.* New York: Routledge.

Sontag, S. (1989). *AIDS and its metaphors.* New York: Farrar, Straus and Giroux.

UNAIDS. (2014). *90-90-90: An ambitious treatment target to help end the AIDS epidemic.* Retrieved from http://www.unaids.org/en/resources/documents/2014/90-90-90.

UNAIDS. (2021). UNAIDS board adopts new global AIDS strategy which paves the way to end AIDS by 2030. Retrieved from https://www.unaids.org/en/resources/presscentre/pressreleaseandstatementarchive/2021/march/20210325_new-global-aids-strategy

Walker, L. (2020). Problematizing the discourse of "post-AIDS." *Journal of Medical Humanities, 41*(2), 95–105.

Wilson, K., Bleasdale, J., & Przybyla, S. M. (2020). Provider-patient communication on pre-exposure prophylaxis (PrEP) for HIV prevention: An exploration of healthcare provider challenges. *Health Communication.* Advance online publication. https://doi.org/10.1080/10410236.2020.1787927

World Health Organization. (2015). *Guideline on when to start antiretroviral therapy and on pre-exposure prophylaxis for HIV.* Retrieved from http://www.who.int/hiv/pub/guidelines/earlyrelease-arv/en/.

Part I

Debate, Discourse, Politics

1 Revisiting "Post-AIDS"

Understanding Gay Community Responses to HIV Then and Now

Gary W. Dowsett, Richard Parker and Peter Aggleton

When the first author of this chapter coined the term "post-AIDS" in 1996 (see Dowsett & McInnes, 1996a) and presented a paper on the idea to the XI International AIDS Conference in Vancouver in 1996 (Dowsett & McInnes, 1996b), the goal was to examine growing division in the responses of Australia's gay communities to their continuing HIV epidemics. This idea was an attempt to re-read the everyday experience of the epidemic at a time when investigating the natural history of HIV infection preoccupied biomedical science. That growing division was configured partly by HIV serostatus but also by diverging priorities between HIV prevention and care and support for people living with HIV (PLHIV).

The Vancouver conference also saw the announcement of the first effective or highly active antiretroviral treatment (HAART, later ART) for HIV infection, which within a decade was to convert HIV infection from a terminal illness ending in AIDS to a chronic manageable condition, at least for those with access to good quality medical care and ART. This announcement is sometimes called the "Protease Moment." The news of effective medications – at least in the short term – was momentous, as it marked the beginning of a new phase of responding to the global epidemic, a phase characterized by the first real treatment successes, but also by divisions and conflicted positions on the dramatic turn in the epidemic that ART produced.

At the time those two papers on post-AIDS were presented, some commentators thought the term post-AIDS was intended to mean that the epidemic was over. This interpretation was buttressed by the arrival of ART. Importantly, the idea of post-AIDS did *not* and was never intended to mean an end to the epidemic. Indeed, the epidemic continues to this day. Others thought the term was calling an end to AIDS as a "crisis." This too was incorrect, although there was a gesture in the papers – drawing in part on the psychological work of Odets (1995) on the situation facing HIV-negative gay men in the U.S.A. at that time – towards a need to rethink the singularity of the ongoing experience of those affected by the epidemic and, in particular, HIV-negative Australian gay men. It was no longer a crisis for all gay men, but it did *not* refer to an end to the crisis.

More recently, some have seen the term post-AIDS as a precursor to slogans such as the "end of AIDS" or an "AIDS-free generation," which emerged early

DOI: 10.4324/9781003000945-3

in the second decade of the new millennium. The term did not mean that, nor was it intended to contribute to the development of these kinds of slogans. These catchphrases derive from a dynamic in the global response to the epidemic that arose first with the establishment of the International AIDS Society (IAS) and the World Health Organization's Global Programme on AIDS (WHO/GPA) in the late 1980s – which sought to encourage rapid governmental responses to the epidemic around the world – and later the Joint United Nations Programme on HIV and AIDS (UNAIDS) in the mid-1990s, which succeeded WHO/GPA and sought to coordinate the responses of various United Nations (UN) agencies and other global nongovernmental organizations. These agencies, positioned at the peak of the global response in terms of policy coordination and communication over the life of the epidemic, have played an increasingly central role in shaping how we see, understand, and, therefore, respond to the epidemic (Seckinelgin, 2017).

Finally, some commentators have applied the term "post-AIDS" to groups and populations affected by HIV other than gay men. The term originally referred very specifically to Australian gay communities. It is undoubtedly the case that the Australian gay communities' responses to HIV were deeply influenced by those in the U.S.A. and, to a lesser extent, the U.K. There were, however, significant differences that emerged in the 1980s and continued to do so well in the new millennium. Not the least of these was the early and rapid, federally coordinated, national response to the epidemic in Australia from 1984 onwards, something that did not occur as readily elsewhere. For example, little by way of a national response developed in the U.S.A. until very late in the second term of President Reagan, being finally encoded into a national strategy only decades later under the Obama administration.

That said, the term "post-AIDS" was quickly taken up and used in the U.S.A. after the first author met the late Eric Rofes, a prominent gay activist and leading HIV/AIDS educator from San Francisco, at the Vancouver conference. Rofes took up the term and reconfigured it to the situation facing U.S. gay communities in the second of his influential books – *Dry Bones Breathe: Gay Men Creating Post-AIDS Identities and Cultures* (1998), which argued for an end to seeing the epidemic as a crisis and contributed much of that particular meaning to the term as a result.

What Did "Post-AIDS" Really Mean?

As originally employed in Australia, the term "post-AIDS" described a widening divide between HIV-positive and HIV-negative Australian gay men, starting in the early 1990s. It began from a discussion on what was happening within gay sexual cultures and could only have happened after the development of PLHIV as a distinct community of interest and circumstance in the late 1980s. A seminal moment in this development occurred at the second Australian National AIDS Conference in Hobart, Tasmania, in 1988. Gay community activists attended this conference in large numbers and, during the final plenary session, a call was made for people living with AIDS (the term then used) to come to the stage to be seen. Many people living with AIDS left the audience for the stage and thereby "came out" publicly. Arms linked and to tremendous applause, they claimed a collective place in the center of the epidemic and national HIV politics.

This period is analyzed in the late Ariss' posthumously published book *Against Death: The Practice of Living with AIDS* (1997). Ariss was a leading and founding member of the first PLHIV organization in Sydney – PLHWA, New South Wales (NSW). He drafted its constitution and became its first convener. Ariss had a canny eye for the politics of the period, including the concatenation of HIV with longer-standing forms of gay activism that had developed since the early 1970s with the rise of gay liberation theory and politics and the "sexual revolution" inspired by it and second-wave feminism. During this period, PLHIV became a collectivity that constituted

> a discursive systematization of the experience of HIV positivity into a strategic "anti-discipline." This new identity, frail because built on the anticipation of death, drew on the established identity formations of gay identity and the "empowered patient", the latter formulated within women's groups and groups of the disabled."
>
> (Ariss & Dowsett, 1997, p. 135)

Gay Communities and the Politics of AIDS

The epidemic in Australia was and has always been largely confined to gay men, with relatively small numbers of infections among women, sex workers, and people who inject drugs. As a result, the model for PLHIV politics derived much from gay community politics and the struggles for equality and social justice within them. While the epidemics in some high-income countries are different in the proportion of infected people who were and are men infected through sex with other men, the centrality of the contribution of gay activism in almost all high-income countries to shaping the politics of and responses to their epidemics is incontrovertible. It is for this reason that we use the example of Australia to provide a context for the development of post-AIDS as a concept at that time.

Sex between men was still illegal in most of Australia when HIV struck, and anti-gay forces opposed any movement toward social equality for gay (and lesbian) people. While some progress had been achieved by the early 1990s, and the politics of gay civil rights were still active, they had dovetailed with HIV politics to the extent that, in the minds of many, HIV-positive people and gay men became synonymous. It is in this climate of progressive gains but continuing opposition that HIV politics and gay politics fused.

By the early 1990s, as the death rate from AIDS was heading towards its peak, and the politics of AIDS increasingly featured the voices of PLHIV, issues of discrimination added fuel to fire among HIV-positive gay men. Stigma and, to a lesser extent, discrimination were to develop into an important political framework that captured a wide range of HIV-related issues over the next 20 years, acting as a growing "hold-all" for struggles over treatments provision and access, approaches to HIV prevention, and legal responses to the epidemic (see Parker & Aggleton, 2003).

Cracks in the façade

This arena was ripe for reframing issues that arose early in the epidemic. Such issues were reliant not just on external stimuli; they soon turned inward. One that became clear in the early 1990s among Australian gay men was that of sex partner selection and the discriminatory selection of HIV-negative partners by men who were also HIV-negative. To our knowledge, no social or behavioral research evidence confirmed that this was occurring on a wide scale, but anecdotal reports of partner selection practices were rife and caused significant resentment among PLHIV who had already been subjected to mainstream anti-gay criticism of their sexuality based on their HIV serostatus. This was the first of emerging divisions among gay men related to their differing experiences of the epidemic.

One response to this issue of sex partner selection was to advocate for HIV-positive people to select only other HIV-positive partners – the discriminatory aspect of which went largely unnoticed. This kind of partner selection was eventually termed "serosorting," and the practice was even advocated by some PLHIV activists as a form of infection control to prevent onward HIV transmission. In a study of the social impact of HIV/AIDS with Australian HIV-negative men, which the first author and Ariss conducted in Sydney and Adelaide in the early 1990s (and which gave birth to the term "post-AIDS"), the selection of partners of the same serostatus was seen as an acceptable strategy to remain uninfected. Furthermore, in Adelaide with its small epidemic, it was clear that a sense of crisis was hard to find. Most gay men there did not even know anyone infected and the representations of the devasting epidemic in Sydney (and the rest of the world for that matter) just did not resonate with local experience. It seemed that after 10 years of the epidemic, some HIV-negative men were no longer well-served by HIV prevention education programs that continued to represent AIDS as a crisis for everyone all the time.

By that time, related research had revealed further sophistication in gay men's sexual responses to the epidemic. Social researchers in Sydney, to some alarm from their colleagues in the U.S.A., had published on what was termed "negotiated safely" in the sexual practices of Australian gay men (Kippax, Crawford et al., 1993). These findings confirmed those of an earlier study (Kippax, Connell et al., 1993) in which agreements on using condoms and other safe sex practices had been assessed. Negotiated safety referred to HIV-negative gay men in regular (or primary) relationships making clear agreements on safer sex with their similarly HIV-negative partners, e.g., not using condoms inside the relationship, but restricting sex practices in various ways with other partners outside the relationship (condoms always, no anal sex, etc.). HIV-positive men had already worked out that condoms were not needed in same HIV-status sex, so it was not a surprise to find the emergence of a parallel strategy among HIV-negative men.

The surprise lay in the fact that HIV prevention education had only ever advocated using condoms every time for everyone and was still doing so. Gay men, irrespective of serostatus, had clearly moved on from any singular experience of the epidemic. As the first author commented in 1995 at the second National Gay Educators Conference in Sydney:

> Segregated partner choice is already happening; how…it is to be configured is up to us. We can decide to retain some outdated notion of blanket safe sex education. We can classify such choices as discriminatory, thus exacerbating an artificial divide based on serostatus which obscures our much greater commonalities. Or we can embrace the ingenuity involved in gay men's evolving sexual practice and re-incorporate it into our collectivity, into our safe sex culture.
>
> (Dowsett, 1995, p. 71)

What these discussions of gay sex revealed was a fissure in the, until then, unified experience of and response to the epidemic in Australian gay communities. There was still a crisis unfolding for HIV-positive people as treatments at that time, though growing in number, were still toxic, partial, and sometimes ineffective. Those who were infected were still facing a foreshortened life and were often regarded as "diseased pariahs" (Long, 2000) in a still largely unsupportive and stigmatizing society. Yet, HIV-negative men, not only those who had known their status for quite a while and those who had very little direct experience with HIV-positive people, but also those who had lost many lovers, friends, and family members, could no longer live lives on a knife's edge, even if infection might always be proximate – only one unsafe sex event away. This division in the sexual experiences and unfolding futures of gay men, based on serostatus, could only widen – and it did so with the arrival of ART. It was the combination of these issues that "post-AIDS" as a concept sought to frame.

The "Protease Moment"

The arrival of ART added weight to these changes already in motion. Hitherto, most efforts internationally had focused on HIV prevention. That is not to say that the search for vaccines or treatment, or better clinical practice to forestall death, were not priorities. However, the absence of effective treatment meant that classical biomedical responses took a back seat to HIV prevention, the latter supported by both significant epidemiological and social/behavioral research that had arisen to inform it.

What the protease moment did was change the balance between prevention, treatment, and care to one in which treatment, and the possibilities of it, became a larger focus, thereby transforming the politics of AIDS globally. It created two clear but different priorities. For PLHIV, treatment and its politics, advocacy, science, effectiveness, cost, access, and availability were to become the focus. For those not infected, these issues were also of major concern, but prevention remained the priority. As treatment changed – and as its costs rose with every new treatment drug – the increasing allocation of public health resources toward treatments became another fissure. This first substantive success for HIV treatment began a new process of "re-biomedicalizing" the epidemic, which was to lead to a reconceptualization of many aspects of the epidemic over the next 10–20 years, including but not restricted to the contribution of gay communities and PLHIV. Post-AIDS flagged a number of these issues and noted these fissures and the fracturing of any singular conception and experience of the epidemic in a linear sense, suggesting diverse and multiple strategies were needed instead.

Almost immediately after the protease moment, however, two things became clear. The first was that the then-available drugs were not perfect. Despite great success in some cases, many drugs had serious side effects and were not suited to every individual. New drugs were developed between 1996 and 2006 by the global pharmaceutical industry with breathtaking speed to deal with this issue. The second challenge was that the high cost of ART revealed significant problems of affordability (and profiteering) for HIV-positive people and public health systems (where these were supposed to provide or subsidize such drugs) playing into the unacceptable social inequalities that underpinned the epidemic. These inequalities were not just between wealthy and poorer citizens in any given country; global inequality between countries was exposed in starker terms that had been talked about for many years in international discourses of neoliberal-inflected international development. The demand for equal access to ART came to the fore at the XIII International AIDS Conference held in Durban, South Africa, in July 2000 – the first time the conference had been held in the Global South. There, in another signal post-AIDS moment, activists from the Global South exposed not just the inequality, but also the *lack* of access to ART and the privilege of Global North PLHIV who already had access, demanding better and cheaper drugs as their main agenda. It is possible to trace from this moment a rapid increase in the growing global treatment access movement that began not long after the protease moment occurred.

South Africa was to provide a graphic example of this kind of activism in its Treatment Action Campaign, which finally forced the post-Apartheid government to provide ART as part of a constitutionally guaranteed right to health. Such activists and their allies in various agencies, e.g. UNAIDS, built a global treatment access and equity movement during this period that came to a head at the UN General Assembly Special Session on HIV/AIDS in 2001. From that moment, a massive scale-up of treatment was initiated throughout the 2000s, producing various global health initiatives such as WHO's 3 × 5 (3 million HIV-positive people in treatment by 2005); the creation of the Global Fund to fight HIV/AIDS, Tuberculosis and Malaria (a new global financing organization to fund the world's response to the epidemic); and new large-scale programs such as the U.S. government's PEPFAR (President's Emergency Plan For AIDS Relief) initiative with its mammoth increase in funding.

However, while these extraordinary efforts recognized both the need for more affordable and effective drugs and began to address global inequalities in treatment access, the scale-up in activity also stimulated the re-biomedicalization of the epidemic, convincing many scientists, public health professionals, and activists that a biomedical silver bullet would not only be effective but could also constitute *the* answer to HIV and AIDS. By 2010, this re-biomedicalization, driven by treatments development and activism, overtook prevention as the central strategy to slow and stop the epidemic. Attention soon turned to other "technologies" as the new buzzword for action. Condoms became a prevention technology, not just a safer-sex adjunct; medical male circumcision was rolled out, mainly in sub-Saharan Africa, despite considerable skepticism and ongoing global criticism (Aggleton, 2007; Dowsett & Couch, 2007; Earp, 2015; Parker et al., 2015). Prevention education and community-based health promotion became the subject of "prevention science," with an insistence that all prevention research adopt randomized control trial methodology, irrespective of population or context or whether the methodology was appropriate for the research questions being asked.

The next step in this process of re-biomedicalization came as disease prevention itself shifted from a broad-based public health approach to a narrower biomedical prevention framework, best exemplified in advocacy for the use of HIV treatments to prevent incident infections. The strategy was to deploy ART for HIV-positive people to reduce the onward transmission of HIV to uninfected others, as a result of achieving viral suppression at individual and community levels ("treatment as prevention," or TasP), and combine this with the use of ART for uninfected sexual partners of HIV-positive people to prevent their infection ("pre-exposure prophylaxis," or PrEP). For this strategy to even be contemplated, a decisive discursive shift had to occur in the longstanding framing of the epidemic as an ongoing emergency and crisis. This was to arrive in the "end of AIDS" narrative, which soon came to dominate the fourth decade of the epidemic.

From the "Protease Moment" to the "End of AIDS"

By the late 2000s, with the perceived success of ART signaling the value of biomedical approaches to HIV prevention, and hot on the heels of significant advances in the scale-up of treatment access, the protease moment began to give way to a new era of optimism about the possibility of the imminent "end of AIDS."

Globally, the seeds of what would later come to be the "end of AIDS" discourse were planted in a 2010 UNAIDS document that defined the agency's strategic plan for the 2011–2016 period (United Nations, 2011). In something of a reversal of UNAIDS' messaging to date, which had tended to stress the growing seriousness of the epidemic but begun to lose traction, this strategic plan focused on "getting to zero," meaning the intentionally aspirational goals of achieving zero new infections, zero AIDS-related deaths, and zero discrimination. The strategy was formally articulated in the "Political Declaration on HIV and AIDS: Intensifying Our Efforts to Eliminate HIV and AIDS," adopted by the UN General Assembly on June 10, 2011 (UN Resolution 65/277), committing to the goal of "getting to 50%" (on the road to zero) by 2015. As Michel Sidibé, then Director of UNAIDS, wrote in his preface to the media material for the launch of the 2001 World AIDS Day Report, issued on December 1, 2011:

> Just a few years ago, talking about ending the AIDS epidemic in the near term seemed impossible, but science, political support and community responses are starting to deliver clear and tangible results.
>
> (UNAIDS, 2010, p. 5)

The Political Declaration adopted by the General Assembly committed the UN to a set of new targets with "with a focus on clear, time-bound goals designed to bring about the end of HIV and also improve human health across diverse communities" (UNAIDS, 2010, p. 5). To reach these targets, the Declaration also argued that the world would need to "step on the accelerator" and adopt "a new framework for AIDS investments, focused on high-impact, high-value strategies" that had been mapped out by UNAIDS.

This new approach was rolled out for primetime publicity in the media frenzy surrounding the XIX International AIDS Conference in Washington, D.C., in 2012. This was the first conference to be held in the U.S.A. since 1990. Counting on significant involvement of the U.S. administration – and with former President Clinton and the former First Lady (by this time U.S. Secretary of State) Hillary Clinton in attendance – the conference announced an end to mother-to-child transmission in the District of Columbia (hence the claim of an "AIDS-free generation"). The announcement was accompanied by a show of optimism from the biomedical research establishment with the launch of the International AIDS Society's "Toward an HIV Cure" initiative (Deeks & Barré-Sinoussi, 2012).

On the heels of the 2012 international conference, with the government of the U.S.A. and its PEPFAR project on board, and the international scientific community, as well as the pharmaceutical industry as willing partners, came the development of the UNAIDS "Fast Track Strategy" (UNAIDS, 2014a, 2014b). Now the goal was to become "90–90–90" (90% of people with HIV diagnosed, 90% of diagnosed people on treatment, and 90% of treated people with fully suppressed viral load) by 2020. This strategy was formally launched, again with an elaborate media campaign, in a 2014 UNAIDS document that explicitly articulated the goal of ending AIDS by 2030 (UNAIDS, 2014c). The new goal was first announced at the XX International AIDS Conference held in Melbourne in 2014, where the emerging "success story" was heralded by the global scientific community and increasingly amplified in the mainstream media (The Economist, 2014). In October 2014, the "Fast-Track Strategy" was published as "an ambitious treatment target to help end the AIDS epidemic" (UNAIDS, 2014c). On December 1, 2014, it became the focus for World AIDS Day media coverage, with the "90–90–90" targets for 2020 marketed as a necessary step to be able to end the epidemic in 2030 on schedule to achieve the UN's Sustainable Development Goals, in which the epidemic received specific mention (Kenworthy et al., 2018a).

As soon as the Fast Track Strategy was issued, most major donor agencies began to endorse it, and key players such as PEPFAR, the Global Fund, and UNICEF (the United Nations Children's Fund) issued statements that articulated the "end of AIDS in 2030" as the global AIDS movement's overarching goal (The Global Fund, 2014; The Office of the U.S. Global AIDS Coordinator, 2014; UNICEF, 2015). By 2015, private donor buy-in was increasingly evident, noted in statements by well-known figures such as Sir Elton John and his husband David Furnish for the Elton John AIDS Foundation (Furnish, 2015; The Guardian, 2015). Civil society organizations were also encouraged to rally around the slogan through UN-sponsored events such as large civil society organizations meetings that UNAIDS organized in Bangkok in 2015, which aimed to mobilize support for the "90–90–90 by 2020" and the "end of AIDS by 2030" goals (amFAR, 2015; Equal Eyes, 2015).

In the echo chamber of both the international development industry and the mainstream media of the digital age, the speed and ubiquity with which this policy goal was embraced began to make it seem something of a *fait accompli* (Kenworthy et al., 2018a, 2018b). Indeed, it came almost as an anti-climax when, in June 2016, the UN General Assembly held a High-Level Meeting on Ending AIDS and officially adopted the new "Political Declaration on HIV and AIDS: On the Fast-Track to Accelerate the Fight against HIV and to End the AIDS Epidemic by 2030" (UNAIDS, 2016). Just a month later, the Declaration had been endorsed by the scientific and policy communities of the international AIDS movement in both the scientific sessions and the media briefings at the XXI International Conference on AIDS, held for the second time in Durban, South Africa, in 2016.

It is important to stress just how different this "end of AIDS" narrative was from the post-AIDS understandings of increasing separation and division described earlier in this chapter. While the concept of post-AIDS was strongly informed by grassroots, community-initiated responses to the epidemic, in contrast, the "end of AIDS" story was a top-down, deliberate manipulation of the epidemic narrative in the face of clear evidence that all was not well in the epidemic. Paradoxically, the international AIDS conferences that were used to herald the "end of AIDS" narrative provided the very same platform for literally hundreds of scientific papers and plenary presentations that made it clear how deeply problematic the "end of AIDS" story was when confronted with the reality of the epidemic for affected individuals and communities. As just two examples, we might point to Filipino, HIV-positive, gay man Laurindo Garcia's final plenary address to the same 2012 conference on the still-pervasive discrimination experienced by gay and other men who have sex with men, and incoming IAS President and Nobel Prize winner Françoise Barré-Sinoussi's plenary challenge to all with its list of "unacceptable" things still occurring in the global response. Both contrasted sharply with former U.S. President Clinton's "Energizing Call to Action" in closing that conference.

Looking beyond the sloganeering of administrators and bureaucrats and listening to those most affected by the epidemic, what was soon evident was a rapid multiplication of relations to the epidemic in the form of greater inequalities in access and outcomes, old epidemics reviving (among gay and other men who have sex in Brazil or Thailand, for example), small epidemics exploding (among men who have sex with men and people who inject drugs in the Philippines), deteriorating social responses (such as the passing of anti-gay laws in Nigeria and Uganda, the continuing criminalization of HIV transmission, sex work legalization, etc.), and vastly different, poorly articulated legal and governmental frameworks in abundance revealed by the Global Commission on HIV and the Law report (2012) *Risks, Rights and Health* and the WHO report (2015) *Sexual Health, Human Rights and the Law*. The epidemic was increasingly multifaceted, occurring in many parallel versions rarely in step. At the very same time, there was clear evidence of a heterogeneous post-AIDS-like multiplicity being discursively homogenized (as an "end of AIDS") in a manner that insulted the intellect of and marginalized those most affected.

In one way, this discursive maneuvering amounted to serious misuse of science, contributing to and covering up the progressive fracturing of affected communities. A reification of scientific expertise not only reproduced Paulo Freire's (1970) "banking theory" of pedagogy – in which experts deposit supposedly true information (the epidemic is ending) into the deficit accounts of the objects of their knowledge who were assumed to know nothing – but actually intensified the stigma experienced by, and its effects on, those directly affected by the epidemic. Inadvertently or not, the "end of AIDS" narrative further fractured affected communities (so-called "key populations"), reinforcing HIV-positive and HIV-negative divisions and creating numerous other social categories (Truvada "whores," PrEP "refusers," circumcision "denialists," and so on), now seen as traitors to the epidemic. These new post-AIDS effects contributed to the conflation (and misreading) of prejudice, hate, vitriol, injustice and other forms of oppression as a singular "stigma," while at the same time combatting stigma and discrimination has increasingly fallen beneath policy priorities and outcome indicators, now reduced to biomedical markers of success such as "90–90–90." Taken together, all this made any coherent community-conceived and initiated response to HIV much more difficult, perversely promulgating the conceit that the "end of AIDS" would be possible only through the enlightened leadership of global administrators and bureaucrats who would take the necessary steps paternalistically to ensure that no one would be "left behind."

Crucially, unlike this contemporary vision of an "end of AIDS," the post-AIDS analysis originally emerged precisely from the context of (gay) communities' responses to the epidemic, and never suggested that the epidemic was close to ending. Rather, it sought to understand and interpret the fracturing and fragmenting of an epidemic as it impacted the changing experiences of those affected by it. The "end of AIDS" story, in contrast, was invented and articulated first and foremost from the top down by administrators and bureaucrats. It posited a kind of biomedical Potemkin Village – a fantasy world that almost completely ignored the grim reality on the ground, largely disconnected from grassroots experience and invented in conferences and boardrooms. As just one example, 30 years on from the protease moment, only 62% of PLHIV globally currently have access to HIV treatment (UNAIDS, 2019), and a significant percentage of those who do have access to medication in low- and middle-income countries only have access to first- and second-generation medications with significantly greater side effects. An "end to AIDS"? Well, no, these events typify the division and fracturing that first characterized post-AIDS that is with us still in 2020.

****

The period between 2001 and 2010 also saw a significant shift of power from affected communities to large global institutions and an increasing sidelining of the social response to the epidemic. Until the protease moment, the prevention of HIV infection had been largely a community-initiated activity underpinned by health education and promotion principles and social and community research. As ART improved, the process of re-biomedicalization was accompanied by a "scientization" of the social aspects of the global responses. The notion of "prevention technologies" shifted the focus of prevention (and the funding streams) away from the socially created and sub-culturally derived responses to HIV that had so successfully managed the epidemic in the earlier years. For example, the invention of safer sex by gay men in the early 1980s was based on gay men's understanding of sexual practices and relationships well before HIV had been isolated and identified as the cause of AIDS. Likewise, later strategies of negotiated safety and serosorting had their origins, not in public health and prevention science, but in the creative responses of affected individuals and communities – again, gay men – as did the safer drug use practices among people who inject drugs, which eventually led to widespread syringe and needle programs and the safer sex and drug use strategies adopted by sex workers with their clients early in the epidemic.

For affected communities worldwide, this marginalization and progressive loss of control were masked by the urgency of a solution to AIDS and formed a trap of their own making. Since the epidemic had begun, community-based prevention programs and care and support for HIV-positive people had adopted culturally appropriate language and imagery. Prevention education materials often featured colloquial phrases, slang terms and attractive images to promote safer sex – in essence, slogans in their own right, e.g., "You'll never forget the feeling of safe sex," "Condoms are cheaper than AIDS," "AIDS: prevention is the only cure," and ones related to supporting PLHIV such as "Hate the disease, but not the diseased!" and "Silence = Death." Collectively, these programs and resources amounted to an extraordinary catalogue of cultural creativity over 38 years, and international AIDS conferences have long celebrated and promoted this ingenuity in the global villages, filled with activists and community-based organizations still doing grassroots prevention and supporting PLHIV, which accompany the scientific program.

However, this use of catchy phrases and colloquial terms was easily colonized as re-biomedicalization proceeded. In a bizarre twist, the slogans developed by international agencies began to attract affected communities' support. For example, worldwide treatment supply problems became a conference theme – "Access for all." Its companions – "Breaking the silence," "Time to deliver," "Knowledge and commitment for action," "Turning the tide together," "Access equity rights now," "Breaking barriers, building bridges," and "No one left behind" – quickly followed, each ever-more glib and each reducing complex and intractable economic, political, and social issues and inequalities to the clever use of the English language. There are numerous other examples, but the point is that affected communities were co-opted into the process, as these goals, phrases, and slogans increasingly informed the priorities and cultures of community-based action. The "end of AIDS" was just another moment in this successive co-option, despite the fact the end of the epidemic was nowhere in sight, even in those countries where HIV incidence rates were dropping.

Even re-biomedicalization itself had become a victim of this sloganeering. The success that ART achieved in controlling HIV infection in those in treatment and reducing viral load to undetectable levels provided grounds for a new slogan: "U=U" (undetectable viral load equals untransmissible HIV), now heavily promoted by affected community activists. The science behind this assertion is very strong. However, there are caveats in viral load assessment (e.g., treatment effectiveness and adherence, medication supply and access, drug resistance, sex partner susceptibility to infection like having STI lesions, patient misunderstandings of viral load status, and so on). As just one example, a recent report from three U.S. cities (Atlanta, Boston, and Chicago) found that, while 72.5% of 314 HIV-positive gay and bisexual men accurately reported their viral load, 7.5% thought their viral load was detectable when it was suppressed, and 20% said their viral load was undetectable but tests indicated this was not the case (Stephenson et al., 2020). The current science tells us that undetectable is very likely to be untransmissible, but as scientific paradigms evolve, so does the "truth" or facticity of scientific certainty. The virus mutates; treatments can become less effective over time; ART does not work equally well in everyone; health systems change; global funding for treatment is never certain and rarely grows despite the need. While the use of ART not just to keep HIV-positive people healthy, but also to prevent onward transmission of HIV (the underlying premise behind "U=U") is a major step forward in prevention, it remains dependent on potentially confounding social and contextual factors. Yet, like the "end of AIDS," these discursive maneuvers now drive affected community action as if they were incontrovertible truths.

The second issue underpinning post-AIDS had been "discrimination" based on HIV serostatus. This issue, framed by the notion of "stigma," was to provide a platform for a second major arena of leadership by PLHIV and affected communities. We noted earlier the origins of the politics of stigma and discrimination in 1970s–1980s gay liberation activism and its centrality to PLHIV identity formation. From the late 1990s onwards, the agenda in this politics expanded to include an array of issues drawing on human rights, legislative changes to decriminalize sexual activity of various sorts and protect other minorities, health service provision and access, race/ethnicity and socioeconomic status, education and employment issues, and many more (AVERT, 2020). As a "hold-all" term, HIV stigma has travelled a fair distance from stigma's original meaning as defined by Goffman (1963). While providing a successful rallying cry and focusing attention on an increasingly wide range of issues, there must be doubt that all that is regarded as occurring under its banner is, indeed, stigma and/or discrimination. It is distinctly possible that these terms mask more complex underlying social processes that prevent the global response to HIV from addressing the real structural and political drivers of the epidemic.

Just two examples of these drivers may suffice: the extraordinary profiteering of multinational pharmaceutical companies that underpins ongoing problems in ART access and supply; and the profound effects of neoliberal economic policies at international and national levels that are exacerbating poverty and marginalization, driving mass migration and the disenfranchisement of millions of people, and placing the planet in peril for the many to guarantee the profit of the few. The increasing vulnerability of huge numbers of people provides a near-perfect ecology for disease development and HIV infection is one of these. Indeed, as UNAIDS (2020, online) admits: "The pace of progress in reducing new HIV infections, increasing access to treatment and ending AIDS-related deaths is slowing down." Put quite simply, the "end of AIDS" is nowhere in sight.

Earlier in the epidemic, responses to some of these issues began to be framed as human rights, especially via the "right to health," as a way of registering the structural forces driving the HIV epidemic yet almost invisible in the dominant biomedical framing through which the epidemic was largely conceived. Human rights issues have become increasingly prominent over the last 30 years. Issues such as women's vulnerability and the illegal status of sex between men are just two examples. The WHO report (2015) on *Sexual Health, Human Rights and the Law* is just one of many more recent attempts to position human rights as central in the global response. This is a signal achievement of HIV in transforming global health. Hitherto, there had never been any attempt during the twentieth century to frame malaria or tuberculosis (or other medical conditions) in this way until their coming together with HIV/AIDS with the advent of the Global Fund. That said, one important concern is that efforts to tackle stigma and discrimination during the first two decades of the epidemic were largely driven by affected communities fighting for themselves (derived initially from gay liberation politics as we noted earlier), whereas current discourse on these issues is increasingly disconnected from reality on the ground and practical actions that address its root causes. The work of research scientists and institutions endlessly measuring and monitoring "stigma" and the production of ever more complex expert documents such as the WHO report mentioned above provide but two examples of this process. As a result, human rights and stigma have become other slogans just like an "end of AIDS," a kind of "must-have" tag line always to be mentioned, or at the least nodded to, but very few real or effective programs or policies have been developed specifically to combat these issues on the ground.

This gulf between the expert discourse and the real experience of the HIV epidemic marks a new aspect to the post-AIDS epidemic, which is no longer just a dispersal and fracturing of focus or diverging futures among those most affected. Notions such as having "partnership" with affected communities as government policy, or the Greater Involvement of PLHIV (the GIPA Principle), and other phrases in many and varied forms have become smokescreens. Together, they mask the actions of a neoliberal cartel of UN agencies, international NGOs and development aid organizations, huge philanthropic foundations such as the Gates Foundation, and the global pharmaceutical industry seeking to manage both the epidemic ***and its narrative*** for themselves. We noted earlier that only 62%, or 24.5 million (range: 21.6–25.5 million), of HIV-positive people, were accessing ART as of June 2019. While the rates of new infection and deaths from AIDS-related conditions have dramatically declined since the worst days of the epidemic, in 2018 1.7 million (range: 1.4–2.3 million) people became newly infected with HIV and 770,000 (range: 570,000–1.1 million) PLHIV died from AIDS-related illnesses (UNAIDS, 2019). This is not the "end of AIDS" by any stretch of the imagination. Such is the current governmentality of the epidemic.

Finally, the irony for gay men, whose activism has been so central to understanding and framing the epidemic, is that the crowning achievement of this governmentality and its entourage of administrators, the ascendency of re-biomedicalization, and the marginalization and co-option of affected communities has been to insert gay men's sexuality firmly back into and under the surveillance of the "clinic" (Dowsett, 2017). By this, we mean that, with the advent of TasP for HIV-negative or untested men, and affected community advocacy for "90–90–90" and TasP for HIV-positive men, all gay and other homosexually active men find themselves and their sexual activities firmly back under the scrutiny of biomedicine, reliant on ART provision by physicians' prescriptions; dependent on public health subsidies (where they exist) for supply, access, and affordability; and subject to public debate as to why diminishing government resources for HIV and other pressing health issues should be spent to facilitate sex between men. One hundred and fifty years of the pathologization of homosexuality resisted and fought so successfully by the gay liberation movements of the world in the late twentieth century have, indeed, come full circle. In a paradoxically post-AIDS fashion, we are now all patients again!

References

Aggleton, P. (2007). "Just a snip?" A social history of male circumcision. *Reproductive Health Matters*, *5*(29), 15–21.

amfAR. (2015). *UNAIDS holds civil society meeting on fast-tracking the end of AIDS*. Retrieved from http://www.amfar.org/UNAIDS-Holds-Civil-Society-Meeting/

Ariss, R. M., & Dowsett, G. W. (1997). *Against death: The practice of living with AIDS*. Amsterdam: Gordon and Breach.

AVERT. (2020). *Global information and education on HIV and AIDS*. Retrieved from https://www.avert.org/professionals/hiv-social-issues/stigma-discrimination

Deeks, S. G., & Barré-Sinoussi, F. (2012). Towards a cure for HIV. *Nature*, *487*(7407), 293–294.

Dowsett, G. W. (1995). Emerging issues, current dilemmas and persistent problems in HIV prevention among gay communities. In Australian Federation of AIDS Organisations (Ed.), *Living in an epidemic: A report from the 2nd national gay educators conference 1995* (pp. 62–72). Sydney: Australian Federation of AIDS Organisations.

Dowsett, G. W. (2017). Abjection. Objection. Subjection: Rethinking the history of AIDS in Australian gay men's futures. *Culture, Health and Sexuality, 19*(9), 935–947.

Dowsett, G. W., & Couch, M. (2007). Male circumcision and HIV prevention: Is there really enough of the right kind of evidence? *Reproductive Health Matters, 15*(29), 33–44.

Dowsett, G. W., & McInnes, D. (1996a). Gay community, AIDS agencies and the HIV epidemic in Adelaide: Theorising "post-AIDS." *Social Alternatives, 15*(4), 29–32.

Dowsett, G. W., & McInnes, D. (1996b, July). *"Post-AIDS:" Assessing the long-term social impact of HIV/AIDS in gay communities.* Paper presented at the XI International Conference on AIDS, Vancouver, BC.

Earp, B. D. (2015). Do the benefits of male circumcision outweigh the risks? A critique of the proposed CDC guidelines. *Frontier in Pediatrics, 3*, 18.

The Economist. (2014, July). *Is an end in sight? Campaigners are now talking openly of beating the AIDS epidemic.* Retrieved from http://www.economist.com/news/science-and-technology/21608568-campaigners-are-now-talking-openly-beating-aids-epidemic-end

Equal Eyes. (2015). "Bangkok: UNAIDS holds civil society meeting on fast-tracking the end of AIDS. Retrieved from http://equal-eyes.org/database/2015/12/13/bangkok-unaids-holds-civil-society-meeting-on-fast-tracking-the-end-of-aids

Freire, P. (1970). *Pedagogy of the oppressed.* New York: Continuum.

Furnish, D. (2015, February). We can make 'Ending AIDS' more than just a slogan. *The Independent.* Retrieved from http://www.independent.co.uk/voices/we-can-make-ending-aids-more-just-than-a-slogan-10050840.html

Global Commission on HIV and the Law. (2012). *Risks, rights & health.* New York: UNDP HIV/AIDS Group. Retrieved from https://hivlawcommission.org/wp-content/uploads/2017/06/FinalReport-RisksRightsHealth-EN.pdf.

The Global Fund. (2014). *Private & NGO partners: (RED).* Retrieved from https://www.theglobalfund.org/en/private-ngo-partners/red/

Goffman, E. (1963), *Stigma: Notes on the management of spoiled identity.* Harmondsworth: Pelican.

The Guardian. (2015, May). *Elton John tells U.S. Congress it has the power to end AIDS.* Retrieved from https://www.theguardian.com/music/2015/may/07/elton-john-us-congress-senate-hearing-hiv-aids

Kenworthy, N., Thomann, M., & Parker, R. (2018a). From a global crisis to the "end of AIDS": New epidemics of signification. *Global Public Health, 13*(8): 960–971.

Kenworthy, N., Thomann, M., & Parker, R. (2018b). "Ending AIDS" or scaling down the HIV response? In R. Parker & J. García (Eds.), *Routledge handbook on the politics of global health* (pp. 276–284). London and New York: Routledge.

Kippax, S., Connell, R. W., Dowsett, G. W., & Crawford, J. (1993). *Sustaining safe sex: Gay communities respond to AIDS.* London: Falmer Press.

Kippax, S., Crawford, J., Davis, M., Rodden, P., & Dowsett, G. W. (1993). Sustaining safe sex: A longitudinal study of a sample of homosexual men. *AIDS, 7*, 257–263.

Long, T. (2000). Plague of pariahs: AIDS 'zines and the rhetoric of transgression. *Journal of Communication Inquiry, 24*(4), 401–411.

Odets, W. (1995). *In the shadow of the epidemic: Being HIV-negative in the age of AIDS.* Durham, NC: Duke University Press.

The Office of the U.S. Global AIDS Coordinator. (2014). *PEPFAR 3.0: Controlling the epidemic: Delivering on the promise of an AIDS-free generation, December 2014.* Retrieved from https://aidsfree.usaid.gov/resources/prevention-update/editions/december-2014/pepfar-30-controlling-epidemic-delivering

Parker, R., & Aggleton, P. (2003). HIV and AIDS-related stigma and discrimination: A conceptual framework and implications for action. *Social Science & Medicine*, *57*(1), 13–24.

Parker, R., Aggleton, P., & Rochel de Camargo, Jr., K. (2015). Circumcision and HIV prevention: Emerging debates in science, policies and programmes. *Global Public Health*, *10*(5–6), 549–551.

Rofes, E. (1998). *Dry bones breathe: Gay men creating Post-AIDS identities and cultures.* Binghamton, NY: Haworth Press.

Seckinelgin, H. (2017). *The politics of global AIDS: Institutionalization of solidarity, exclusion of context.* Switzerland: Springer International Publishing.

Stephenson, R., Bratcher, A., Mimiaga, M. J., Garofalo, R., Hidalgo, M. A. ... Sullivan, P. S. (2020). Brief report: Accuracy in self-report of viral suppression among HIV-positive men with HIV-negative male partners. *Journal of Acquired Immune Deficiency Syndromes*, *83*(3), 210–214.

UNAIDS. (2010). *UNAIDS strategy 2011–2015: Getting to ZERO.* Geneva: UNAIDS. Retrieved from https://www.unaids.org/sites/default/files/media_asset/JC2034_UNAIDS_Strategy_en_1.pdf

UNAIDS. (2014a). *Fast-track: Ending the AIDS epidemic by 2030.* Geneva: UNAIDS. Retrieved from http://www.unaids.org/sites/default/files/media_asset/JC2686_WAD2014report_en.pdf

UNAIDS. (2014b). *UNAIDS reports that reaching fast-track targets will avert nearly 28 million new HIV infections and end the AIDS epidemic as a global health threat by 2030* [Press release]. Retrieved from http://www.unaids.org/en/resources/presscentre/pressreleaseandstatementarchive/2014/november/20141118_PR_WAD2014report

UNAIDS. (2014c). *90-90-90: An ambitious treatment target to help end the AIDS epidemic.* Retrieved from https://www.unaids.org/sites/default/files/media_asset/90-90-90_en.pdf

UNAIDS. (2016). *Political declaration on HIV and AIDS: On the fast track to accelerating the fight against HIV and to ending the AIDS epidemic by 2030.* Retrieved from https://www.unaids.org/sites/default/files/media_asset/2016-political-declaration-HIV-AIDS_en.pdf

UNAIDS. (2019). *Global HIV & AIDS statistics—2019 fact sheet.* Geneva: UNAIDS. Retrieved from https://www.unaids.org/en/resources/fact-sheet

UNAIDS. (2020). *AIDS by the numbers.* Retrieved from https://www.unaids.org/en

UNICEF. (2015). *UNAIDS, UNICEF and partners launch "All In" campaign to end the AIDS epidemic among adolescents.* Retrieved from https://www.unicef.org/media_23613.html

United Nations. (2011). *Political declaration on HIV and AIDS: Intensifying our efforts to eliminate HIV and AIDS.* Retrieved from http://www.unaids.org/sites/default/files/media_asset/JC2216_WorldAIDSday_report_2011_en_1.pdf

World Health Organization. (2015). *Sexual health, human rights and the law.* Geneva: World Health Organization. Retrieved from https://www.who.int/reproductivehealth/publications/sexual_health/sexual-health-human-rights-law/en/

2 Biocommunicability and the Biopolitics of "Post-AIDS"

Nicola Bulled

Mass media has successfully increased people's general knowledge about HIV transmission (Bertrand, O'Reilly, Denison, Anhang, & Sweat, 2006; Wilson, Bonevski, Jones, & Henry, 2009). Media messages have also proved successful at promoting favorable attitudes towards voluntary counseling and testing for HIV and at offering information on where to access medical and treatment services (Mckee, Bertrand, & Becker-Benton, 2004). A ten-year systematic review of HIV/AIDS mass communication campaigns focused on sexual behavior, HIV testing, or both (1998–2007) found that campaigns increasingly use strategies that include targeted defined audiences and behavior change messaging using behavioral theories rather than knowledge promotion (Noar, Palmgreen, Chabot, Dobransky, & Zimmerman, 2009). These campaigns achieved high message exposure. Media campaigns also used stronger research designs for outcome evaluations and included measures of behavior (or behavioral intentions) in outcome assessments as compared to campaigns conducted in years prior (Myhre & Flora, 2000). An assessment of 16 unique sexually transmitted infection testing and prevention mass media campaigns found that nearly all showed a difference between exposed and unexposed individuals on one or more key behavior outcomes (Friedman, Kachur, Noar, & McFarlane, 2016). Several campaigns found dose-response relationships and sustained effect. For example, an assessment of the New York City Department of Health and Mental Hygiene's "It's Never Just HIV" campaign revealed that among 447 self-reported HIV negative or unknown status National HIV Behavioral Surveillance study participants, more than one-third had seen the campaign and recalled its message (Reilly et al., 2016). Almost 10% of those who saw the campaign reported having changed their sexual or health behaviors in response, suggesting that thousands had been reached by the prevention media, although the impact on behavior remains unknown.

Beyond explicit health promotion media campaigns, media (including newspapers) routinely disseminate information on health and disease, framing how the public should understand health issues of concern, as well as reflecting public opinion. For example, a risky billboard advertisement by the Ghana Social Marketing Foundation wrote out, "Use a Condom" with sexually explicit stick figures reenacting the Kama Sutra. An article in the local newspaper, the

DOI: 10.4324/9781003000945-4

Daily Graphic, condemned the billboard, sparking significant public debate regarding suppressed issues of sexuality and condoms (McDonnell, 2016). News media frame the social organization of the human experience (Goffman, 1974), having a significant impact on contextualizing experiences that are beyond an individual's direct involvement and acting as a window on the world. News media also provide cues concerning which event should be regarded as important through its selections, omissions, and interpretations, intentionally or otherwise (McCombs, 2004). News media do so with superficial characteristics including choice of words, images, sources, and style, such as the fear and urgency promoting statement, "AIDS Kills" and images of the grim reaper popular in newsprint press early in the HIV pandemic. Media also frame issues in more fundamental ways, including how questions of life and death, relationships between men and women, sexuality in general, caregiving, and values such as honesty and openness are articulated (Johnson, Flora, & Rimal, 1997). Media also work with biomedical authorities to co-produce health messages (Briggs & Hallin, 2016). The media thereby puts a "face" on issues such as HIV, both "mediat[ing] and partially construct[ing] people's understandings of health and health-related issues" (Hodgetts & Chamberlain, 2006, p. 317; Rimal, Johnson, & Flora, 1997). As noted by McCombs (1993, p. 65), "[T]he media not only tell us what to think about, but also how to think about it, and consequently what to think."

This chapter explores the content of recent newsprint reporting (2012–2019) on Pre-Exposure Prophylaxis (PrEP) for HIV prevention, which was hailed as a "game changer" when it received U.S. Federal Drug Administration (FDA) approval in 2012. PrEP is a once daily pill, sold commercially under the name Truvada® (emtricitabine/tenofovir disoproxil fumarate), that offers 90% reduction in HIV infection risk when taken consistently. Three diverse responses to this new biomedical HIV prevention strategy are examined: campaigns to promote consumer demand in the U.S., activism to obtain access to PrEP in the U.K., and highly restricted PrEP distribution in South Africa. Evidence is offered in the form of excerpts from accessible articles published in the *New York Times* (U.S., n=27), *The Telegraph* (U.K., n=14), and *The Star* (South Africa, n=28) using the search terms "HIV," "prevention," and "PrEP."

The assessment likely does not include all related articles published in these periodicals within the specified period. The search relied on the search engines of the periodicals, not all articles were open access, and articles that were not reflective of the society in which it was published were excluded. For example, I excluded articles published in *The Star* (South Africa) about study results announced in Washington, D.C.

I draw on the concept of "biomediatization" which recognizes the media as a "co-produc[er] of medical objects and subjects through complex entanglements between epistemologies, technologies, biologies, and political economies," (Briggs & Hallin, 2016, p. 5) to examine the content of news reports, the origin of the information, and the impact of the message on efforts to move towards a "post-AIDS" era. Drawing from the concept of mediatization, biomediatization reflects on the role that media plays in shaping and framing the processes of biomedical knowledge communication. As described above, media are regarded as active players in the construction of biomedical knowledge and central to meaning making. Media are not viewed as passive transmitters of information. Furthermore, given the centrality of and our increasing dependence on media in our modern world, media have become instrumental in sociocultural shifts, not necessarily causing transformations, but co-constitutive for the articulation of politics, economics, and health.

Biomediatization emerged from work on biocommunicability, the critical examination of the circulation of biomedical knowledge from producers to consumers via various forms of translators and distributors. Biocommunicability models identified by Briggs and colleagues (Briggs & Hallin, 2007, 2010, 2016) include the biomedical authority, patient-consumer, public sphere, and social movement.

The ***biomedical authority or doctor knows best model*** imagines a hierarchical ordered linear trajectory of knowledge and agency, whereby knowledge is produced by biomedical authorities, codified in texts, translated in popular discourse, disseminated (via the media), and received by the passive public or patients. Briggs and Hallin (2016) argue that "the intensification of political, economic, and cultural conflicts over biomedicine have transformed this model of biocommunicability and eroded its dominance" (p.29). However, they argue that it continues to illustrate the centrality of biomedical professionals as sources of knowledge, the "primary definers," and the linear assumptions of injecting knowledge into an ill-informed populous. Prior work examining HIV discourse in print media during the early years of the HIV epidemic revealed the prominence of this model (Bulled, 2015). The ***patient-consumer model*** shifts the relationship between health professionals and the public, positioning laypersons as making informed decisions independently from the direct supervision of health authorities. A slight shift further, the ***public sphere model*** positions media consumers as citizen-spectators, as opposed to passive patients or consumer agents, interpreting biomedical information based on social values and collective decisions. Most of the articles presented in this analysis fall into this latter category. Finally, the ***social movement model*** recognizes the role of social movements in challenging biomedical authorities, including researchers, policy makers, and media representation. Briggs and Hallin's (2016) examination of health news reveals that social movement stories are only present in a limited extent. However, they recognize the significant role of social movements in shaping biocommunicability, and specifically point to social mobilization around HIV/AIDS in the 1980s. Activists, privileging forms of personal witnessing, intervened in HIV/AIDS knowledge production, challenged the processes of biomedical research, pushed forward the treatment agenda, informed government policy, and shifted media representation (Epstein, 1996).

This view that media is a co-producer of medical objects and subjects is informed by the work of Michel Foucault, who examined the manner in which state power mutated and developed new strategies and technologies to exercise sovereignty. As a co-producer of health news in collaboration with technocrats and biomedical authorities informed by knowledge that is evidenced by highly codified and institutionalized procedures such as scientific studies, the media channels the directives of State institutions. The media is a form of what Foucault describes as "governmentality," a mechanism for the State to exert control over populations, accomplished through stories that target, describe, and seek to regulate populations (Burchell, Gordon, & Miller, 1991; Dean, 1999; Foucault, 1997, 2003; Rose, 2006). I present an overview of recent newsprint media on PrEP, noting the shifting positions of actors involved in the circulation of biomedical knowledge and the role of the media in co-producing medical objects and subjects serving as a form of biopower.

Newsprint on PrEP in the "Post-AIDS" Era

Initial considerations of an HIV treatment drug as a prevention option surfaced in the 1990s as anecdotal evidence mounted of uninfected men who have sex with men (MSM) taking the antiretroviral Tenofovir in combination with Viagra and Ecstasy, a practice known as "taking the T" or "MTV" (Costello, 2005). The practice appeared to reduce the chance of HIV infection despite condomless sex. Drug trials on once-daily combination therapy Truvada revealed 42%–75% efficacy in preventing HIV infection among study participants assigned to Truvada as compared to placebo groups (Baeten et al., 2019; Grant et al., 2010). These studies included trials with MSM (Baeten et al., 2012), transgender women (Grant et al., 2018), serodiscordant couples (Baeten & Celum, 2011), women (Hanscom et al., 2016; Thomson et al., 2016), and people who inject drugs (Alistar, Owens, & Brandeau, 2014). However, PrEP effectiveness (HIV protection in general use) has proven higher than efficacy (protection seen in clinical trials) (Pyra et al., 2019). What might explain this unusual outcome? Closer examinations of clinical trial data revealed that of the study participants with detectable levels of the drug in their blood (a sign that Truvada was taken regularly), rates of HIV transmission dropped by as much as 92%. In general use, PrEP is proving 99% effective, indicating that people who choose to use PrEP use it consistently (Donnell et al., 2014).

Nevertheless, adherence challenges, stigma, concerns regarding behavioral disinhibition (no longer using condoms), costs, and healthcare capacity have limited the impact of this "game changing" disease prevention approach in reducing population-level HIV incidence (Bulled, 2019; McAllister, 1992; Rivet Amico & Bekker, 2019; Watts, 1993). Global estimates from 2018 suggest that between 300,000 and 380,000 individuals are prescribed PrEP, falling far short of the UNAIDS goal of 3 million PrEP users by 2020 (UNAIDS, 2019b). As noted in 2018 by Dawn Smith of the U.S. Centers for Disease Control and Prevention (CDC), speaking of PrEP use in the U.S., "After six years, we're nowhere near tapping the full potential of PrEP as a hugely powerful HIV prevention tool" (cited in Highleyman, 2018). Even in the U.S., which accounts for 75% of the global use of PrEP, the CDC estimates indicate that only a fraction of the at-risk population is taking advantage (cited in Buchbinder, 2018).

PrEP in the U.S.: Uncertainty, Acknowledgement, Access

Examining recent U.S. newsprint reports on PrEP reveals a contemporary social response that echoes the history of HIV concerns, as described above. Early accounts of PrEP exposed the fear and uncertainty surrounding the approach as experienced by the intended target audience, mainly MSM. These early articles reflect on social values that privilege biomedical expertise and marginalize individuals that are perceived to engage in risk behaviors. In a 2013 article, reporter Tuller (2013, para. 3) describes a "resisted pill to preventing HIV" as despite hopes that PrEP would be "exuberantly embraced by HIV-negative gay men … Truvada has been slow to catch on …. [and] In some quarters, the idea that healthy gay men should take a medication to prevent infection … has been met with hostility or indifference." Articles discussed a "backlash" against PrEP. Among MSM, "Truvada whores" became a commonly used trope, stigmatizing gay men who used PrEP to inspire a "sexual revolution" – engaging in condomless sex given the limited threat posed by HIV (McNeil, 2014; Tuller, 2013).

These concerns of risk compensation or behavioral disinhibition were amplified in the general population, revealing the continued stigmatization of HIV and the behaviors, lifestyles, and identities of those most burdened. An article by McNeil published in 2013, offers the most jarring evidence of HIV-stigma. Announcing the results of a study that proved the effectiveness of PrEP in people who inject drugs, McNeil repeatedly uses stigmatizing language – "new studies must work out how best to motivate *unpredictable drug users* to take [PrEP]," "*promiscuous* gay male patients," "*addicts* both share needles and *sell their bodies*," etc. (McNeil, 2013, para. 12; para. 17; para. 18). McNeil draws on official voices to indicate that these are not his opinions alone, but perceptions he shares with established biomedical authorities, stating "some researchers thought it *unlikely* that [PrEP] would protect *drug addicts*, and they were *pleasantly surprised it worked fairly well*" (McNeil, 2013, para. 20 emphasis added). Such language both reflects and establishes publicly held stereotypes of people who inject drugs being unreliable and MSM being licentious.

This media representation of MSM and people who inject drugs as erratic consumers of the new prevention technology further influenced how providers perceived their patients and consequently influenced PrEP access. Reporting the following year, McNeil (2014, para. 8) writes of men "being 'slut-shamed' by their own doctors, who are reluctant to write prescriptions." Similar accounts reveal men "receiving negative reactions from their healthcare providers when they brought [PrEP] up" (Tuller, 2013, para. 13). Survey studies revealed that U.S. primary care practitioners evaluated patient PrEP eligibility based on relationship stability and sexual health (as cited in Buchbinder, 2018). HIV-care providers were less willing to prescribe to people who inject drugs and high-risk heterosexuals (Adams & Balderson, 2016). U.S. medical students' willingness to prescribe PrEP was inconsistent with patient risk, as assessed by patients' current and planned condom use and engagement with multiple sexual partners (Calabrese et al., 2018). Black patients were perceived as more likely to engage in unprotected sex, which was associated with a reduced willingness to prescribe PrEP (Calabrese, Earnshaw, Underhill, Hansen, & Dovidio, 2014). Pushing on in his agenda to position MSM and people who inject drugs as non-compliant, undeserving risk-takers, the journalist McNeil (2015, para. 16) notes that these concerns are valid as studies show that "after starting PrEP, half of [the patients] became infected with syphilis, gonorrhea, or chlamydia within a year."

As information surfaced about the value of PrEP in moving towards a "post-AIDS" era, media reports began surfacing about the negative implications of such biased provider behavior. Offering a rare first-hand account of the challenges to taking PrEP, Hannah, as a member of an "at-risk" group, writes a compelling piece describing when he finally worked up the courage to ask his doctor for a prescription: "I'll never forget the look of disgust on her face as she told me why I wasn't a candidate for the drug: I didn't engage in 'reckless sex' and I wasn't a 'druggie'" (Hannah, 2017, para. 7). In 2016, the CDC was cited as explaining that, among doctors who are familiar with PrEP, "some are reluctant to prescribe it, fearing that it could encourage risky behavior that could lead to other infections" (Editorial Board, 2016, para. 6).

Media reports, such as those offered by Hannah, flipped claims of biomedical authority or expertise faulting biomedical authorities for not utilizing this new tool of prevention appropriately. In 2016, the CDC acknowledged that "many doctors and nurses are not familiar with [PrEP]" (Editorial Board, 2016, para. 6). Even an article published three years later noted that "doctors may not have heard of Truvada" as a reason for the slow uptake (Albeck-Ripka, 2019, para. 13). Hannah (2017, para. 7; para. 8), speaking as a Black male MSM who grew up in poverty in the southern U.S. (where the challenges of HIV are particularly acute), describes the discriminatory practice of providers as "unfortunate, but not surprising," placing the HIV epidemic within the broader U.S. social condition. Reflecting on his first attempt to acquire PrEP he describes his female doctor as "white and her tone so thick with judgement that it made my skin crawl." Five years later, he discussed PrEP with a new doctor, "He was a gay man of color and he initiated the conversation. Instead of telling me why I wasn't right for the drug, we spent the time talking about why I felt that I needed it." Hannah's personal journey with PrEP reveals the ongoing experiences of racism at the doctor's office, deep rooted suspicions held by Blacks about the healthcare industry, and strong stigmatization of sex between men in Black and Latinx communities that places them at heightened risk for HIV. Hannah also reveals a slow shift in the social consciousness regarding PrEP.

The initial uncertainty surrounding PrEP that motivated fear and brought to the fore stigma and discrimination has been replaced by an acknowledgement of the value of the product. Drawing on scientific evidence, PrEP is now considered a "data-driven, sex-positive approach" (McKinley, 2019, para. 15). In a rather rare turn for the media (Briggs & Hallin, 2016), more recent articles begin describing the structural barriers limiting PrEP access, rather than positioning HIV risk engagement as a conscious individual choice. In 2019, the conversation shifted to the high cost of the drug (McNeil, 2019b). In February 2019, the U.S.

government announced a goal to "end the H.I.V. [sic] epidemic in America" by 2030 (Victor, 2019, para. 3), with PrEP central to this goal. However, "critics have said that the drug's lofty price tag has limited its accessibility to high-risk people with low incomes, thwarting the government's efforts" (Victor, 2019, para. 3). Truvada can cost patients up to $20,000 a year (drugs.com/price-guide/truvada). As of June 2019, most private health insurers were required to offer the medication "at no out-of-pocket cost to their policyholders" (Albeck-Ripka, 2019, para. 12). Cities including New York and San Francisco provide free or subsidized access to PrEP. Gilead Sciences, the maker of Truvada, promised to supply 200,000 uninsured patients with the pill or "picks up insurance co-pays for patients who qualify" (McNeil, 2019a, para. 4) for 11 years. Gilead released Descovy® (emtricitabine and tenofovir alafenamide), a safer[1] Truvada replacement approved by the FDA, in October 2019, also available through insurers at no or limited out-of-pocket cost. A new program launched in December 2019, "Ready, Set, PrEP," "marks the first time the federal government is supplying PrEP to patients not enrolled in Medicaid, the Veterans Health Administration or any other federal health program" (McNeil, 2019a, para. 5). In November 2019, the Trump administration filed a legal suit against Gilead Sciences, "accusing the company of earning billions from research funded by taxpayers without paying taxpayers back" (Victor, 2019, para. 1), claiming that the federal government, and not the pharmaceutical company, owns the Truvada and Descovy patents.

These announcements on efforts to lower the cost of Truvada to improve PrEP access spark conversations on ongoing public concerns regarding structural challenges with healthcare in general. Drawing on official voices, the media highlight the debate regarding inequitable access to healthcare in the U.S., that includes high costs of healthcare visits, limited public transportation options, and high rates of being un- or underinsured among certain demographics (Flash, 2019). Quoting James Krellenstein, founder of the advocacy group PrEP4All Collaboration, and Dr. Rochelle P. Walensky, leader of a team at Massachusetts General Hospital who has analyzed the cost of the HIV plans of the Obama and Trump administrations, McNeil (2019a, para. 20) makes the argument that simply reducing the price of Truvada does not reduce the financial costs of PrEP to consumers. Krellenstein is quoted as saying "the government's plan 'is poised to repeat the errors of Gilead's own medication assistance program'" as patients get "no help paying for the medical exam and laboratory tests needed to get and keep renewing the prescription, which can cost up to $1,000 a year." Dr. Robert Grant, a professor of medicine at the University of California, San Francisco, who led the development of Truvada, is quoted in another article as saying that many patients find it impossible to navigate the "byzantine [healthcare] system" and that "costs for doctor's appointments themselves might be prohibitive" (Albeck-Ripka, 2019, para. 13). Speaking specifically of challenges facing communities in the American south, the new epicenter of the HIV epidemic there, Charlene Flash (2019, para. 13), an infectious-disease doctor and associate chief medical officer at Legacy Community Health and a clinical assistant professor at Baylor College of Medicine, concludes her article that details some of the distressing cases she sees of patients with advanced HIV diagnosed too late in their illness, by stating, "[Y]es, we can meet the president's goal of ending AIDS in a decade, but only if we race to get our new tools more efficiently and equitably to those who need them."

PrEP in the U.K.: Ethical Debates of Consequentialism

In the U.K., PrEP discussions have pondered the ethical quandary of consequentialism – less about whether PrEP is the right approach than whether PrEP has the right consequences. Media accounts of PrEP in the U.K. began surfacing in 2016 as activists began to confront the National Health System (NHS) England regarding PrEP access. Patients in England can purchase PrEP online and import the drug for private use, but cannot obtain PrEP for free through the NHS. A 30-day supply ranges in cost between £20 and £80. PrEP is, however, available through the NHS in Scotland and Northern Ireland. Early in 2016, Dr. Michael Brady, medical director of the Terrence Higgins Trust (a charity supporting HIV and sexual health services) was quoted in *The Telegraph* as saying, "[T]he reality is that the U.K. is now lagging well behind other countries on its approach to HIV prevention and its investment in successful interventions such as PrEP" (Graham, 2016, para. 4). These comments were made in response to a *Lancet HIV* mathematical modeling study indicating that PrEP alone could prevent almost 10,000 new HIV infections by 2020 when aimed at the entire MSM population in the U.K. (Punyacharoensin et al., 2016). Upfront costs of PrEP were estimated to offset treatment costs with every infection averted saving an estimated £360,000 (US$440,000) in lifetime treatment costs (Donnelly, 2016b; Graham, 2016). In August and again in November 2019, reports announced court rulings that rejected NHS England's claims that they could not afford to fund PrEP (Donnelly, 2016a; Telegraph Reporters, 2016). The NHS offered a utilitarian argument that funding PrEP at £20 million (US$24.4 million) a year meant that patients with costly diseases such as cancer and cystic fibrosis would be refused treatment (Telegraph Reporters, 2016).

Speaking out against the ruling requiring NHS England to pay for PrEP, spokesman for the Christian Medical Fellowship said, "We will need much more evidence that PrEP is truly effective in practice before embarking on a strategy that seems to have more to do with political correctness than medical science" (Telegraph Reporters, 2016, para. 5). Echoing sentiments of behavioral disinhibition from the U.S., James Mildred from the Christian Organization CARE raised fears of the drug "promoting promiscuity and more hedonistic, but risky lifestyles" (Donnelly, 2016a, para. 9). Presenting such viewpoints as biomedical authorities, the media reveal the perpetuation of prejudiced attitudes that existed towards HIV and its victims during the early days of the epidemic when little was known and the "mysterious new disease seemed to be spiraling out of control" (Gulland, 2019a, para. 1). Reflecting back on the epidemic in an article published in 2019, Lord Norman Fowler, a long-standing member of the U.K.

parliament, described a time of hysteria and misinformation. Attitudes towards gay people and to the disease were "backwards" – "The chief constable of Manchester, James Anderton, said that gay people, prostitutes or drug addicts who had contracted the disease were 'swirling in a cesspit of their own making'" (Gulland, 2019c, para. 5). Fowler describes a proposal circulating at the time to corral all people living with HIV into an isolation camp.

A staunch advocate for the provision of PrEP through NHS England, Deborah Gold, National AIDS Trust chief executive, stated that the court rulings compelling the NHS to provide PrEP were "vindication for the many people who were let down when NHS England absolved itself of responsibility for PrEP … over 4,000 people are getting HIV every year in the U.K. – we desperately need further prevention options" (Donnelly, 2016a, para. 6). Any delays to commissioning PrEP she described as "unethical and expensive" (Donnelly, 2016a, para. 6). Reporter Michael Segalov made a personal appeal writing that "as the arguments drag on in the corridors of Whitehall [government], members of my community are dying. Opponents say making such medicine available encourages promiscuity and reckless behavior" (Segalov, 2016, para. 2). He adds that these debates regarding whether or not to supply PrEP draw on past homophobic fears, in that "once again the sex lives of gay men [are] being judged and policed by the state" (Segalov, 2016, para. 2).

Following the court rulings, instead of providing PrEP, health officials again drew on their utilitarian arguments and announced a large three-year trial to "work out the best way to ensure take-up of the drug, examine the impact on HIV levels – and whether it increased rates of other sexually transmitted infections" (Donnelly, 2016b, para. 1). The PROUD trial is estimated to cost £10 billion and provide 26,000 men with PrEP (McCormack et al., 2016). Speaking out in 2019, Debbie Laycock, head of policy at the Terrence Higgins Trust, argued against the trial approach, stating that "we know PrEP works … there have been cases of people getting HIV because they haven't been able to access PrEP. It's such an important preventive tool and we haven't got it into the hands of those who need it" (Gulland, 2019a, para. 6). A report in 2019 estimated that this approach has left 25% of men desiring PrEP unable to access it (Gulland, 2019b).

By 2017, PrEP was no longer being hailed as the "promiscuity pill" (Telegraph Reporters, 2016), but as a significant component of the combination of strategies that led to a 21% decline in new cases of HIV infection among gay and bisexual men in the U.K. (Bodkin, 2017). This success, of which PrEP is recognized as making a "substantial contribution," is noted by Dr. Fitzpatrick as "reflect[ing] a welcome shift in the public health strategy, away from the moralizing and scaremongering of the notorious 'Don't Die of Ignorance' campaign of 30 years ago, to the discreet focus on groups at high risk of infection and the development of effective medications" (Fitzpatrick, 2017, para. 3). Despite the media shifting the presentation of PrEP, drawing on biomedical authorities to argue for the provision of PrEP via the NHS, the PROUD trial continued through 2019. Lord Fowler noted in an article published in November 2019 that the prevailing attitudes of the Margaret Thatcher administration of the 1980s that resisted telling young people about risky sex for fear of promoting promiscuity was partly behind the failure of the current government to fully fund access to PrEP (Gulland, 2019c). Moralizing and making ethical determinations about who has the right to health based on sexual identity and lifestyle choices clearly influenced PrEP access and consequently HIV risk in the U.K. The media's positioning of certain voices as biomedical authorities allowed for the co-production of public sentiments regarding PrEP. Initially, the media presented PrEP as an unproven strategy that valued the life of a gay man over the life of cancer victim. Later, PrEP was portrayed, evidenced by scientific research, as an effective disease prevention tool that not only saves lives but also lowers healthcare costs.

PrEP in South Africa: Ethical Allocation of Scarce Resources

In 2015, the World Health Organization and UNAIDS endorsed the global distribution and use of oral PrEP as an additional HIV prevention strategy. UNAIDS offered the endorsement with caution, noting that "PrEP can be a cost-effective addition, depending on how well it is integrated into comprehensive HIV programmes and given priority for people who are at highest HIV risk and want PrEP" (UNAIDS, 2015, p. 10). The South African Health Products Regulatory Authority approved PrEP that same year. The South African Department of Health first adopted the use of PrEP in 2016.

South Africa currently has the largest HIV epidemic in the world, with 7.7 million people living with HIV and an HIV prevalence of 20.4% (UNAIDS, 2017, 2019a). The denialist stance[2] of former President Thabo Mbeki during the 1990s and his refusal to allow treatment access is generally agreed to be the primary contributor to the HIV-burden experienced today (Fassin, 2007). However, South Africa currently boasts the largest anti-retroviral treatment program in the world, with 68% of people aware of their status on treatment and 87% of those virally suppressed, putting South Africa close to the UNAIDS 90–90–90 target.[3] Clear successes of the treatment program, including a rise in national life expectancy of seven years between 2010 and 2015 (SANAC, 2017), have not translated into prevention. In 2018, there were an estimated 240,000 new infections (SANAC, 2017). While high-risk groups include sex workers, MSM, and people who inject drugs, HIV prevalence among young women aged 15–24 years made up 37% of new infections in 2016. HIV prevalence in young women in South Africa is four times greater than that of men their age – a consequence of biology, gender-based socioeconomic disparities, gender power dynamics, and a lack of female controlled HIV prevention options (Harrison, Colvin, Kuo, Swartz, & Lurie, 2015).

South Africa was the first country in sub-Saharan Africa to fully approve PrEP (UNAIDS, 2017), but the roll-out was limited only to high-risk groups. Responding to the FDA approval of PrEP in 2012, Dr. Francesca Conradie, president of the Southern African HIV Clinicians Society, was quoted in *The Star* as being in favor of the new approach, stating that "there was no one single answer to the prevention of HIV infection, no 'one size fits all'" (Thom, 2012a, para. 4), but that PrEP is an "ideal intervention" in cases where people are unable to negotiate safer sex (Thom, 2012b). Yet, adding a note of caution, Conradie stated, "[W]e would like to stress that the efficacy of Truvada is linked to adherence. The risks of taking this medication erratically are great. Like the use of condoms, consistent use to prevent infection is mandatory" (Thom, 2012a, para. 5). The president of the South African Medical Research Council, Glenda Grey, rather than placing responsibility on individual consumers, presented the structural challenges to including PrEP in South Africa's national strategy. Beyond just concerns of ensuring high individual adherence to PrEP, budget and healthcare resource capacity limitations make providing treatment to already infected individuals a challenge. Offering treatment to people not yet infected, in the form of PrEP, would significantly increase costs and capacity needs. Grey laid out these challenges and argued for a continued focus on treatment (Thom, 2012a, para. 6):

> First-line therapy now includes [Truvada], at a cost of $11 billion (R90bn). The implementation of antiretroviral therapy in [South Africa] has been further stressed by the increase in the threshold for initiating treatment to a CD4 count of 350 cells per cubic millimeter [a product of the test-and-treat approach]. In addition, the frequent lack of availability of antiretroviral drugs suggests that existing antiretroviral treatment programmes are already overwhelmed. ... Giving effective antiretroviral treatment to HIV-infected persons earlier and enhancing the use of proven strategies should be the current mainstays for preventing HIV transmission.

Here, Grey articulates the ethical quandary facing South Africa – prioritizing the lives of people who have not yet been infected by providing PrEP, or prolonging the lives of those already infected through treating them.

The question surrounding PrEP in South Africa reflects the central tension of public health: whose life is more important? If resources are spent on preventing someone from getting HIV, ensuring they can be a healthy contributor to the economy and not ultimately saving the state money in lifelong HIV treatments, does that deny HIV treatment to a person living with HIV? And given that treatment is a form of prevention (an undetectable viral load reduces the likelihood of transmission), is investing in treatment saving more lives? Which approach is ultimately more cost-effective? Writing an opinion piece in 2012 titled, "HIV could become retro," Alex Welte, director of the South African Centre for Epidemiological Modelling and Analysis at Stellenbosch University, provoked readers by asking (Welte, 2012, para 23–24):

> How easy is it to pay a huge up-front cost for long-term saving that accrue only beyond the technical planning horizon? Are there effective, and ethical, ways of prioritizing treatment across for key groups where the epidemiological impact would be more efficient? How do we administer an audaciously bigger programme of drug distribution and chronic patient care than the impressive one SA [South Africa] has set up in recent years?

These conversations regarding the structural challenges of public health and healthcare are rare in health news. Considering who deserves the drug (for treatment or for prevention), how to prioritize among vulnerable risk groups (sex workers, MSM, young women), and how to provide high quality care in an already burdened health sector, let alone expand services to people who are not yet ill, ultimately resulted in South Africa electing to go with a highly regulated PrEP distribution plan. Media accounts of PrEP returned to a primary focus on individual responsibilities. Following the announcement of South African approval of PrEP in 2015, Dr. Joey Gouws, registrar of the Medicines Control Council, stated, "[T]he drug won't be dispensed willy-nilly. We hope that medical practitioners will be a guard against abuse of the drug" (Fokazi, 2015, para. 7). Gouws' comments hint at critics' concerns that Truvada "may promote unsafe sex and promiscuity" (Fokazi, 2015, para. 4), as well as recognizing the concerns of the "ethical allocation of scarce resources" (Gostin, 2016, para. 15). These articles are clear examples of the public sphere model of biocommunicability, where citizens are regarded as active participants in the discussion. The politics of access are discussed, with concerns raised regarding structural and resource limitations. However, these are coupled with concerns regarding individual responsibility and deservingness. The media presents the rationale behind limited PrEP distribution as concerns regarding an inability to control consumer use of the product and the potential for misuse of a valuable technology by members of society already considered incompetent to maintain their own health.

By 2017, between 30,000 and 35,000 individuals were being targeted with PrEP in ongoing and planned projects across South Africa (PrEP Watch, 2018). A news article published in 2017 stated that if "South Africa plan[s] to reduce new infections from the estimated 270,000 new HIV infections a year to less than 100,000 by 2022, it is imperative that we offer PrEP to those most at risk" (Isaacs, 2017, para. 17). The 2017–2022 National Strategic Plan aims to expand PrEP access to all those who are most likely to benefit, including adolescents, sex workers, MSM, and people who inject drugs (SANAC, 2017). An estimated 85,858 more people from the most affected groups should be initiated onto PrEP by 2022 (SANAC, 2017). However, by 2018, the Department of Health estimated that only 3,011 young people (15–24 years) were using PrEP, a statistic described as a "woefully low figure" by Professor Francois Venter from the Wits Reproductive Health and HIV Institute (Green, 2018, para. 4). Venter adds, "It's not clear why something that clearly works is not being rolled out aggressively." Published on World AIDS Day 2018, the article notes, "South Africa is sleeping on the most successful weapon against HIV in recent history."

The "Face" of AIDS and "Post-AIDS" in Newsprint

By virtue of its sociological involvement in public opinion (Dearing & Rogers, 1996) and its role in disseminating information to the people, news media plays a central role in contextualizing, negotiating, shaping, and defining power relationships between stakeholders in the HIV epidemic (Bulled, 2015; Clarke, 1992;

Grube & Boehme-Deurr, 1989; Lester, 1992; Lim, 1995; Lupton, 1993; Netter, 1992; Princeton Survey Research Associates, 1996; Semetko & Goldberg, 1993; Traquina, 1996). Assessing historical media coverage of the HIV pandemic reveals shifting public opinions regarding the threat of HIV (Bulled, 2015; Watts, 1993). During the early phase of the global pandemic, when little was known in the scientific and medical communities about the virus and politicians offered little support, media coverage of HIV was marked by fear, ignorance, and blame attribution. This was replaced by a phase of exploration, understanding, and acceptance as science began to determine transmission routes and political will ensured the funding necessary to promote risk prevention and develop biomedical diagnostics and treatments (McAllister, 1992). From the 1990s onwards, the focus of news media has been on routine events such as World AIDS Day and the annual AIDS conference. This is likely because there have been few significant advancements to report in the progression of HIV control beyond the most recent PrEP. It can be argued that this phase reflected by routine media coverage has generated a false sense of security, recasting the urgency of HIV as a life-long debilitating disease or certain death into a mold of routine (Sepulveda, Fineberg, & Mann, 1992). As a consequence of this routine reporting, or reporting only on announcements of trial and study results, policies, and approvals, "official" sources including biomedical researchers, practitioners, and policy makers have come to control and shape the contours of the HIV narrative (Bardhan, 2002; Gans, 1979) in collaboration with the media.

The "face" of "post-AIDS" as presented by the news media is that of a highly controlled and easily managed disease that poses little threat to individuals or society. In 2019, numerous news reports in the U.S. focused on announcements from many large cities including New York, Philadelphia, San Francisco, and Chicago, all reporting historic falls not only in AIDS, but also in new cases of HIV infection. In June 2019, a headline in the *New York Times* read, "'If we do this right' maybe HIV will be forgotten" (Dubin, 2019); later that same year, the article "New York Says End of AIDS Epidemic Is Near," (McKinley, 2019, para. 2) announced an 11% drop in reported AIDS cases, on target to meet a goal to "end the AIDS epidemic in the state [of New York] by 2020." In March, *The Telegraph* reported of a London man cured of AIDS, only the second individual to be cured of the HIV infection (Knapton, 2019). In July, *The Telegraph* reported on new gene editing technology to "snip" viral DNA out of the chromosomes of individuals infected with HIV, as a future cure for infection.

But post-AIDS, as presented by the news media, is duplicitous. On the one hand it appears that the epidemic is moving to a point of control, even eradication. On the other, the epidemic remains a significant problem. Despite triumphs in big cities in the U.S., rural American is seeing rising cases of HIV as a result of the opioid crisis, inaccessible healthcare, lack of prevention services, and poverty (Thrasher, 2019). The South African newspaper, *The Star*, centered its 2019 World AIDS Day stories on the impact to communities (Byanyima, 2019) in "the *battle* against HIV/AIDS" (Jasson Da Costa, 2019, emphasis added, para. 1). Jasson Da Costa (2019) writes of the Gogo Support Group program, providing economic and social support, education, and skills training to *gogos* (grandmothers) who have nursed their dying children, raised the orphaned grandchildren, and provided an income to support the family. Byanyima (2019) introduces the Ritshidze Project, people living with HIV actively monitoring HIV and TB service delivery to improve health services and advocate for change. Articles also reported on government officials getting tested for HIV to "encourage people to take responsibility for their health" (Staff reporter, 2019, para. 1). As these less abundant reports suggest, AIDS remains a very real and current challenge for many marginalized communities.

Examining newsprint media reports of PrEP since its approval in 2012 in the U.S., U.K., and South Africa reveals unique yet overlapping concerns. Researchers, providers, and policy makers have offered their thoughts through the media, as quoted officials, or opinion piece writers, driving public opinion. In all three spaces, the historical trajectory of the media's projection of AIDS is repeated through PrEP, with language of fear, skepticism, and resistance, eventually replaced by acceptance and celebration. Media on PrEP initially privileged biomedical expertise, then shifted towards to patient consumers, and finally began presenting a public sphere model of biocommunicability that has allowed readers to make judgements about collective actions and social values. On occasion, these accounts raise the structural challenges of healthcare, positioning the burden of HIV on society rather than select individuals. Media accounts more often highlight the social stigma and discrimination that continues to thwart progress in HIV control. Racial discrimination limits access to PrEP by those most in need, namely Black and brown men and women in the U.S.' southern states, as doctors resist prescribing PrEP, costs of healthcare are prohibitive to adhere to PrEP check-up requirements, and many are under- or uninsured. NHS England's determination that it is not required to provide PrEP reflects globally held perceptions that gay lifestyles are hedonistic, that PrEP as a "party drug" is the cause of increased rates of sexually transmitted infections among MSM, that responsible individuals can prevent HIV through behavior modification, and, consequently, that the state is justified in placing greater value on the lives of others (SAPA-AP, 2014). Conversations of PrEP as a vital tool in the goal to end AIDS in South Africa reveal structural challenges that continue to drive the epidemic. These include laws, policies, and practices that discriminate against and stigmatize people living with HIV and key risk populations as well as socially embedded inequalities that render young women and girls particularly vulnerable to HIV infection (Bekker, 2018; Mngoma, 2016). The official mediatization of PrEP in all contexts, as co-produced by media, policy makers, researchers, and practitioners, privilege biomedical expertise and position the patients that stand the most to benefit from PrEP as either unlikely to be adherent or use PrEP as a reason to take greater risks (Bulled, 2019).

Ethical quandaries are also presented in each case. Recent reports of the Trump administration suing Gilead Sciences, maker of Truvada, over their right to profit off the U.S. public given that their product was developed using taxpayer money raises questions about the profiteering of the pharmaceutical industry. In the U.K. and South Africa, the public health challenge of scare resource allocation raises questions of whose lives are worth saving. In the U.K., the argument is against "AIDS exceptionalism" – that AIDS should no longer be prioritized over other health conditions. This is a notable shift in AIDS discourse, remarks Lawrence Gostin, Professor of Global Health at Georgetown University, in an opinion piece published in *The Star*, who states, "[T]he issue is [no longer] so much that public health and civil liberties are in tension but rather that AIDS has captured a disproportionate amount of political attention and economic resources" (Gostin, 2016, para. 14). In England, while the state may not want to assume responsibility to supply the prevention drug, it remains accessible to many at risk of infection through private means. On the other hand, in South Africa, not only do unaddressed social structures increase risk of HIV in select populations, most individuals at greatest risk for HIV and best served by PrEP could never afford to access it otherwise. Furthermore, there is little evidence, and none presented in the news media examined for this study, of civil action to compel the South African state to assume greater responsibility in saving lives.

As a window framing the issue of PrEP and the "Post-AIDS" agenda, the media reveals that despite 40 years of major advancements in HIV control, structural challenges, resource limitations, and continued discrimination remain barriers to "HIV becom[ing] retro" (Welte, 2012). Yet the media offers more than merely a passive reflection of societal views. Journalists have become central figures in the co-production of knowledge, central in controlling the body politic. Biomediatiziation recognizes the power of media to co-produce understandings of biomedical objects (PrEP) and subjects (potential consumers of PrEP). The centrality of media in our modern lives and our increasing dependence on media, allow it to shape social perceptions. Furthermore, health news is often treated as political, although active participants are primarily biomedical insiders and rarely citizens, and structural causes of illness are often avoided with focus shifted towards technology and individual responsibility for health (Briggs & Hallin, 2016). Directing consciousness and changing bodily practice are governmentalities directed at the biological existence of those living with or potentially at risk for HIV (Nguyen, 2009). Greater attention, therefore, should be paid to the presentation of PrEP and PrEP consumers by media, as media play a vital role in either perpetuating stigma and discrimination or, alternatively, stimulating a progressive movement towards an inclusive society. As biopolitical agents, media mediate public opinion about who is deserving of access to PrEP and assist government regulators in justifying restrictive and discriminatory access policies

Notes

1 Truvada and Descovy are combination drugs. Both contain the drug emtricitabine, but Truvada also contains tenofovir disoproxil fumarate (TDF), while Descovy contains a newer version of the medication called tenofovir alafenamide (TAF). TAF is less likely to cause bone loss and kidney problems than TDF. However, Descovy has implications for cardiovascular risk as a result of changes in blood fat levels.

2 Former South African President Thabo Mbeki argued that HIV did not cause AIDS, and therefore drugs for HIV would not prevent people from dying from AIDS. These perspectives were supported by the radical view of University of California biologist Peter Duesberg (Duesberg, 1992). Duesberg claimed that HIV is harmless and that AIDS is actually caused by illicit drug abuse, poverty, and antiretroviral medications (Duesberg, Nicholson, Rasnick, Fiala, & Bauer, 2009).

3 In 2014, UNAIDS set out new targets for reducing the burden of HIV by 2020, this included getting 90% of people living with HIV to know their status, 90% of all people living with HIV on antiretroviral therapy, and 90% of all people receiving antiretroviral therapy to have viral suppression (UNAIDS, 2017).

References

Adams, L. M., & Balderson, B. H. (2016). HIV providers' likelihood to prescribe pre-exposure prophylaxis (PrEP) for HIV prevention differs by patient type: a short report. *AIDS Care, 28*(9), 1154–1158. doi:10.1080/09540121.2016.1153595

Albeck-Ripka, L. (2019, July). How Australia could almost eradicate HIV transmissions. *New York Times.* Retrieved from https://www.nytimes.com/2019/07/10/world/australia/hiv-aids-prep-prevention-drug.html?searchResultPosition=7

Alistar, S. S., Owens, D. K., & Brandeau, M. L. (2014). Effectiveness and Cost Effectiveness of Oral Pre-Exposure Prophylaxis in a Portfolio of Prevention Programs for Injection Drug Users in Mixed HIV Epidemics. *PLoS One, 9*(1), e86584. doi:10.1371/journal.pone.0086584

Baeten, J., & Celum, C. (2011, July). *Antiretroviral pre-exposure prophylaxis for HIV-1 prevention among heterosexual African men and women: The Partners PrEP Study.* Paper presented at the 2011 International AIDS Society Conference on HIV Pathogenesis, Treatment and Prevention, Rome, IT.

Baeten, J., Donnell, D., Ndase, P., Mugo, N. R., Campbell, J. D., Wangisi, J., …Partners Pr, E. P. S. T. (2012). Antiretroviral prophylaxis for HIV prevention in heterosexual men and women. *New England Journal of Medicine, 367*(5), 399–410. doi:10.1056/NEJMoa1108524

Baeten, J., Palanee-Phillips, T., Mgodi, N., Ramjee, G., Gati, B., Mhlanga, F., …MTN-025/HOPE Study Team. (2019, July). *High adherence and sustained impact on HIV-1 incidence: Final results of an open-label extension trial of the dapivirine vaginal ring.* Paper presented at the 2019 International AIDS Conference, Mexico City, MX.

Bardhan, N. R. (2002). Accounts from the field: A public relations perspective on global AIDS/HIV. *Journal of Health Communication, 7*(3), 221–244.

Bekker, L. G. (2018, July). The 2018 World Aids conference - reflecting on the HIV pandemic. *The Star.* Retrieved from https://www.iol.co.za/lifestyle/health/the-2018-world-aids-conference-reflecting-on-the-hiv-pandemic-16206401

Bertrand, J., O'Reilly, K., Denison, J., Anhang, R., & Sweat, M. (2006). Systematic review of the effectiveness of mass communication programs to change HIV/AIDS-related behaviors in developing countries. *Health Education Research, Theory and Practice, 21*(4), 567–597.

Bodkin, H. (2017, October). HIV cases among gay and bisexual men drop for the first time as experts hail 'significant advance'. *The Telegraph.* Retrieved from https://www.telegraph.co.uk/news/2017/10/03/hiv-cases-among-gay-bisexual-men-drop-first-time-experts-hail/

Briggs, C., & Hallin, D. (2007). Biocommunicability: The neoliberal subject and its contradictions in news coverage of health issues. *Social Text, 25*(4), 43–66.

Briggs, C., & Hallin, D. (2010). Health reporting as political reporting: Biocommunicability and the public sphere. *Journalism, 11*(2), 149–165.

Briggs, C., & Hallin, D. (2016). *Making health public: How news coverage is remaking media, medicine, and contemporary life*. New York: Routledge.

Buchbinder, S. P. (2018). Maximizing the benefits of HIV Preexposure Prophylaxis. *Topics in Antiviral Medicine, 25*(4), 138–142.

Bulled, N. (2015). *Prescribing HIV prevention: Bringing culture into global health communication*. Walnut Creek, CA: Left Coast Press.

Bulled, N. (2019). Public health's social contract: An obstacle in the advancement of effective HIV technologies. *Glob Public Health, 14*(9), 1264–1274. doi:10.1080/17441692.2019.1585468

Burchell, G., Gordon, C., & Miller, P. (Eds.). (1991). *The Foucault effect: Studies in governmentality*. Chicago, IL: University of Chicago Press.

Byanyima, W. (2019, November). Communities are making the difference in SA's HIV response. *The Star*. Retrieved from https://www.iol.co.za/news/opinion/communities-are-making-the-difference-in-sas-hiv-response-38170327

Calabrese, S. K., Earnshaw, V. A., Underhill, K., Hansen, N. B., & Dovidio, J. F. (2014). The impact of patient race on clinical decisions related to prescribing HIV Pre-Exposure Prophylaxis (PrEP): Assumptions about sexual risk compensation and implications for access. *AIDS and Behavior, 18*(2), 226–240. doi:10.1007/s10461-013-0675-x

Calabrese, S. K., Earnshaw, V. A., Underhill, K., Krakower, D. S., Magnus, M., Hansen, N. B., …Dovidio, J. F. (2018). Prevention paradox: Medical students are less inclined to prescribe HIV pre-exposure prophylaxis for patients in highest need. *Journal of the International AIDS Society, 21*(6), e25147. doi:10.1002/jia2.25147

Clarke, J. N. (1992). Cancer, heart disease, and AIDS: What do the media tell us about these diseases? *Health Communication, 4*(2), 105–120.

Costello, D. (2005, December 19, 2005). AIDS pill as party drug? *The Los Angeles Times*. Retrieved from http://articles.latimes.com/2005/dec/19/health/he-hiv19

Dean, M. (1999). *Governmentality: Power and rule in modern society*. London: Sage.

Dearing, J. W., & Rogers, E. (1996). *Agenda-setting*. Thousand Oaks, CA: Sage.

Donnell, D., Baeten, J. M., Bumpus, N. N., Brantley, J., Bangsberg, D. R., Haberer, J. E., …Celum, C. (2014). HIV protective efficacy and correlates of tenofovir blood concentrations in a clinical trial of PrEP for HIV prevention. *Journal of Acquired Immune Deficiency Syndromes, 66*(3), 340–348. doi:10.1097/qai.0000000000000172

Donnelly, L. (2016a, August). AIDS charity wins battle over funding for HIV preventative treatment. *The Telegraph*. Retrieved from https://www.telegraph.co.uk/news/2016/08/02/aids-charity-wins-battle-over-funding-for-hiv-preventative-treat/

Donnelly, L. (2016b, December). Trial for HIV prevention drug approved. *The Telegraph*. Retrieved from https://www.telegraph.co.uk/news/2016/12/04/trial-hiv-prevention-drug-approved/

Dubin, S. (2019, June). 'If we do this right' maybe H.I.V. will be forgotten. *New York Times*. Retrieved from https://www.nytimes.com/2019/06/12/health/demetre-daskalakis-hiv-aids.html

Duesberg, P. (1992). AIDS: The alternative view. *Lancet, 339*(8808), 1547.

Duesberg, P. H., Nicholson, J. M., Rasnick, D., Fiala, C., & Bauer, H. H. (2009). HIV-AIDS hypothesis out of touch with South African AIDS–A new perspective. *Population, 45*, 50.

Editorial Board. (2016, February). HIV's toll on black and Latino men. *New York Times*. Retrieved from https://www.nytimes.com/2016/02/29/opinion/hivs-toll-on-black-and-latino-men.html?searchResultPosition=37

Epstein, S. (1996). *Impure science: AIDS, activism, and the politics of knowledge*. Berkeley: University of California Press.

Fassin, D. (2007). *When bodies remember*. Berkeley: University of California Press.

Fitzpatrick, M. (2017, July). Doctor's diary: The end of AIDS? *The Telegraph*. Retrieved from https://www.telegraph.co.uk/health-fitness/doctors-diary/doctors-diary-autism-medication-hindrance-help/

Flash, C. (2019, March). San Francisco is beating H.I.V. why can't Houston? *New York Times*. Retrieved from https://www.nytimes.com/2019/03/01/opinion/hiv-aids-south.html?searchResultPosition=32

Fokazi, S. (2015, December). New HIV prevention drug welcomed. *The Star*. Retrieved from https://www.iol.co.za/lifestyle/health/new-hiv-prevention-drug-welcomed/1958244

Foucault, M. (1997). The birth of biopolitics. In P. Rabinow (Ed.), *Ethics: Subjectivity and truth* (pp. 73–80). New York: New Press.

Foucault, M. (2003). *'Society must be defended': Lectures at the Colle ̀ge de France 1975–1976*. London: Picador.

Friedman, A. L., Kachur, R. E., Noar, S. M., & McFarlane, M. (2016). Health communication and social marketing campaigns for sexually transmitted disease prevention and control: What is the evidence of their effectiveness? *Sexually Transmitted Diseases, 43*(2 Suppl 1), S83–S101. doi:10.1097/olq.0000000000000286

Gans, H. J. (1979). *Deciding what's news*. New York: Pantheon.

Goffman, E. (1974). *Frame analysis: An essay on the organization of experience*. New York: Harper & Row.

Gostin, L. (2016, February). Advances made in HIV/AIDS fight. *The Star*. Retrieved from https://www.iol.co.za/dailynews/opinion/advances-made-in-hivaids-fight-1987808

Graham, C. (2016, January). Daily HIV pill for men 'would prevent 10,000 new cases in UK by 2020'. *The Telegraph*. Retrieved from https://www.telegraph.co.uk/news/health/news/12098835/Daily-HIV-pill-for-men-would-prevent-10000-new-cases-in-UK-by-2020.html

Grant, R. M., Lama, J. R., Anderson, P. L., McMahan, V., Liu, A. Y., Vargas, L., ...iPrEx Study, T. (2010). Preexposure chemoprophylaxis for HIV prevention in men who have sex with men. *New England Journal of Medicine, 363*(27), 2587–2599. doi:10.1056/NEJMoa1011205

Grant, R. M., Mannheimer, S., Hughes, J. P., Hirsch-Moverman, Y., Loquere, A., Chitwarakorn, A., ...Holtz, T. H. (2018). Daily and nondaily oral preexposure prophylaxis in men and transgender women who have sex with men: The Human Immunodeficiency Virus Prevention Trials Network 067/ADAPT study. *Clinical Infectious Diseases, 66*(11), 1712–1721. doi:10.1093/cid/cix1086

Green, A. (2018, December). #WorldAIDSDay: State ignoring key weapon in fight against HIV. *The Star*. Retrieved from https://www.iol.co.za/news/politics/worldaidsday-state-ignoring-key-weapon-in-fight-against-hiv-18344073

Grube, A., & Boehme-Deurr, K. (1989). AIDS in international magazines. *Journalism Quarterly, 66*, 686–689.

Gulland, A. (2019a, March). The AIDS endgame: How the UK and US are committed to wiping out HIV. *The Telegraph*. Retrieved from https://www.telegraph.co.uk/global-health/science-and-disease/aids-endgame-uk-us-committed-wiping-hiv/

Gulland, A. (2019b, October). Half a million gay men across Europe miss out on HIV prevention tool. *The Telegraph*. Retrieved from https://www.telegraph.co.uk/global-health/science-and-disease/half-million-gay-menacross-europe-miss-hiv-prevention-tool/

Gulland, A. (2019c, November). The minister for AIDS: How an establishment figure helped avert the HIV crisis. *The Telegraph*. Retrieved from https://www.telegraph.co.uk/global-health/science-and-disease/minister-aids-establishment-figure-helped-avert-hiv-crisis/

Hannah, D. (2017, September). My struggle to take anti-HIV medicine. *New York Times*. Retrieved from https://www.nytimes.com/2017/09/21/opinion/sunday/-truvada-gay-hiv-aids.html?searchResultPosition=33

Hanscom, B., Janes, H. E., Guarino, P. D., Huang, Y., Brown, E. R., Chen, Y. Q., ... Donnell, D. J. (2016). Brief report: Preventing HIV-1 infection in women using oral preexposure prophylaxis: A meta-analysis of current evidence. *Journal of Acquired Immune Deficiency Syndromes, 73*(5), 606–608. doi:10.1097/QAI.0000000000001160

Harrison, A., Colvin, C. J., Kuo, C., Swartz, A., & Lurie, M. (2015). Sustained high HIV incidence in young women in southern Africa: Social, behavioral, and structural factors and emerging intervention approaches. *Current HIV/AIDS Reports, 12*(2), 207–215. doi:10.1007/s11904-015-0261-0

Highleyman, L. (2018). PrEP use growing in US, but not reaching all those in need. *NAM AIDSMAP*. Retrieved from http://www.aidsmap.com/PrEP-use-growing-in-US-but-not-reaching-all-those-in-need/page/3222068/

Hodgetts, D., & Chamberlain, K. (2006). Developing a critical media research agenda for health psychology. *Journal of Health Psychology, 11*(2), 317–327.

Isaacs, L. (2017, September). Boost in fight for those at high risk of HIV exposure. *The Star*. Retrieved from https://www.iol.co.za/capetimes/news/boost-in-fight-for-those-at-high-risk-of-hiv-exposure-11397551

Jasson Da Costa, W. (2019, December). These gogos are heroes in the battle against HIV/AIDS. *The Star*. Retrieved from https://www.iol.co.za/sunday-tribune/news/these-gogos-are-heroes-in-the-battle-against-hivaids-38445015

Johnson, D., Flora, J. A., & Rimal, R. N. (1997). HIV/AIDS public service annuncements around the world: A descriptive analysis. *Journal of Health Communication: International Perspectives, 2*(4), 223–234.

Knapton, S. (2019, March). London man becomes only second person to be 'cured' of HIV as scientists hail breakthrough. *The Telegraph*. Retrieved from https://www.telegraph.co.uk/news/2019/03/05/british-man-may-second-cured-hiv/

Lester, E. (1992). The AIDS story and moral panic: How the Euro-African press constructs AIDS. *Howard Journal of Communications, 7*(1), 1–10.

Lim, K. (1995). Reporting AIDS: News representations in the Malaysian newspapers. *Journal of Development Communication, 7*(1), 79–86.

Lupton, D. (1993). AIDS risk and heterosexuality in the Australian press. *Discourse and Society, 4*, 307–328.

McAllister, M. P. (1992). AIDS, medicalization, and the news media. In T. Edgar, M. Fitzpatrick, & V. Freimuth (Eds.), *AIDS: A communication perspective* (pp. 195–221). Hillsdale, NJ: Lawrence Erlbaum Associates.

McCombs, M. (1993). The evolution of agenda-setting research: 25 years in the marketplace in ideas. *Journal of Communication, 43*, 58–67.

McCombs, M. (2004). *Setting the agenda: The mass media and public opinion*. Cambridge: Polity.

McCormack, S., Dunn, D. T., Desai, M., Dolling, D. I., Gafos, M., Gilson, R., ...Gill, O. N. (2016). Pre-exposure prophylaxis to prevent the acquisition of HIV-1 infection (PROUD): effectiveness results from the pilot phase of a pragmatic open-label randomised trial. *Lancet, 387*(10013), 53–60. doi:10.1016/s0140-6736(15)00056-2

McDonnell, T. E. (2016). *Best laid plans: Cultural entropy and the unraveling of AIDS media campaigns*. Chicago, IL: The University of Chicago Press.

Mckee, N., Bertrand, J., & Becker-Benton, A. (2004). *Strategic communication in HIV/AIDS epidemic*. New Delhi: Sage.

McKinley, J. (2019, October). New York Says end of AIDS epidemic is near. *New York Times*. Retrieved from https://www.nytimes.com/2019/10/02/nyregion/aids-hiv-epidemic-ny.html

McNeil, D. G. J. (2013, June). Study shows pill prevents HIV among drug addicts. *New York Times*. Retrieved from https://www.nytimes.com/2013/06/13/health/pill-prevents-hiv-among-drug-addicts-in-a-study.html?searchResultPosition=44

McNeil, D. G. J. (2014, May). Are we ready for H.I.V.'s sexual revolution? *New York Times*. Retrieved from https://www.nytimes.com/2014/05/24/opinion/sunday/ready-for-hivs-sexual-revolution.html?searchResultPosition=50

McNeil, D. G. J. (2015, September). Insurer says clients on daily pill have stayed HIV-free. *New York Times*. Retrieved from https://www.nytimes.com/2015/09/03/health/insurer-says-clients-on-daily-pill-have-stayed-hiv-free.html?searchResultPosition=29

McNeil, D. G. J. (2019a, December). 200,000 uninsured Americans to get free H.I.V.-prevention drugs. *New York Times*. Retrieved from https://www.nytimes.com/2019/12/03/health/truvada-prep-hiv-gilead.html?searchResultPosition=1

McNeil, D. G. J. (2019b, May). Gilead will donate Truvada to U.S. for H.I.V. prevention. *New York Times*. Retrieved from https://www.nytimes.com/2019/05/09/health/gilead-truvada-hiv-aids.html?searchResultPosition=12

Mngoma, N. (2016, July). Action focus shifts to steps to eradicate HIV/AIDS. *The Star*. Retrieved from https://www.iol.co.za/dailynews/news/action-focus-shifts-to-steps-to-eradicate-hivaids-2049237

Myhre, S., & Flora, J. (2000). HIV/AIDS communication campaigns: Progress and prospects. *Journal of Health Communication, 5*(supl), 29–45. doi:10.1080/108107300126731

Netter, T. (1992). The media and AIDS: A global perspective. In J. Sepulveda, H. Fineberg, & J. Mann (Eds.), *AIDS prevention through education: A world view* (pp. 241–253). New York: Oxford University Press.

Nguyen, V. K. (2009). Government-by-exception: Enrolment and experimentality in mass HIV treatment programmes in Africa. *Social Theory & Health, 7*(3), 196–217.

Noar, S. M., Palmgreen, P., Chabot, M., Dobransky, N., & Zimmerman, R. S. (2009). A 10-year systematic review of HIV/AIDS mass communication campaigns: Have we made progress? *Journal of Health Communication, 14*(1), 15–42. doi:10.1080/10810730802592239

PrEP Watch. (2018). *South Africa*. Retrieved from https://www.prepwatch.org/country/south-africa/

Princeton Survey Research Associates. (1996). Covering the epidemic: AIDS in the news media, 1985–1996. *Columbia Journalism Review, 35*(supplement), 1–12.

Punyacharoensin, N., Edmunds, W. J., De Angelis, D., Delpech, V., Hart, G., Elford, J... White, R. G. (2016). Effect of pre-exposure prophylaxis and combination HIV prevention for men who have sex with men in the UK: A mathematical modelling study. *Lancet HIV, 3*(2), e94–e104. doi:10.1016/s2352-3018(15)00056-9

Pyra, M. N., Haberer, J. E., Hasen, N., Reed, J., Mugo, N. R., & Baeten, J. M. (2019). Global implementation of PrEP for HIV prevention: Setting expectations for impact. *Journal of the International AIDS Society, 22*(8), e25370–e25370. doi:10.1002/jia2.25370

Reilly, K. H., Neaigus, A., Shepard, C. W., Cutler, B. H., Sweeney, M. M., Rucinski, K. B., ...Hagan, H. (2016). It's never just HIV: Exposure to an HIV prevention media campaign and behavior change among men who have sex with men participating in the National HIV Behavioral Surveillance System in New York City. *LGBT Health, 3*(4), 314–318. doi:10.1089/lgbt.2015.0016

Rimal, R., Johnson, D., & Flora, J. (1997). *International HIV/AIDS public service announcements: An assessment of behavior and social content.* Unpublished manuscript.

Rivet Amico, K., & Bekker, L. G. (2019). Global PrEP roll-out: Recommendations for programmatic success. *Lancet HIV, 6*(2), e137–e140. doi:10.1016/s2352-3018(19)30002-5

Rose, N. (2006). *The politics of life itself: Biomedicine, power and subjectivity in the twenty-first century.* Princeton, NJ: Princeton University Press.

SANAC. (2017). *Let our actions count: South Africa's National Strategic Plan for HIV, TB and STIs 2017–2022.* Retrieved from https://sanac.org.za//wp-content/uploads/2017/06/NSP_FullDocument_FINAL-1.pdf

SAPA-AP. (2014, April). Experts divided on AIDS drug. *The Star.* Retrieved from https://www.iol.co.za/dailynews/news/experts-divided-on-aids-drug-1671967

Segalov, M. (2016, October). If Theresa May is serious about LGBT equality, she needs to offer more than pardons. *The Telegraph.* Retrieved from https://www.telegraph.co.uk/news/2016/10/21/if-theresa-may-is-serious-about-lgbt-equality-she-needs-to-offer/

Semetko, H., & Goldberg, E. (1993). Reporting AIDS in the US and Britain. In R. Spitzer (Ed.), *Media and public policy* (pp. 171–186). Westport, CT: Praeger.

Sepulveda, J., Fineberg, H., & Mann, J. (Eds.). (1992). *AIDS prevention through education: A world view.* New York: Oxford University Press.

Staff reporter. (2019, November). WATCH: Cape Health MEC administers HIV test to premier ahead of World AIDS Day. *The Star.* Retrieved from https://www.iol.co.za/capeargus/news/watch-cape-health-mec-administers-hiv-test-to-premier-ahead-of-world-aids-day-38111458

Telegraph reporters. (2016, November). NHS to consider funding 'game-changer' HIV drugs as Court of Appeal upholds High Court ruling. *The Telegraph.* Retrieved from https://www.telegraph.co.uk/news/2016/11/10/nhs-to-consider-funding-game-changer-hiv-drugs-as-court-of-Appeal-upholds-High-Court-ruling/

Thom, A. (2012a, July). HIV drug offers hope. *The Star.* Retrieved from https://www.iol.co.za/pretoria-news/hiv-drug-offers-hope-1344189

Thom, A. (2012b, July). New hope in AIDS war. *The Star.* Retrieved from https://www.iol.co.za/the-star/new-hope-in-aids-war-1343701

Thomson, K. A., Baeten, J. M., Mugo, N. R., Bekker, L.-G., Celum, C. L., & Heffron, R. (2016). Tenofovir-based oral preexposure prophylaxis prevents HIV infection among women. *Current Opinion in HIV and AIDS, 11*(1), 18–26. doi:10.1097/COH.0000000000000207

Thrasher, S. (2019, December). H.I.V. is coming to rural America, and rural America is not ready. *New York Times.* Retrieved from https://www.nytimes.com/2019/12/01/opinion/hiv-aids-rural-america.html

Traquina, N. (1996, August). *Portuguese journalism and HIV/AIDS: A case study in news.* Paper presented at the 1996 Association for Education in Journalism and Mass Communication convention, Anaheim, CA.

Tuller, D. (2013, December). A resisted pill to prevent H.I.V. *New York Times.* Retrieved from https://www.nytimes.com/2013/12/31/health/a-resisted-pill-to-prevent-hiv.html?searchResultPosition=27

UNAIDS. (2015). *Oral pre-exposure prophylaxis: Putting a new choice in context.* Retrieved from Geneva: http://www.unaids.org/sites/default/files/media_asset/UNAIDS_JC2764_en.pdf

UNAIDS. (2017). *Ending AIDS: Progress towards 90-90-90 targets.* Retrieved from Geneva:https://www.unaids.org/sites/default/files/media_asset/Global_AIDS_update_2017_en.pdf

UNAIDS. (2019a). *AIDSInfo.* Retrieved from http://aidsinfo.unaids.org/

UNAIDS. (2019b). *Global HIV & AIDS statistics - 2018 fact sheet.* Retrieved from https://www.unaids.org/en/resources/fact-sheet

Victor, D. (2019, November). Trump administration sues Gilead, maker of H.I.V. prevention drugs. *New York Times.* Retrieved from https://www.nytimes.com/2019/11/07/business/gilead-truvada-hiv-lawsuit.html?searchResultPosition=3

Watts, L. (1993). Coverage of polio and AIDS. *Ohio Journalism Monographs, 4.*

Welte, A. (2012, July). HIV could become retro. *The Star.* Retrieved from https://www.iol.co.za/dailynews/opinion/hiv-could-become-retro-1351347

Wilson, A., Bonevski, B., Jones, A., & Henry, D. (2009). Media reporting of health interventions: Signs of improvement, but major problems persist. *PLoS One, 4*(3), e4831.

3 Last People Standing

People Living with HIV after the "End of the Epidemic"

Andrew Spieldenner, Laurel Sprague, Robert Suttle, Ariel Sabillon, and Bre Rivera

Dear 2030,

You promised us this would be over. That the HIV epidemic would end by 2030.

We have been living with HIV for much of our lives. HIV has brought us together and driven us out of other places. We have been marked in our interactions with family, friend,s and potential lovers as different, sometimes excluded. We found each other though and we built a community.

As states and countries take up "End the HIV Epidemic" plans, we recognize that these are built on advances in science and knowledge. We understand that HIV treatment saves lives, that new prevention tools like PrEP will prevent HIV acquisition for HIV-negative individuals, that resources could be better used for more targeted efforts.

We take notice that an HIV cure has not been part of the "End the HIV Epidemic" plans. We acknowledge that there are no plans to end HIV stigma and criminalization of sex work, drug use, and HIV non-disclosure. What about fighting for racial justice and sexual and reproductive health and rights? There is nothing about the role of capitalism in limiting our economic, health, mobility, and social possibilities.

In 2030, have the HIV service organizations shut down? What about the advocacy groups? Or did they transform themselves into other kinds of groups, as they had already started to by the 2010s?

We did learn something as HIV became less visible in our own service and advocacy groups: just because they removed "HIV" or "AIDS" from their names, our needs did not change.

You promised this would be over, but it's only over for you. You wanted us to be compliant patients, taking our pills. But some of us do not have healthcare, some of us are dealing with jobs and housing and mental health and discrimination.

Your vision of the "End of the HIV Epidemic" is not the same as ours.

Sincerely,

A community of people living with HIV

DOI: 10.4324/9781003000945-5

******

"Ending the Epidemic" (EHE) plans have emerged throughout the United States (Cuomo, 2014). Due to multiple advances in HIV science and technologies, several jurisdictions believed that the HIV epidemic could be curtailed. Knowledge about the impact of viral suppression – where a person living with HIV cannot transmit the virus – spurred Treatment as Prevention (TasP) programs (Wilson, 2012). HIV Pre-Exposure Prophylaxis (PrEP), where taking one anti-retroviral medication daily can prevent the acquisition of HIV in an HIV-negative person, has been lauded by health departments who see it as a viable means of stopping new HIV transmissions (Grant et al., 2010). Scientists and HIV advocates began envisioning an end to the HIV epidemic if these technologies could be encouraged at the community level (Diffenbach & Fauci, 2011). These were initially state-by-state; the federal Centers for Disease Control and Prevention (CDC) has funded all public health jurisdictions to engage in EHE plans (Azar, 2019). Many of these have already developed their own "Getting to Zero" or EHE plans so we will categorize these plans as EHE for the sake of this chapter.

We focus on the reality and rhetoric of EHE in this chapter by engaging the context of the HIV movement in the U.S., where people living with HIV first organized as a community in the early 1980s. We entered the U.S. HIV movement at various points, depending on our year of diagnosis (from 1991 at the earliest to 2015 at the most recent). Treichler (1999) notes, "[E]xploring the diversity of meanings do not tell what the 'truth' about AIDS and HIV is ... they do help us understand the rules ... by which truth in a given context, community, or culture is generated, accepted, or rejected" (p. 323). This chapter will explore the truths and meanings of EHE. With many EHE initiatives declaring 2030 as the arbitrary end of HIV as a public health epidemic, we challenge this discourse with different visions of what EHE could be. The authors are all people living with HIV, with a range of racial (African American, White, Latinx, and Asian), ethnic (American, Honduran, and Vietnamese), sexual (gay, lesbian, and queer), gender (cis and trans men and women), and family migration identities (immigrant, refugee, and U.S.-born). We range in age from 22 to 49 years old. The HIV movement differed over time, and our entry also frames our knowledge and experience with HIV care, stigma, and community.

HIV Movement in the U.S.

Historically, the HIV movement in the U.S. began in the early 1980s and was built off the framework of Gay and Lesbian Liberation, a social movement begun in the 1960s; by the 1970s, in some cities, gay and lesbian neighborhoods emerged. Out of these neighborhoods, gay and lesbian businesses and other institutions, including political and social service groups, formed (Brier, 2009). The first communities impacted by HIV in the U.S. were the lesbian, gay, bisexual, transgender, and queer (LGBTQ) communities; people who inject drugs;

immigrants (particularly Haitians); and people with hemophilia. While people engaged in sex work as well as those who were erratically housed also experienced a disproportionate impact in the HIV epidemic, these were not categories within the epidemiological markers (Hollibaugh, 2000; Treichler, 1999). One early lesson of the HIV epidemic in the U.S. that continues to be relevant is that epidemiology often overlooks bodies that are not already within the categories set up in public health surveillance (Casper & Moore, 2009). The HIV movement had early success in identifying structural challenges as well as advancing HIV policy at the institutional and social levels, but struggled with media and organizational approaches to the diversity of the epidemic.

The 1983 Denver Principles defined the early HIV movement. A manifesto of the rights of people living with AIDS, the Denver Principles outlines language and participation as integral to moving the HIV movement forward. It begins, "We condemn attempts to label us as 'victims,' a term which implies defeat, and we are only occasionally 'patients,' a term which implies passivity, helplessness, and dependence upon the care of others. We are 'People With AIDS'" (People with AIDS Coalition, 1983, para. 2). The importance of language and self-determination was recognized early, as the community struggled with an unknown and deadly disease. HIV organizations and groups lauded the leadership of people living with HIV.

HIV has always disrupted clear ideas of borders and populations, as it often spreads across these easy categories. Advocates have long recognized the need to act strategically across global movements and moments. In 1989, HIV activists took over the opening session of the International AIDS Conference to read the "Montreal Manifesto" (Brier, 2009). The manifesto explicitly asked the governments for military spending to be redeployed for global healthcare. While this was an open call, it was understood that the U.S. had the largest military expenditures globally. It recognized that HIV treatment was contingent on ending poverty. These kinds of actions were typical of the AIDS Coalition To Unleash Power (ACT-UP) and other HIV activist groups in the world at the time. Through engaged communication in regular meetings, coalition members were able to identify key barriers in the HIV epidemic. Rather than focus solely on HIV, much of this activism recognized that HIV occurs on a body and within a socio-political context. Understanding the complex interplay of race, gender, sexuality, nationality, and poverty was the integral to comprehending the epidemic. In large part, people of color, people who use drugs, immigrants, and White cis and trans women held the largely White cisgender gay male leadership of ACT-UP and other activist groups accountable (Bordowitz, 1988). Specific to HIV, this included identifying and dealing with: how racism persisted in healthcare service delivery (Mumford, 2016), how homophobia framed public health discourse (Treichler, 1999), how sexism excluded women from HIV surveillance (Casper & Moore, 2009), how government structures impeded HIV treatment research and availability (Brier, 2009), and how stigma prevented public health practices like needle exchanges from being implemented (Treichler, 1999). HIV activists pushed for more than just health service delivery.

ACT-UP and other HIV activists had several political accomplishments. They made media companies cover HIV, and critiqued salacious and stigmatizing news coverage (Treichler, 1999). They forced the federal Food and Drug Administration to change their bureaucracy in order to facilitate HIV treatment research (Brier, 2009). They built community organizations to advocate and provide services to people living with HIV and those most vulnerable to HIV, including people of color, people who use drugs, women, and LGBTQ people (Cohen, 1999). The HIV movement forced politicians to pass laws to protect people living with HIV, fund HIV prevention and services, provide HIV treatment when it became available, and even resource housing for people living with HIV (Brier, 2009). These accomplishments occurred amidst a staggering death toll (Brier, 2009; Mumford, 2016).

Although the HIV movement had many accomplishments, there were challenges, especially with diversity. Mumford (2016) points out that "[r]esearchers and activists alike understood AIDS as racially inflected by the mid-1980s" (p. 172) which led to "black activists charg[ing] that mainstream AIDS organizations had failed to recruit people of color to help care for HIV-positive black men" (p. 173). The HIV movement built organizations but seemed to replicate the social reality of the U.S. – i.e, failing to account for racism, transphobia, and other exclusionary practices. These challenges remain in the current HIV movement, as organizations have focused more and more on clinical services and concerns, especially with the advent of effective HIV treatment. This shift has largely – and ironically – relegated people living with HIV to being patients within the same organizations that the community helped found. EHE plans are being developed, implemented and assessed between government institutions and these HIV service organizations. These present powerful actors in determining HIV discourse, but fail to include the community of people living with HIV.

Communities of People Living with HIV

While the HIV movement has consisted of a vibrant coalition including a diversity of straight and LGBTQ people, people who were HIV-negative and people living with HIV, people of color and White people, as well as various professions and organizations, the community of people living with HIV has occupied a slightly different space. People living with HIV have come together in informal and formal ways through community-based organizations, social media and other social networks, and businesses like bars, coffee shops, and gyms.

For decades, after getting diagnosed with HIV, people were often referred to their local HIV support group (Jolivette, 2016; Strub, 2014; Watkins-Hayes, 2019). In these groups, people would gain social interaction, medical information, and referrals from other people living with HIV. Some of these groups were specific to particular identities, such as women or people of color. In the past decade, this model has shifted as more onus is put on getting newly diagnosed individuals into clinical care rather than connecting them with community (CDC, 2015). While healthcare and treatment are clearly vital in the HIV response, it is not the sum total of why people living with HIV build together. Instead, we will focus here on the benefits of engaging the communities of people living with HIV. In particular, we will highlight how the communities of people living with HIV become part of healthcare and interpersonal relationships. We will also discuss how the communities of people living with HIV continue to struggle from both internal and external forces.

Since the beginning of the epidemic, people living with HIV have come together to share medical information, health regimens, and support. Before effective HIV treatment was available, people searched for information about opportunistic infections, harms and benefits of various treatments, and good and bad healthcare providers (Adelman & Frey, 1997; Strub, 2014). They found it in support groups, through community media, and social networks (Brouwer, 2005; Strub, 2014). The HIV community valued embodied knowledge as personal expertise and this was reflected in its early activism and organizations. In a study of women living with HIV, Watkins-Hayes (2019) notes that "[e]ngagement with the HIV safety net accounts for a sizable portion of the variation between those who thrive and those who do not following an HIV diagnosis" (p. 142). This HIV safety net includes information-sharing, social support, healthcare, and support services such as childcare, food pantries, housing, and mental health and harm reduction services.

While much of the early HIV work focused on the needs of cisgender White gay men, the epidemic itself was much more diverse. People of color, women, and people who use drugs all created parallel (though often less-resourced) community groups and organizations to better meet their needs. These individuals "face difficulties not just around coming to accept the various aspects of their identities, but also in facing and accepting their HIV-positive status and the stigmas that come from living with the disease" (Jolivette, 2016, p. 89). As such, the common ethnicity, cultural roots, and needs that are part of these identities expand HIV services so that they are more relevant. In building these homes, community members are able to connect with others who face similar challenges and are potentially able to offer solutions.

These connections could evolve into deeper relationships. Communities of people living with HIV offer space for friendships and sexual partners (Adelman & Frey, 1997; Strub, 2014). These relationships provide opportunities to obtain resources and strategies in dealing with a sometimes overwhelming medical care system, obtaining social support services, and managing discrimination (Chase, 2011; Watkins-Hayes, 2019). Within these friendships, people living with HIV commiserate about common feelings like frustration, loss, anger, and isolation (Adelman & Frey, 1997; Jolivette, 2016; Spieldenner et al., 2019). In addition, these relationships can lead to taking on advocacy roles in the community (Ramirez-Valles, 2011). At other times, these deep relationships spur creative work and art collectives (Bost, 2019; Rodríguez, 2003). Friendships develop within the HIV community as the result of a shared diagnosis. These multiple outcomes reflect the changing support needs after diagnosis: not just access to healthcare and treatment, but access to each other in meaningful ways.

Within the community of people living with HIV, sex and other intimate relationships have also been a central concern. Serodiscordant relationships (where one person is living with HIV and the other is not) often have to deal with complex negotiations with disclosure, intimacy, prevention, and healthcare. When both partners are living with HIV, there is a shared knowledge of stigma and healthcare. In addition, there is no need to disclose nor use prevention technologies. When people living with HIV get together, sex and sexual relations are a possibility. In the early years of the epidemic, some of these relationships were an intense response to the disease and the death toll; for some, it was a means of connecting along common politics and experiences (Strub, 2014). Serosorting – when people living with HIV deliberately choose another person living with HIV for sex – is still a practice (Spieldenner, 2017).

The various communities of people living with HIV in the U.S. continue to face challenges. At the start of the epidemic, HIV organizing was almost entirely community-led, and now the HIV industry includes pharmaceuticals; governments; healthcare providers; and international, national, and regional non-governmental organizations and community groups. These larger structures involve multiple decision-makers and priority-setting that occurs outside of people living with HIV. Healthcare providers and public health agencies often refer to people living with HIV as "consumers," indicating that people living with HIV are passive recipients of service (Spieldenner et al., 2019). More problematic is the way that "consumer" is configured in a capitalist healthcare system. Rather than being able to provide any meaningful inputs or recognizing our labors in healthcare processes, people living with HIV are relegated to objects whose sole purpose is to consume the services being made available. The meaningful involvement of people living with HIV (MIPA), once a central tenet of the HIV responses, has become a much less integral part of building EHE plans. While there is rhetoric in the EHE plans, there is very little substantive prioritizing or planning about MIPA – where people living with HIV identify priorities and needs that may be different from clinical care. In the Illinois plan, for instance, "Linkage to Care" is a clinical goal, with two strategies that include percentage increases and time-phased benchmarks (Illinois Department of Public Health, 2019, p. 35). In the same plan, the MIPA goal is vaguely worded as "Support People with Lived Experiences" and one strategy (of 11 oddly grouped strategies) is to "decriminalize sex work" without any benchmarks or specific targets (Illinois Department of Public Health, 2019, p. 43). This vision for MIPA is unclear, where the clinical goals are clear priorities.

The diversity challenges and racism that trouble the HIV movement are also part of the community of people living with HIV. Even documentaries about HIV activism spend more time creating a heroic figure of able-bodied, White cisgender gay men than examining the collective action and strategic organizing of the early HIV movement (Shahani, 2016). The representational issues reflect the policy and organizational ones: where organizations dedicated to people of color living with HIV are often marginalized and under-resourced (Cohen, 1999; Jolivette, 2016; Mumford, 2016). Where people living with HIV gather, there are different issues that people prioritize across communities. For instance, people of color living with HIV might prioritize dealing with HIV decriminalization since these laws are part of systemic racism, which readily deploys the police, while White cisgender gay men living with HIV might not see it as a priority since their experience with law enforcement differs (Strub, 2014). People of color living with HIV might be struggling to maintain social and familial support, while White cisgender gay men living with HIV have valorized an independence separate from biological family structures (Ferguson, 2019; Jolivette, 2016). Women living with HIV continue to have to fight for a space at the table, even amongst people living with HIV groups (Adelman & Frey, 1997; Hollibaugh, 2000; Watkins-Hayes, 2019). These have both been internal and external forces that have minimized community-building and divided people living with HIV.

We describe the community of people living with HIV as distinctive, with particular issues and ways of engaging. While people living with HIV are central to the HIV movement and its activism, we want to differentiate between the activism and the wider community. In this way, we want to start to tease apart the nuances between how EHE could move forward without us, and what we envision when we consider the End of AIDS.

Conversations about the End of the HIV Epidemic

In choosing to work together on this chapter, we recognized that we did not have a clear method or even a language to approach this discussion. As people living with HIV, we wonder at what the "End of the HIV Epidemic" means. As a signifier, it proposes that the epidemic is finally over. Would this herald an effective, affordable and available vaccine and cure? In practice, many health departments are describing this moment as a reduction in HIV transmission as measured by HIV diagnoses and an increase in people living with HIV on treatment and virologically suppressed. For us, this would be a facade. We grow concerned that there will be a shutdown of the broad range of HIV services we fought so hard for as a means of demonstrating the "End of the HIV Epidemic."

We grapple with developing a language about the "End of the HIV Epidemic" for two reasons. First, the actors who are constructing this discourse are government entities and HIV service organizations, both of whom have complicated and extended relationships with communities of people living with HIV. The government has been neglectful, but eventually came to be a partner and primary funder for many HIV organizations. These same groups have provided us essential services and employment over the course of our lifetimes. In addition to our complex relationships, government agencies and HIV service providers both hold institutional power in determining HIV discourses.

Secondly, we struggle with the paucity of language concerning the "End of the HIV Epidemic." The rhetoric of these plans provide extensive space for clinical interventions, but remain thin when it comes to larger issues. The very vulnerabilities and structural barriers that inculcated and enabled the HIV epidemic to spread and remain centered amongst some groups in the United States go largely untouched in any meaningful way. Housing, socioeconomics, racism, sexism, homophobia, and transphobia, as well as the rampant criminalization of HIV, drug use, and sex work, constitute parts of these larger structures. It is almost as if the clinical EHE plans cannot envision these structures. Law (2004) notes that a particular notion of reality in social science cannot manage multiplicity well, and that the "multiple or the fractional, the elusive, the vague, the partial and the fluid are being displaced into Otherness" (p. 137). EHE plans acknowledge that these factors exist, but do little to address them. In order to develop this language, we turn to more creative and iterative processes.

As a group of people living with HIV, we seek to expand the "End of HIV Epidemic" discourse and extend the visions of what it might look like. Rather than recreating a singular voice or vision, we embrace the multiplicity. Law (2004) suggests finding "new ways of knowing and reality-making that allow the creation of many possible, more or less real, worlds" (p. 153). As such, we have structured this chapter as a conversation between us. This is an intervention in the public health plans about our lives, our healthcare, and our community-building. While HIV has been a global epidemic, it is also an industry with far more reach and material influence than the five of us from our various positions. Collectively, this dialogue is meant to illustrate what the end of the epidemic would mean to us.

What Does the Idea of the End of the HIV Epidemic by 2030 Mean to You Personally?

LAUREL: I never wanted to die of AIDS. So I want the end of AIDS to mean a cure – one that works in this body and every other body. Since 1991, I have been trying my hardest to survive AIDS and not leave my son without his mother.

But even a cure would not feel like the end of AIDS to me. The physical manifestations of AIDS some time ago came to represent to me the visible edge of the deep inequalities and violence that shape the AIDS epidemic. AIDS is the consequence of gender-based violence, racism, homophobia, transphobia, misogyny, poverty, and hatred and bias toward anyone seen as smaller, weaker, less well-off, disposable. It is a disease that has been inflicted and allowed to flourish by those who have power against those who are bullied, devalued, marginalized. There should be no right to claim the end of AIDS while these inequalities remain.

ARIEL: I think medicine itself will be transformed. It means we will have a cure. It means that there will be a cure to the condition and HIV will be similar to syphilis. Back in the day, you would die from syphilis but now it's rare that people die from it. I just want it to be gone.

ROBERT: I don't necessarily believe there will be a cure, but that HIV will be something that will be treated like any other disease. HIV will no longer be enforced as another way to disenfranchise minoritized communities, nor as an offensive form of state-sponsored discrimination that creates a viral underclass in the law, defining people living with HIV as an inherent danger to society.

BRE: Ending AIDS to me is a short-sighted goal. Even if we are able to cure HIV/AIDS in my lifetime, I don't believe that we could effectively eradicate it, without causing more harm to community. Ending AIDS using the current framework looks like more criminalization, mandatory testing, care and mentoring, resources shifting to surveillance. It implies more stigma. "Why wouldn't you want a cure as someone who has been living with this virus?" I am healthy, comfortable, and wouldn't want to risk my health and well-being for a cure that hasn't been monitored for long-term effects. I have too many close friends and comrades who would rather not be cured. Would it be a choice for folks? Would we be forced to wear a scarlet letter? Stigma is like racism; eradicating racism hasn't worked despite policy and law.

ROBERT: The End of AIDS by 2030? It would mean that there would be no more criminalization of HIV. Period! No more people living with HIV out of fear of having to disclose their status anywhere in the U.S., facing an arrest, or incarceration for an unjust prosecution. Black gay men would no longer be targets within the U.S. criminal justice system based upon their HIV status, race, or sexual orientation.

LAUREL: Even in the most difficult years for people living with HIV, there was the possibility that, even if sometimes for the wrong reasons, country after country would become a safer place for the groups of people most affected by HIV – as we gathered and used better and better evidence about the positive effects on the HIV response of anti-poverty efforts, education for girls, decriminalization of sex work, drug use, same sex relationships, and transitions in gender identity. Networks gained valuable skills in monitoring health service delivery and holding governments accountable for their commitments to their people. While the HIV response overall has sought to become biomedicalized, people living with HIV still have these skills and experience in fighting for social justice.

ARIEL: HIV organizations are made up by people. That's what fuels the organizations and activism. And I don't think that will just stop. We make up such an important network on a global scale. I don't think they will dissipate, they will transform. Because people care about people. People come out in the HIV response because they want to change society to be more responsive. There are other issues to work on: housing, healthcare, racial inequalities, anti-war movements.

LAUREL: In the AIDS response, we saw how people – people who sometimes shared nothing more in common than a stigmatized virus – forged movements of solidarity that changed how health is understood, governed, funded, and provided globally.

And we had some power because governments were scared of the disease we had and, therefore, were willing to put aside some of their discriminatory policies in order to feel they had some control over the AIDS epidemic.

ANDREW: This brings up an interesting point, for me. What is – exactly – ending? We hold the disease in our bodies, and barring a cure, this will not change. Many of us are marginalized across identities and these produce particular vulnerabilities. How do these end?

LAUREL: Over the years of our movements as people living with HIV, the intersections between violence, oppression of women, hatred of LGBTI people, sex workers, and people who use drugs, experience trauma, displacement, and more became ever clearer. Networks of people living with HIV, sex workers, gay men, people who use drugs, women, and young people affected by HIV emerged and took on these issues, increasingly doing so together, across networks. Funding was made available, never enough, but some, because the fear of the epidemic made funding for networks of affected groups a higher priority – in the belief, largely accurate, that they held the key to ending the epidemic.

At the same time, anti-retroviral drugs (ARVs) became more effective at keeping people alive and preventing new infections – kept under patent by any and every means possible. Discussions started on "epidemic control" and "epidemic transition" as steps on the road to end AIDS, focused on two numbers only: numbers of new infections and numbers of people living with HIV per country.

Now what? Is everyone just supposed to take a pill and go home?

What Does the Idea of the "End of AIDS" by 2030 Mean to Your Community?

ARIEL: I have multiple communities I belong to. I can't have a blanket statement because, for instance, not all gay men are part of my community.

ROBERT: To my HIV community, it means we are thriving and living openly as HIV-positive Black gay or Same Gender Loving (SGL) men, engaging in meaningful and lasting relationships with those we choose to love and those who choose to love us back without any reservation, shame, or resentment about HIV status.

LAUREL: My HIV community: people living with HIV (PLHIV) networks, PLHIV activists, women living with HIV, and especially those long term survivors who learned the hard way not to trust the promises of pharmaceutical companies or to believe that all stakeholders in the HIV response have the same interests at heart. We have common goals at times – for example, getting the best ARVs into the bodies that need them – but our overall struggle for health for ourselves and our communities as we define it, is seldom shared by those with power. This overall struggle is the struggle to end the violence against us, which includes the violence of unaffordable medicines; of quality health care reserved only for those who can afford it; of poverty; and of legal and policing systems that systematically discriminate against – and often physical abuse against – members of our communities.

BRE: Ending AIDS wouldn't do much for Black trans women but extend our lives without impacting its quality.

ANDREW: That's my biggest worry – that some parts of the HIV community believe that if some of them are okay, then everyone is.

ARIEL: The people that I know living with HIV ... there's the day-to-day, the picking up medication, the doctor visits, the discrimination in dating and on apps. The "End of AIDS" should mean that those things will no longer be present. No longer taking meds for HIV, no more doctor visits for HIV, no more stigma because there would be a cure. That also means having access to those cures. This means not just in the U.S., of course, but transnational communities. Rural communities. A global effort to make sure that everyone has access to quality medicines – that is, a cure – by 2030.

Not having a cure means it's not the end of AIDS. That is handing the baton down from this global network that was required to address the epidemic to a more localized response. To do that it would require a governmental and societal change to address – like for instance in Honduras, with the privatization of medicine, doctors, if global organizations stopped working there, the government would not necessarily fill in that role. What's required is for imperialism to stop, for companies to stop having so much influence over the government, for Western transnationals to stop dictating policy, requires entire societies to care about gay men, trans women, and people in general, and we just don't have the tools and the environment required for that just yet. Without the aid from a global transnational community, I fear that many communities – my community – will be left to die because the dominant cisgendered heterosexual patriarchal society does not deem us worthy of saving. This is especially true for black, Indigenous, rural, and *campesino* communities in the U.S., in Honduras, and elsewhere.

BRE: Many trans people still use HIV care as an access point for gender affirming care. What happens to them?

ROBERT: Hopefully, it means others would be non-judgmental, more accepting, and supporting of one another as we are. Embracing the fact that we can be vulnerable and interact with one another without feeling like we are putting ourselves at risk. And we get there by sharing our lived experiences, to hopefully bring us closer together. Leveraging our sphere of influence to encourage one another, motivate one another, and be known as a creditable influence within the Black gay community.

Right now, there are some spaces for people to share their experiences – like on social media and public gatherings. We always need more stories. As more people are finding they are diagnosed with HIV, there will always be stories and experiences that need to be shared. So that more people know they are not alone. What's not happening is more mainstream exposure of Black gay men living with HIV. They might be coming out within their networks but not in mainstream culture. We are not part of the mainstream except in pharmaceutical ads. Whatever it means to see people – music, TV, movies – we are not there yet. Hopefully in the future, we will see more Black gay men living with HIV in the limelight as positive representations.

ANDREW: We definitely need more spaces where we can come together and build community – whatever that looks like. More spaces for cross-generational and the diverse range of PLHIV to come together and learn how to support and listen and engage. It feels like there was more deliberate community-building being done in the early years of the epidemic.

How Would You Know That the HIV Epidemic Was Over? What Would Be the Signs for You?

ROBERT: PLHIV having full access to adequate and comprehensive healthcare. Having their health and insurance needs met without the struggle, whether or not they have enough money. Not having to think twice about who or what you are when getting your care and treatment.

BRE: The end of AIDS means an end to the conditions that facilitate risk – stigma, mental health, lack of healthcare, racism, sexism, transphobia, homophobia, prisons, religion (the church in the U.S.), homelessness, people first treatments.

ARIEL: So there's the traditional way of looking at HIV – it is HIV period. In my head, HIV is a symptom of a network of a lot of illnesses. If you alleviate HIV as a symptom, whether through ARVs or a cure, it does not necessarily mean we have treated the larger illness.

ANDREW: We are all on the same page – treatment access alone is not the sole sign of the end of the epidemic. Nor is a drop in transmission. We are seeing in Covid-19 how quickly pandemics become a way to link public health with law enforcement – and these authorities act on us differently depending on race, gender, sexuality, and socioeconomic class.

LAUREL: I fear we would see news story after story of new anti-gay laws passed, LGBT-friendly clinics closed, patient lists seized, and all of the resulting violence the LGBT communities know to expect when political leaders espouse homophobic and transphobic rhetoric. In many countries, health clinics that are safe and welcoming for LGBT people have only been tolerated in the name of fighting HIV. If HIV is over, then so is this little bit of safety and healthcare that LGBT communities have won for themselves. In the U.S., we would see headlines stating that thousands of people have lost access to health care as ADAP programmes are closed down. We would also see stories about where the billions of dollars in funding to fight AIDS would go next – but where would it go? Healthcare for all? Alleviating poverty? Or to fascist border security plans and additional foreign aid to authoritarian regimes? My hope is that it would go to supporting community-led organizations to monitor health systems and hold their leaders accountable to ensure that what the end of AIDS means is that every person everywhere has good healthcare, from competent providers, in a supportive space.

BRE: We'd need to have the shifting of language around HIV. Around our identities, including gender.

ARIEL: The way that I think of it in my head is an illness of sexuality, as in we don't have a healthy sexuality at a societal level. For one, the separation of the genders – women as separate from men and not complimenting men. Gender as a binary system, where the categories are not seen in relationship. That is the cause of a lot of illnesses. These gender binaries – like trans women being separate from cis women – can keep trans women out of the labor force into survival sex. HIV as a social illness, beyond the sterile "science-y" perspective of it, stems from a deep wound that was created when we reduced the genders and sexes into compartmentalized categories that are not static, subjecting those who exist outside this system (which, considering the majority of the world is not a cisgendered heterosexual man, is most of us) to untold violence.

Second, the idea of repressed sexuality, sexual purity. This repression has pushed gay men into hypersexuality after decades, centuries of repression. This does not mean it's a healthy sexuality, it's just like rebelling. Like if your dad is strict, and you rebel. You run away, you do drugs. And you're free? Of course you're not.

In my experience as a young queer person, I've seen myself and many of my peers engage in unhealthy sexual behavior because there are wounds we have not healed. We should have the option to pursue the paths we want to take without it being a trauma response. If we *want* to engage in sexual behavior, it should be because we really do want to. Not because we are craving intimacy we do not have the tools to access healthily. As children, we are not allowed to have cute crushes the way straight cis kids do. We are in a crisis of healthy role models. We crave healthy male figures. We need to have representation of queer people outside the hypersexualized metropolitan urban core. I pray that, in the future, I will see more queer farmers, queer professors, queer people existing without being reduced to our sexuality. We deserve that. We need that.

Third, we're so separated from each other, so isolated. For HIV to be over and not just have any disease – drug abuse, for instance – take its place. It requires us to go into our communities – a community that will take care of you, a real community that will keep you safe and have your back. People who are homeless, for instance, show us a lack of connection. People walk by and don't even notice. This is inhumane and a society that allows for this to occur is a deeply wounded society. If we cure HIV, we don't just pack up and go home. If I were to get into a car crash, a doctor who merely treats my broken arm without addressing head damage, cuts and scratches, etc. would be negligent. The same applies to the HIV response. In this way, HIV is inextricably linked to other diseases – environmental racism, oppression against women, orientalism, etc.

ANDREW: Looking to the world that we want to be in is integral to managing some of the dismal systems we live in.

ROBERT: I'm living so hard right now in the present that I rarely have time to consider the future. All I have is today, so let me see what hopes and dreams I have I can make happen today, this coming year, but not 20 years from now. We walk day-to-day where I come from. You don't always have enough independent means to think about the future.

Looking Ahead

We can see an end coming, but to what? Ending the epidemic seems to signal many ends. This is not just an epidemiological end, it also affects the community resistance and organizing, relationship building, as well as various ways of being. This policy and rhetorical device – "Ending the HIV Epidemic" – impacts heavily our everyday lives. We are – rightfully – fearful of premature declarations that leave us with less support and protections than before. The shift towards relegating HIV to solely a medical problem with clinical solutions ("take your pills") has meant overlooking the structural violence that frames so many of the health disparities. Will there be a pill to solve homophobia or transphobia or misogyny or racism? Will there be an injection that resolves massive disparities in wealth and resources?

They can say they ended AIDS, but they have not – not the AIDS that we know. Even if they stop new infections, they won't be able to stop people dying, people suffering from unjust criminalization laws and other kinds of structural violence. We insist on activism and resistance. It is not enough to be the last people standing and a lot of the battles we are fighting are not just HIV. The HIV movement's position will be even more precarious if it does not retool, orient resources, and build alliances towards addressing the structural violences that we face.

References

Adelman, M. B. & Frey, L. R. (1997). *The fragile community: Living together with AIDS.* Mahwah, NJ: Lawrence Erlbaum Associates.

Azar, A. (2019). *Ending the HIV epidemic: A plan for America.* Washington, DC: Department of Health and Human Services. Retrieved from https://www.hhs.gov/blog/2019/02/05/ending-the-hiv-epidemic-a-plan-for-america.html

Bordowitz, G. (1988). Picture a coalition. In D. Crimp (Ed.), *AIDS: Cultural analysis, cultural activism* (pp. 183–196). Boston, MA: MIT Press.

Bost, D. (2019). *Evidence of being: The Black gay cultural renaissance and the politics of violence.* Chicago, IL: University of Chicago Press.

Brier, J. (2009). *Infectious ideas: U.S. political responses to the AIDS crisis.* Chapel Hill: University of North Carolina Press.

Brouwer, D. C. (2005). Counterpublicity and corporeality in HIV/AIDS zines. *Critical Studies in Media Communication, 22*(5), 351–371.

Casper, M. J. & Moore, L. J. (2009). *Missing bodies: The politics of visibility.* New York, NY: New York University Press.

Centers for Disease Control & Prevention. (2015). *HIV infection: Detection, counseling, and referral.* Retrieved from https://www.cdc.gov/std/tg2015/hiv.htm

Chase, S. M. (2011). *Surviving HIV/AIDS in the inner city: How resourceful Latinas beat the odds*. New Brunswick, NJ: Rutgers University Press.

Cohen, C. J. (1999). *The Boundaries of Blackness: AIDS and the breakdown of Black politics*. Chicago, IL: University of Chicago Press.

Cuomo, A. M. (2014, June 29). *Governor Cuomo announces plan to the AIDS epidemic in New York State* [Press release]. Retrieved from https://www.governor.ny.gov/press/06292014-end-aaids-epidemic

Diffenbach, C. W. & Fauci, A. S. (2011). Thirty years of HIV and AIDS: Future challenges and opportunities. *Annals of Internal Medicine, 154*(11), 766–771.

Ferguson, R. A. (2019). *One-dimensional queer*. Medford, MA: Polity Press.

Grant, R. M., Lama, J. R., Anderson, P. L., McMahan, V., Liu, A. Y., Vargas, L.,… Glidden, D. V. (2010). Preexposure chemoprophylaxis for HIV prevention in men who have sex with men. *New England Journal of Medicine, 363*, 2587–2599. doi:10.1056/NEJMoa1011205

Hollibaugh, A. L. (2000). *My dangerous desires: A queer girl dreaming her way home*. Durham, NC and London: Duke University Press.

Illinois Department of Public Health. (2019). *Getting to Zero Illinois, 2019–2023 Plan*. Springfield: Illinois Department of Public Health.

Jolivette, A. J. (2016). *Indian blood: HIV and colonial trauma in San Francisco's two-spirit community*. Seattle, WA: University of Washington Press.

Law, J. (2004). *After method: Mess in social science research*. New York: Routledge.

Mumford, K. J. (2016). *Not straight, not White: Black gay men from the March on Washington to the AIDS crisis*. Durham, NC: University of North Carolina Press.

Ramirez-Valles, J. (2011). *Compañeros: Latino activists in the face of AIDS*. Urbana, Chicago and Springfield: University of Illinois Press.

Rodríguez, J. M. (2003). *Queer latinidad: Identity practices, discursive spaces*. New York: New York University Press.

Shahani, N. (2016). How to survive the whitewashing of AIDS: Global pasts, transnational futures. *QED: A Journal in GLBTQ Worldmaking, 3*(1), 1–33.

Spieldenner, A. R. (2017). Infectious sex?: An autoethnographic exploration of HIV prevention. *QED: A Journal in LGBTQ Worldmaking, 4*(1), 121–129.

Spieldenner, A. R., Sprague, L, Hampton, A., Smith-Davis, M., Peavy, D., Bagchi, A.,… Brewer, R. (2019). From consumer to community-based researcher: Lessons from the PLHIV Stigma Index. In P. Kellett (Ed.), *Narrating patienthood: Engaging diverse voices on health, communication, and the patient experience* (pp. 151–166). New York: Lexington Press.

Strub, S. (2014). *Body counts: A memoir of politics, sex, AIDS, and survival*. New York: Scribner.

Treichler, P. A. (1999). *How to have theory in an epidemic: Cultural chronicles of AIDS*. Durham, NC: Duke University Press.

Watkins-Hayes, C. (2019). *Remaking a life: How women living with HIV/AIDS confront inequality*. Oakland: University of California Press.

Wilson, D. P. (2012). HIV treatment as prevention: Natural experiments highlight limits of antiretroviral treatment as HIV prevention. *PLoS Medicine, 9*(7), e1001231. doi:10.1371/journal.pmed.1001231

4 A Dramatization of Post-AIDS Stigma

A Pentadic Analysis of the CDC's "Let's Stop HIV Together" Campaign

Jaime S. Robb

Health campaigns have traditionally crafted messages aimed towards influencing an audience's health knowledge, attitudes, and behavior. Such campaigns tend to be strategically designed to reach specific target audiences with the goal of altering behavioral practices. According to Rogers and Storey (1987), these campaigns often focus on specific outcomes, in a substantial number of individuals, within a given time frame, which is achievable through an organized set of communication activities. For many communication scholars, the "organized set of communication activities" that is involved in health campaigns tends to be understood as some type of a rhetorical construct. In traditional health campaigns, rhetorical practices tend to be overlooked or taken for granted, or simply dismissed as persuasion designed "to produce noncommercial benefits to individuals and society" (Atkin & Rice, 2012, p. 14). For example, the Centers for Disease Control and Prevention's (CDC) 2018 flu vaccination campaign utilized rhetoric in multiple ways (such as animation, emotional and logical appeals, jingles, etc.) to stress the importance of vaccination in protecting "yourself, your family, your friends, and your community" (CDC, 2018). Another rhetorical feature of the campaign is the use of Black animated bodies to represent the message, which indicates that the message was designed and intended to reach Black audiences. Health campaigns like the CDC's flu vaccination campaign rely on rhetorical techniques in order to promote their messages in a way that connects with the target audience. While the rhetoric used in health campaign messages can be impactful for those who are part of the target audience, it can also create limitations for those segments of a particular population that have limited resources, such as Black audiences, who lack the resources needed to get vaccinated.

The media plays a significant role in promoting health messages to influence behavioral changes using various mediums. The typical model for mediated health campaigns tends to go through four stages, which starts with the planning and designing of the campaign (McGuire, 2013). This leads to the implementation, and later the evaluation of the campaign. The fourth and final stage deals with improving the message design and implementation to reach and connect with a wider audience base. The process of designing and re-designing the campaign

DOI: 10.4324/9781003000945-6

message is an inherently rhetorical act because of the obvious intent to influence. Media outlets are important for helping to inform, persuade, and shape public perception of cultural norms about health, and rhetorical strategies are necessary for information to connect with the target audience (Wakefield, Loken, & Hornik, 2010). YouTube has become a popular media outlet for sharing health campaign messages due to the platform's low cost and its diverse audience base. This was one of the platforms (in addition to billboards, social media, and buses) the CDC used to promote its 2018 "Let's Stop HIV Together" campaign. It was a campaign that aimed to "shape public perception" about the cultural beliefs surrounding individuals diagnosed with HIV (CDC, 2018). The campaign was designed to promote awareness about HIV survival rates and reduce cultural stigmas about HIV/AIDS. The message was clearly aimed at encouraging change in the public's attitudes towards people living with HIV/AIDS. The CDC drew on a "post-AIDS" frame to present a premise whereby the medical risks related to HIV/AIDS have been surpassed by the negative impact of the stigmas attached to the illness and the people managing it. While the CDC campaign was designed to increase awareness and identify stigma as a central factor that creates negative health outcomes for individuals living with HIV/AIDS, it offers a message that (1) draws on stigmatized identity groups that are already marginalized in the AIDS community to promote this message, (2) flattens the environmental obstacles that exist for local agents from diverse cultural backgrounds, and (3) promotes a neoliberal understanding of "post-AIDS" that suggests the illness is now manageable and preventable, universally, with biomedical intervention.

This essay draws on rhetorical criticism as an approach for investigating the taken for granted and unforeseen effects of health campaign messages (Lundberg, 2013). I begin by critiquing the CDC's use of a single universal approach to situate their message, while showing how such theoretical approaches do not consider the cultural make-up of diverse audiences when crafting a persuasive campaign messages. I draw on Burke's (1945) pentad as a tool for doing rhetorical criticism, which makes note of the subtle strategies that allows meaning to be transformed through dramatic discourse. The aim is to show how the CDC's campaign limits diverse cultural understanding to managing HIV/AIDS stigma, and instead promotes a universal premise that is rooted in a Western ideology of a post-AIDS society.

Health Campaigns, Culture, and Influence

There are many significant health risks individuals face in our current society. From the risks associated with heart disease, diabetes, stroke, HIV/AIDS, etc., a rhetoric of prevention has emerged to promote health practices that combat these health challenges before they begin. The most evident display of such efforts is a public health campaign (Atkin & Rice, 2012). Critical health communication scholars have long problematized the way messages are constructed for public consumption in campaigns of these types (Dutta, 2017). One area of concern that has emerged from critical health research involves the way culture tends to be universalized in Western health campaigns (Lupton, 1994). More importantly, contemporary health communication research has shown that mass-produced health messages tend to be structured with a particularly dominant Western ideology/audience. This has brought to the forefront the impact of persuasive health messages on cultural groups who do not necessarily fit the discursive mold of a Western audience member. A universal frame of culture not only reduces diverse ways of knowing and managing illnesses, but it also creates a space for stigmas to (re)emerge regarding which cultures are seen as most appropriate in their health behavior and knowledge.

Health Campaigns

Traditional health campaigns tend to draw on established behavior change theories derived from psychological concepts to formulate a public health and social scientific approach. Traditional models, such as the Health Belief Model, the Social Cognitive Theory, and the Theory of Planned Behavior, are used as foundations for predicting how groups will respond to new health information. These psychology-based theories are used to help explain how individual attitudes toward healthy behavior affect their willingness to change their own behavior (Fishbein & Cappella, 2006). The problem with starting from these theoretical perspectives is that they treat culture as static and unchanging, as opposed to a dynamic and fluid process that is (re)created through communicative action (Dutta, 2008).

Health campaigns inherently involve persuasion. In general, their goal is to be able to reach an audience in a manner that influences a change in the population's health behavior (Dutta-Bergman, 2005). Campaigns feature thoughtfully designed messages that are broadly disseminated in order to change the understanding level, attitude, and behavior of a targeted population in a given time by using means that can be measured and evaluated (Rogers & Storey, 1987; Silk, Atkin, & Salmon, 2011). These campaigns tend to operate with the Aristotelian attitude that rhetoric and persuasion can and should be used to improve public life. While such practices have garnered much success in getting various populations to change their negative health behaviors, it tends to limit the multiple environmental and individual disparities that marginalized groups must navigate to reimagine their health-related practices (Basu, 2011; Dutta, 2008). For example, undocumented immigrants living in the United States must navigate dominant health information/practices, such as getting a flu vaccination, in ways that are markedly different from U.S. citizens. This population is subjected to the same health campaign massages as citizens, but they lack the means to participate in the same way due to structural factors such as limited resources, political fears, and related stigmas.

Kreps and Sparks (2008) highlight how health campaigns can contribute to or help prevent risky attitudes towards health. In order for campaigns to achieve such impact, Kreps and Sparks (2008) suggest that it is of critical importance for campaign planners to examine the cultural backgrounds and orientations of their target population before distributing campaign messages. Understanding a groups' beliefs, values, and attitudes offer more nuanced possibilities for reaching and educating various at-risk communities. The problem tends to lie in the design of messages, whereby one cultural perspective tends to dominate the rhetorical strategies used to reach a diverse audience (Kreps & Sparks, 2008). In short, the more diverse the target audience, the less effective the message becomes. Dutta speaks to the importance of critical health scholarship that is involved in "interrupting the theory and practice of health communication in the mainstream, bringing to the forefront questions of social justice, equity, participation and structural transformation" (p. 534). Dutta argues that health discourses tend to be taken as all-inclusive without questioning who gets left out of the conversation. This in turn creates a dominant health narrative that suggests one cultural understanding of health is best, while limiting possibilities for marginalized groups' ways of knowing (Lupton, 1994).

Similar to Kreps and Sparks (2008), Viswanath and Ackerson (2011) articulate how environmental inequalities affect cancer information dissemination based on race, class, and ethnicity. They highlight the disparities in information that appear among people seeking cancer-related information from different socioeconomic positions (Viswanath & Ackerson, 2011). Their quantitative study used national survey data from the National Cancer Institute to investigate how the same cancer information being given by the CDC was being received differently by various minority groups. The researchers found health communication, cancer knowledge, and beliefs about cancer-related behaviors to be key areas for investigating how minority groups were receiving various public health messages about cancer (Viswanath & Ackerson, 2011). The authors showed that the discourse used by the cancer institute to give information to the public drew on a universal understanding of cancer patients that removed any sense of cultural difference. The flattening of cultural identities has long been a feature of HIV/AIDS public campaigns, whereby messages run with a single universal perspective that reinforces Western approaches to managing health and illness (Dutta, 2008). This, in turn, leads to negative health outcomes for those marginalized groups. In the following section, I make note of how critical health communication scholars have previously gone about analyzing the way HIV/AIDS campaigns function with a static approach to culture.

HIV/AIDS Campaigns

Basu analyzes HIV/AIDs campaigns aimed at improving sex workers' attitude towards preventative behavior. He makes note of how HIV/AIDs campaigns tend to draw on social-psychological theories to try and impact individual behavior, such as condom use and regular blood testing (Karim, Karim, Soldan, & Zondi, 1995). Basu suggests that these types of campaigns fail to create the type of messages that connect with the marginalized experiences of sex workers; his analysis offers a resistive reading of a stigmatized population, which shows their consciousness and agency as rooted in their cultural environment. Specifically, by focusing on how health campaign messages were created for sex workers, Basu shows that health strategies were generally created with a universalist health philosophy grounded in Western ideology that ignores the discursive location of the audience it seeks to engage. Though messages were aimed towards aiding an at-risk community, they did not incorporate representative information about the group, as campaign mangers created the type of health messages designed for a static culture. Basu's work shows the historic practice involved with health campaigns designed to reach marginalized audiences that tend to mitigate cultural differences. For example, Dillon and Basu's (2014) study on men who have sex with men in African American and Latino communities, showed the impact of these cultural groups' beliefs and values on how they received and interpreted HIV/AIDS-related information. The study aimed to improve the way health campaigns try to connect with these at-risk groups by showing the unique cultural factors that tend to be ignored in national HIV/AIDS prevention campaigns. In effect, Dillon and Basu (2014) further argue that minority groups that are typically left out of consideration when health campaigns design messages with a static interpretation of group culture. In the next section, critical health communication is discussed as an approach by which to investigate the taken-for-granted aspect of health campaign discourses.

Critical Health Communication, Culture, and Rhetoric

"Health communication" refers to the multitude of communication processes that are involved when it comes to shaping understandings of health. This type of scholarship can be understood in two main ways: "[T]he process based perspective and the message based perspective" (Dutta & Zoller, 2008, p. 165). The message-based approach takes into consideration that health-related messages are constructed with a cultural environment in mind. A critical health perspective points to the ways that health campaigns have traditionally used a neoliberal logic that removes the marginalized individual from consideration (Lupton, 1994). This approach takes into account how representations of health function as a source that informs how people make health-related decisions, and what happens when certain groups fail to be effectively represented. Additionally, a focus on communication in general asks how sense-making occurs for marginalized groups, against the backdrop of a dominant health ideology.

Lupton details the role of discourse in shaping public health beliefs and the way health is understood as a concept. She claims that more work needs to be done in the way critical health communication scholars attend to "the discursive nature of health-care process and messages". She goes on to label discourse as a "patterned system of texts, messages, talk, dialogue or conversation which can be both identified in and located in social structures". What she describes is the importance of recognizing cultural ideology and the structures erected by cultural beliefs that shapes local meaning for individuals. Lupton (1994) makes it clear that discourse constructs and is constructed by the context in which it gets articulated. "The line of work on discursive constructions of health suggest that health is constituted and negotiated through discourse. It is in the realm of discourse that meanings of health are articulated, and realms of possibilities are imagined". As such, health messages that are framed for a particular group that leads to other groups being removed from consideration are worthy of critical investigations. Lupton (1994) argues that discourse is an interwoven practice used to define and constrain the scope of social practices. She suggests that dominant messages tend to clash with how marginalized cultures do sense-making in local spaces and, at times, erases prior cultural health knowledge. This, in turn, leads to health disparities among these groups, along with negative health outcomes due to their inability to access the resources available to dominant audiences.

Dutta and Zoller also explore the role of communication theory in deconstructing the taken-for-granted nature of health discourses that are framed with a global perspective. They argue that "discourse is intrinsically connected with the practice of health care as it sets the parameters, norms, and guidelines for expectations, choices, and actions in the domain of health". They explore the role of discourse in the health industry to highlight how media messages relating to health tend to be framed for Western audiences. Their argument speaks to the need to critically engage the taken for granted rhetorical function that language tends to operate within traditional health campaigns.

There is currently little work in the field of health communication that is focused solely on investigating the rhetorical practices employed by traditional health campaigns. Several health scholars have urged the need for more rhetorical investigation in health related spaces. Scott et al. (2013) suggest a rhetorical expertise is needed to show "how specific symbolic patterns structure meaning and action in health and medical contexts and practices" (p. 37). Meloncon and Frost (2017) add that rhetorical scholars needed to explain how "discourses create situations and allow participants and users to act on them" (p. 8). Burke's (1945) pentad is an excellent tool for analyzing the way situations emerge and shift within discourse. In the following section, I position rhetorical criticism as a tool for engaging in critical health communication.

Rhetoric of Health

Rhetorical analysis offers the opportunity to investigate language and the potential forcefulness of discourse in its day-to-day application. Rhetoric can be defined as a "human effort to induce cooperation through the use of symbols". As such, a rhetorical analysis aims to investigate the symbolic elements that humans use to create shared attitudes that help groups act in unison. Rhetorical investigations describe, interpret, and evaluate language that functions to organize humans in certain ways (Black, 1965). According to Brock and Scott, "[T]he process of calling attention to a phenomenon, interpreting it, and judging it, will inevitably result in a product designed to be persuasive" (p. 9). The authors speak to the implicit ways that rhetoric functions in terms of the taken-for-granted nature by which individuals tend to accept health messages.

Rhetorical investigations allow for scholars to ask questions about the presumed effect symbols carry through their use. According to Black (1965), rhetorical discourses are those that are written or spoken with the aim to influence humans; they are persuasive, referring to intent as opposed to accomplishment. "Whether a given discourse actually exerts an influence has no bearing on whether it is rhetorical" (Black, 1965, p.15). Black makes the claim that communication is the most useful source for measuring intent, and as such a rhetorical investigation looks to understand how intent can create influence.

Scholars such as Derkatch and Segal (2005) have suggested that rhetoric in health and medicine should focus on persuasive agents and the function of health and medical discourse to ask: Who is persuading whom of what? In addition, Malkowski et al. (2016) also believes it's important to consider the means of persuasion being used in any given health campaign. This perspective aligns with Segal's claim that critical health researchers need to take a "rhetorical frame of mind that can attune scholars to pose prior questions about discursive practices and explain how they persuade, and asses their persuasiveness" (p. 239).

These central questions are at the root of this investigation of the CDC's "Let's Stop HIV Together" campaign, as to who is meant to be persuaded by the message of this campaign and what the unforeseen effects of such promotions are. Additionally, a rhetorical investigation seeks to highlight how the CDC's rhetorical strategy functions with a universalizing drama that suggests we are now living in a "post-AIDs" environment. To conduct this type of inquiry, I turn to Burke's (1945) pentad as an approach to investigate the rhetorical implications of the CDC's message.

Pentad as Method

Burke's theories of symbolic action argue that humans are distinguished by their symbol-using behavior (Burke, 1950). People have the ability to create, use, and misuse the symbols that work to help them act in unison. Because humans use symbols to name things, situations, and people, they often abuse the way these symbols work to present reality. The reality that people perceive is filtered through some kind of symbolic filter, which Burke (1937) refers to as "a terministic screen." Both the imagined and physical worlds are symbolically filtered according to Burke. As people search for the need to be social and coordinate their actions, the symbolic pieces of language become the vehicle by which individual attitudes are shaped. For Burke (1950), rhetoric involves the use of language as "the symbolic means for inducing cooperation in beings that by nature respond to symbols" (p. 45). The means by which individuals go about constructing and enacting a shared identity depends on their ability to identify with various symbolic signs (Burke, 1950). Health campaigns are designed with this notion of using cultural symbols to get groups to change potentially risky health behavior. The question here is: What happens when campaign planners, in their attempt to reach at risk-marginalized populations, draw on symbols/messages that generalize a group in a manner that limits their cultural agency?

Burke (1945) explains the pentad as a five-point system of rhetorical analysis. As a tool, it shows the dialectic effects within the cultural rules of grammar that structure our language. He uses the pentad as a metaphor for the "dramatic" (drama) by pointing out how a shift in scope, based on symbolic use, not only changes the nature of the situation but also (re)assigns motives for agents involved in the situation. He uses the five key terms of dramatism to ask, "What is involved when we say what people are doing and why they are doing it?" (Burke, 1945, p. 35). What is involved when the CDC promotes HIV/AIDS as a virus of the past? How does this message assign purpose for at-risk cultural groups that lack the resources to prevent contracting the virus according to the information provided by the CDC?

In Burke's pentad, the act names the thing that happened (in thought or action); the scene is the setting/location/background of the act, essentially what the situation gets labeled as; agent points to the individuals or potential persons involved in the performing of such act; agency is the means the agent uses to accomplish the act; and, finally, the purpose is the "why" of the entire process (Burke, 1950). In a reduced way, the pentad lays out motives in five questions; what was done (act), when or where was it done (scene), who did it (agent), how did they do it (agency), and why (purpose). This paper focuses on the scene and agency as a ratio that dictates the CDC's campaign video to show how the scene and agent work together to promote a "post-AIDs" ideology. The scene–agent–agency ratio runs as a dramatic metaphor for showing how both the agent and the scene sustain itself in a process that Burke points to as a function of the rhetoric doing the job of division and merger.

Burke (1945) believed that by situating talk as part of a social drama, and using the pentad of dramatistic terms (act, scene, agent, agency, and purpose) to label the pivotal elements of the drama, the critic gains the language needed to expose how rhetoric operates and how various discursive shifts work to create and exclude identities. Implementing the pentad aids the criticism by pointing out the traps of dominance by asking how dramatic language works to expose the scene and act as interchangeable keys that give life to the rhetoric. This type of criticism problematizes the general acceptance of health campaigns as ethical and informative events. Thus, this analysis questions the way human motives arise and fade within the discursive make-up of the video. Further, by pointing out the dialectics of communication that is overlooked in everyday exchanges, we can start to see how dominant ways of knowing impacts those on the outskirts of the intended audience. Burke (1945) understands a scene-dominated message as pointing to elements of realism while a purpose-dominated rhetoric points to a mystified engagement. The act that fits into said container is the agent's identification with the scene and their efforts to construct a post-AIDS ideology. The pentad will be an effective tool for answering the central research question of this essay: How does the CDC's use of dramatic discourse rhetorically frame the "Let's Stop HIV Together" to promote the notion of a post-AIDS society by situating this campaign video as a drama of de-stigmatization involving localized experiences?

Tonn and Endress utilizes the pentad as a rhetorical tool for investigating how various news media sources framed the death of a new community member (i.e., Karen Wood) who was accidently shot and killed in her backyard by another local community member who was hunting. The authors used the pentad to highlight how the issue of Karen Wood's death was framed for different audiences leading up to the trial, whereby local and regional news media outlets stressed different dominating aspects of the drama (pentad) to rhetorically shape public perception regarding Wood's death as either murder or an accident. The authors noticed that because Karen Wood had recently moved to a historical hunting community while not being a hunter herself, local papers positioned her "agency/act" as the dominant (determining) element dictating the drama surrounding her death. Tonn and Endress noticed that the local media framed the narrative as a failure on Wood's part due to her outsider status and lack of knowledge regarding proper practice during hunting season. This was in stark contrast to the frame regional media outlets took, which positioned the "scene" as the dominant element that shaped Wood's death, framing the issue as rooted in the local community's hunting traditions/practices. The effects of each rhetorical choice were made apparent by the authors, as local audiences were largely in support of the hunter who shot and killed Karen Wood, while more regional audiences called for the hunter to be convicted for the death of Wood, along with pressing for changes to be made to the historic hunting laws and traditions of that Maine community. Ultimately, Tonn and Endress' use of the pentad exposed how the framing and impact of the story was dictated by which element of the drama (what, where/when, how, why) was positioned as the primary source of influence towards the final outcome.

"Let's Stop HIV Together"

The CDC "Let's Stop HIV Together" campaign (formerly known as Act Against AIDS) is aimed at stopping HIV stigma and promoting prevention practices (CDC, 2020). According to the organization, the campaign "empowers communities, partners on the ground, and health care providers to reduce stigma, prevent HIV among the hardest-hit populations, and help people with HIV" (CDC, 2020, para. 1). To try and achieve this, the organization produced and published a ten-minute short film that is used to promote the goals of the campaign. The video was published on YouTube in October 2018 and will be the main source of analysis for this paper. I chose this video to analyze because it brings together the multiple shorter ads that were created to promote this campaign. Each individual ad runs from 30 seconds to 2 minutes and features narratives from individuals currently living with the virus. The video is meant to bring these stories together to create a coherent message against HIV stigma.

The ten-minute video (which can be found on YouTube by searching "Let's Stop HIV Together") features a documentary-style design, which allows the viewer to feel like they are in conversation with each participant. The video begins with individuals (who seem to be in their home or workplace) sharing how long they have been living with HIV/AIDS along with their current location.

Along with individual narratives, the video also features slides with definitions for concepts such as "HIV Stigma," which are used to direct the narratives being shared by individuals. The narratives being shared in the video are segmented so that to the audience, it feels like all the participants are engaging in the same discussion. The video also features a narrator who acts as informational support for the stories being shared by participants, as she provides CDC definitions of the concepts that participants discuss. The overall narrative of the video moves from one focused on HIV stigma to the new medical means of HIV prevention. The video ends with a message from the CDC to learn more about HIV prevention by accessing the CDC's website.

It will be important to start by offering a description of what I understand to be scene and the acts before moving on to analyze the significance of the relationship between the scene, the agent, and the act. The goal is to show how the elements of the drama created by the CDC's campaign work to formulate a rhetoric that suggests participants are taking part in a post-AIDS society due to the introduction of Western medicine.

Scene

Burke (1945) makes the point when discussing the pentad to focus first on scene because that is how the critic interprets the ways that the scene influences how judgements occur in and around it. For instance, if I located the scene of the CDC campaign as being the YouTube page itself, it leads to a different set of relationships with regards to who the actors are and what they are doing in said scene. According to Burke (1950), it is the relationship between the various parts of the drama that highlights the rhetorical move being made. For our purpose, it is important to locate the scene beyond the literal configuration of space and time, and instead locate the scene that is the discursive environment of the campaign's message. Thus, the scene in question starts out as a symbolic U.S., which later shifts to suggest that the scene is actually class-based as opposed to being based on nationality. I interpret the external scene as the U.S. because each participant in the video shares their location, all of which are in the U.S. While everyone's location is varied (as in they live in different states), the discourse used by participants in the video makes it clear that individuals are speaking from a middle-class perspective. This interpretation is based off actions that participants engage in within the video – such as lounging at coffee shops, getting their hair styled, wearing jewelry and smart watches – and off participants' backgrounds, which can be assumed to be their homes and which feature pools, leather couches, foosball tables, and well-manicured landscapes. What is most indicative of a middle-class lifestyle is the way individuals speak about having 100% adherence to medical advice, having steady access to medical information, being able to take their medication every day, and having access to regular checkups (Zoller & Dutta, 2008).

The opening scene of the campaign video starts by showing an individual who is doing work in a coffee shop. He orders a drink, sits, and writes while he shares his story. The next clip shows a woman who shares her experience in Spanish (with English subtitles) where she informs viewers that she is in the southeastern U.S. This is followed by multiple others who also share their location and identify themselves as living in the U.S. with HIV/AIDS. The video then makes a move to expand the scene, symbolically, by having participants share their place of birth. The shift is subtle yet effective. This communicates an idea that the U.S. is a diverse society and, as such, this message is meant to reach a diverse audience. It creates the illusion of a multicultural perspective of concern with this move to have immigrants talk about their place of origin. The young man who opened the scene in the U.S. coffee shop shares that his family originates from El Salvador. This is followed by individuals sharing their location of birth: "Nashville, Tennessee"; "Chicago, Illinois"; "Colombian"; "Broward county"; "Fort Jarvis, New York"; "Savannah, Georgia"; "Hollywood, Florida." Even though each participant is currently located and participating within the United States, the video expands the scene to suggest that this message is also meant to connect with non-American identities who can access similar resources – a global scene manifests from the narratives shared.

The use of Black and brown bodies as the voice of this message creates the sense of this being a multicultural message. In addition, the language and themes used to present this message draws on communicative patterns that are particular to middle-class Americans. This shift is confirmed by the message that followed the naming of birth locations when an individual says, "Everyone can be affected by HIV." This rhetorical move allows the audience to think about HIV stigma as a global issue that affects all types of populations. While this is certainly true, the act being done in this video is one that is concerned with stigmas in middle-class populations, not "everyone." As noted above, most working class and marginalized individuals who are living with this illness face major structural limitations, where they are unable to maintain 100% adherence, or have regular access to a doctor for check-ups and updated health information.

This is to say, that the CDC does not want viewers to limit the scene of HIV stigma to the U.S., while using concepts and themes that are designed to influence a U.S.-centered understanding. Once the scene expands beyond the U.S., a globalized appeal emerges within the act that creates a sense of universality meant to represent those outside of the U.S. The problem lies in that this is an incomplete and culturally inaccurate message for those living outside the U.S., and those living within the U.S. in marginalized positions – to put it simply, the way stigma functions differs in populations based on cultural beliefs and socioeconomic resources.

Act

Burke (1945) sees the act of the drama as being the thing that is being done in the scene. If we are judging this drama based on the stories provided by participants, then the act seems clear when placed in conjunction with the scene. The sharing of narratives runs as an action that is meant to help reduce stigma for individuals living with HIV/AIDS by increasing stories of survival. The participants clearly communicate their "post-AIDS" experiences as evidence for why the social stigma of having AIDS now carries greater threat than the virus itself. One individual who said they have been living with HIV for over 20 years proclaims, "In the beginning it was labeled as a deadly weapon, disease and everything, where, in reality HIV is just a virus, it's the stigma that's the deadly disease." His story becomes a testimony of evidence that suggest that we have long been living in a post-AIDS society. His words suggest that because it is "just a virus" then it can be managed by modern medicine like most known viruses. His comments fit the CDC theme of Western medicine being the vehicle for this post-AIDS era. Further, his narrative gets authorized by the main agent operating within and beyond the scene.

The CDC functions as the agent (with agency) acting within the scene, as a narrator supplies definitions and explanations between participants' narratives. The narrator is the one that moves the act along, while the participants stories act in a supporting role. Following the participants comments on their experience with stigma, a message appears on the screen that offers a working definition of what HIV stigma means. The narrator directs and dictates the act by supplying official definitions and explanations. The participants stories are (non-)agents that work to dramatize and connect the definitions and explanations provided by the narrator.

The CDC's definition of HIV stigma draws on the Western biomedical model of understanding, which explains stigma as "negative attitudes, beliefs, and behavior towards people with HIV" (CDC, 2018, p.1). This definition is general enough to reach a widespread audience without reproach. This interjection by the CDC does two things; first, it creates a sense of universality about HIV stigma without concern for how cultural practices affects beliefs within certain population, which in turn reduces the structural and power dimensions of stigma to "feelings" and "ignorance" (Farmer, 2003). This also creates the perception that HIV stigma has been solely based on risk of infection, which mutes the historic (rhetorical) practice that have stigmatized certain groups based on race and ethnicity, as well as sexual minorities, as the perpetrators of this disease. Secondly, this act shows the CDC as supplying an "official" definition, which tries to define stigma from a Western biomedical perspective. This definition creates the question that can later be answered by the CDC: Why should people no longer be afraid of contracting this virus?

As the video continues and other individuals share their experiences, it becomes clear that the CDC is the only agent with agency propelling this drama while everyone else acts in a supporting role. Towards the end of the video, the narrator returns to explain that "we now have the medicine to prevent exposure," as she goes on to explain Pre-Exposure Prophylaxis (PrEP) as a key resource to a post-AIDS environment. The act itself shifts fully in this moment, from one focused on reducing stigma to one aimed at promoting the idea of a post-AIDS society due to the implementation of this medicine. This move reinforces the idea presented earlier that this is "just a virus," showing that Western medicine has conquered this virus as well. This rhetorical shift occurs subtly but it symbolizes a sense of who the target audience for this message is (or can be), i.e., those who can afford this type of medication. The act, according to Burke's theory, configures the actual scene to be middle-class Westerners (not necessarily people who live in the Western part of the globe, but more to those who live by Western ideological standards, especially with regards to medical beliefs and practices), those with the means to take part in the post-AIDS neoliberal society through the purchasing of preventive medicine.

Agents/Agency

The individuals, who seem to be functioning as agents in the campaign video, do the job of supplying support to the overall message being promoted. These individuals lack agency in regard to shaping the act being done in the drama. Their narratives supply an embodied pathos that works to situate the CDC's message as a moral concern that has material effect. This helps to shape the ongoing drama of de-stigmatization being presented. According to Burke (1945), agents are the connective tissue that brings the scene and act together. Yet, when we interrogate the relationship between the (non-)agents in the scene who are supporting the act, it becomes clear from a rhetorical perspective that the agency to act lies with the narrator. This is the CDC's message, not the participants' stories. The narratives being supplied by individuals must be considered as examples that are meant to offer support to the action being done by the CDC narrator. This begs the question of what kind of stigmas are being reproduced by the CDC as they choose to centralize Black and brown bodies as the symbolic face of HIV/AIDS (again). Before moving to discuss the agency involved with producing the act, it will be important to first discuss the agents involved.

One noticeable aspect of the CDC's campaign video was the diverse range of bodies and identities used to offer testimony. The video featured individuals who are typically considered minorities in the U.S. landscape. This is worthy of note because health campaigns tend to try to represent and connect with who they see as their majority target audience. When considering that over 60% of the U.S. population is white and straight, it becomes noteworthy when an organization aiming to reach the masses limits their representation to minority actors. Out of the 13 individual participants in the group, only 1 identified as both straight and white. There was one white male who did not identify as either gay or straight. The other participants identified as Black, Hispanic, gay, etc. Additionally, four individuals identified as immigrants. The cast of bodies used to present and promote this message shows a tacit intent that is aimed at identifying these minority groups as the face of HIV/AIDS stigma. These (non-)agents inherently operate as the representative bodies of those living with HIV/AIDS. This rhetorical move is meant to frame the drama as inclusive but when analyzing the CDC as the main agent, it exposes the lack of cultural sensitivity in this message.

The diverse bodies in the video do two things rhetorically when considering the scene and the act as relational. First, it stretches the potential scene beyond the U.S. (again) as the lack of white bodies along with the individuals speaking other languages, creates a sense of multicultural awareness. These (non-)agents are meant to show which types of bodies are most affected by the virus according to the CDC, hence which audiences require the most attention. This, in turn, creates a drama that suggests that HIV/AIDS is mostly a non-white issue and, by extension, the stigmatization of HIV/AIDS as largely a non-white concern. Secondly, because the CDC chose to focus on Black, brown, and gay bodies as the main source of testimonial evidence, the campaign video subtly (re)creates the historic stigmas attached to these bodies as the main carriers of the virus. While I do not think this is the aim of the CDC, they nonetheless foster a continuation of the historic idea that HIV/AIDS is a Black, brown, and gay disease even in the "post-AIDS" era. The act then becomes a promotion for the strategies available to Western societies to limit the spread of HIV/AIDS sourced from these populations. The relationship between the scene, the act, and the agent (the narrator) with agency shows a rhetoric of morality meant to reach non-white and non-straight bodies. This also suggests that stigma towards people with HIV/AIDS is most prevalent in these minority communities.

At the 1:23 minute mark of the video, it becomes apparent that the agent operating "behind" the scene held the most agency. The CDC is the only agent with agency in the video. They utilize text and voice overs to offer "official" definitions for what participants' narratives provide evidence for. The CDC's role in this campaign message does the work of authorizing the ideas put forth by the individual participants. This means that the actors in the scene are used as markers for identifying with the potential audience, as opposed to agents directing the distribution of information. This observation supports the criticism presented earlier that suggests that this type of message production inherently (re)stigmatizes certain populations as the culprit of HIV/AIDS and the stigmas surrounding the virus. While (non-)agents speak in the scene, they do not move the act, they offer support and evidence for the "official" message as directed by the CDC's narrator agent. For Burke (1945), agents show agency in a scene by being able to move the act along, which is only done in this campaign video by the narrator. Identifying the agent with agency of this drama as the CDC's narrator creates a different set of rhetorical expectations. The purpose of the message becomes worthy of deeper interrogation. While the overall goal of the campaign is to reduce stigma, attention to the CDC's actions within this drama shows the organization as promoting Western biomedicine as the main source for reducing HIV/AIDS stigma. The CDC, in effect, tacitly states that stigma is unwarranted because HIV is not the same "threat" that it once was (due to biomedical advancements), which suggests that it was warranted in the past (prior to its shift towards being a manageable chronic illness). The message suggests that de-stigmatization is needed and possible due to the implementation of Western medicine, which reduces the idea of stigma from a structural/cultural/social issue to one that is simply a biomedical issue. This reinforces the idea that a post-AIDS society is only possible through the implementation of a Western medical logic.

Scene–Act–Agent/Agency

It is important to note that, under further analysis, the idea of scene, act, and agency run interchangeably and will be important ratios to focus on moving forward. The scene–act–agency–purpose ratio operates in a unique way in the campaign video because of the way they shift, influence, divide, combine, and reduce each other. The video becomes one where agent/agency is featured as the dominant term(s) influencing the way the drama unfolds, but only insofar as the scene and act helps to dictate that purpose. What is being argued here is that, at times, a scenic perspective is the dominant means for engagement, and at other times it is the act or agent, all of which subsequently equals a purpose that is rhetorically framed, based on which element of the drama is most dominant. The idea is that the scene, act, and purpose shifts once the agent is located as the CDC; it exposes a drama that carries multiple conflicting messages. In the video, the agent (CDC) dictates the purpose and direction of the message beyond stigma. What it shows is that the overall purpose of this video is less concerned with reducing stigma and more centered on presenting an argument that centralizes a post-AIDS society through the implementation of Western medicine.

According to Burke (1945), "[I]t is the principle of drama that the nature of acts and agents should be consistent with the scene" (p. 27). Thus, it is a case of agent sees scene, agent acts scene. The point Burke makes is that all the elements of a drama are communicatively constructed, which tends to situate a more dynamic set of motives as opposed to analyzing the physical make-up of the drama. The motive of the drama, hence, lies in the relationship between the communicative parts of a drama, and how they unfold to present a narrative. Thus, if you were to analyze the CDC's campaign video as a physical drama, this would seem like a local-sourced message, with diverse actors communicating multicultural beliefs of inclusion and acceptance. But by analyzing the way the drama unfolds communicatively, the pentad shows how the CDC functions as the main agent delivering this message, which creates a different set of relationships between actors, the scene, and the act. The subtle symbolic transformation that occurs through communicative acts, turns one of the deadliest diseases in human history into "just a virus." This dramatization is meant to alter one's belief that viruses should not be feared as they are things that can be controlled by scientific approaches to medicine. The individual participants in the video become the vehicle for dramatizing this message, their statements need not be taken as "literal" (because the narrator is the authority), but instead are employed to dramatize the point or create an impression that fits the unfolding rhetorical situation.

In the video, identities are transformed from stigmatized individuals living with an incurable disease that requires costly medication and medical intervention. Symbolically, the CDC puts these actors back in the driver's seat through the implementation of PrEP medication. The fear that these individuals previously experienced due to their condition can/should now be levitated and reduced because PrEP has fostered the type of post-AIDS environment that makes the fear of contracting the virus irrational. At the 5:29 minute mark of the video, the narrator returns to explain that advancement in medical treatment has led to better outcomes for those living with HIV/AIDS. This moment, which is situated between participants' narratives of stigma related fears, moves the drama towards its symbolic purpose. The post-AIDS message comes to the fore, as the narrator indicates that the advancement in treatments are allowing individuals with the virus to live healthy and full lives. This is followed by individual stories as evidence of the narrator's message that this virus is under control. Once more, the narrator as agent directs the drama as the actors (participants) supply the communication for dramatizing this message that promotes a post-AIDS society through PrEP.

Purpose

For Burke, the purpose of the drama can only be interpreted from the nature of the relationship between the scene, the act, and the agent. Considering the terminologies of the CDC's campaign video, dramatistically, reveals a systematic way of defining and attributing social solutions through medical advancements, such that when we talk about de-stigmatizing HIV/AIDS we do so through the terms of Western medicine. In effect, the campaign video rhetorically constructs HIV/AIDS stigma as steeped in the fear of not having a medical solution to the virus. The introduction of PrEP becomes the catalyst for a post-AIDS society, but stigma towards the virus can only be reduced once the right populations are made aware of this medical advancement.

At the 6:20 mark, the narrator presents PrEP as the "HIV prevention option for people who are HIV negative. It works by taking one pill every day. When taken daily, it can greatly reduce the risk of getting HIV." This moment marks the purpose of the CDC's video and campaign in general. Reducing stigma is the drama being used to promote PrEP as a potential solution to not contracting the virus. The narrator draws on dramatical language to suggest that this drug "greatly reduces" the risk with getting the virus but offers no literal definition of how this compares to other preventative options. Additionally, the narrator qualifies her statement by framing it as "can," which would indicate that it also cannot work for certain individuals. This, in effect, dramatizes the function of the drug and its potential capabilities. This dramatization is supported once again by individual narratives regarding their experiences with this product. Stigma is transformed through the introduction of this drug.

The narrator, as the agent with agency in the campaign video, offers a final message, which reinforces the central purpose (and potential motive) of this message as being concerned with the promotion of this new drug intervention. This is one of the more sophisticated rhetorical moves made by the CDC, as the narrator translates the message that is written on the screen to dramatically communicate the importance of adherence. The written message she reads states, "People living with HIV who take their HIV medicine as prescribed and achieve and keep an undetectable viral load have effectively no risk of transmitting HIV to their HIV negative sexual partners." This supports the claim of the purpose of this campaign as being motivated by the promotion of this type of preventative medication. While the textualization of this message makes it clear, the narrator manipulates the drama with her verbal utterance. She follows up by saying, "This means that taking HIV medicine as prescribed and getting and keeping an undetectable viral load is one of the BEST ways to prevent sexual transmission of HIV." This is followed by the words fading in the background that say, "[E]ffectively no risk." This subtle rhetorical move where the narrator simplifies the message with "this means" is meant to connect with audiences passively through repetition.

As the agent, she dramatizes the effects and potential benefits of this drug to promote its use. Further, her message gets reinforced and supported by the participants sharing their stories with the camera. Immediately following the narrator's final message, Maria proclaims, "This is going to free us from the stigma of being seen as infectious, it's going to promote adherence." Once again, the (non-)agents' stories in the video work as the main source of dramatization that filters the promotion of PrEP medication through a discourse of stigma. The CDC can avoid questions related to cost and access because this campaign is framed as a drama solely concerned with stigma. For the CDC, the spread of awareness about these drugs and their presumed effect will create the type of post-AIDS society that is free of stigma. The drama presented in this campaign message sees stigma reduction as part of the trickle-down effect afforded by PrEP. This would confirm that this message is meant to reach populations with the resources needed to access this drug.

Conclusion

According to Burke (1950), because the human world is built upon symbolic interpretations, we tend to need greater means of interpretation to recognize the "cultural tangles" beneath our experiences of societal doings. The pentad is one example of the many ways through which scholars can go about illuminating the rhetorical features of a drama and the presumed motive. The CDC's "Let's stop HIV together" campaign is one example of how health campaigns draw on rhetorical strategies to situate a drama that communicates conflicting influential health messages. While the CDC's campaign video starts out as a message of de-stigmatization, a pentadic analysis shows that the drama quickly shifts to promoting PrEP as fostering a post-AIDS society. The pentad shows how dramas are composed of statements and depictions of people's motives for their actions. When considering the CDC as the primary agent directing this drama, it becomes important to interrogate the terminologies that dictate this message. In this case, a focus on Western medicine as the solution becomes the dominant terminology for reducing stigma.

A dramatistic approach is concern with the vocabularies of motive that dominate a drama. This type of investigation is concerned with uncovering the systematic communicative principles whereby people (institutions) ascribe, understand, and communicate their analyses of what human action should look like in particular situations. According to Burke (1945), there are basic "forms of thought" associated with the systematic, communicative operations of a vocabulary, such as those used in health campaigns. This speaks to the historic practices of health campaigns, and campaigns in general, which draw on top down institutional definitions and illustrations to promote health practices. I propose that the CDC move away from using the traditional health campaign models that draw on psychological theories as its frame, which attempts to treat culture as a static state with agency-less actors, and instead move towards the culture-centered approach to health communication. The culture-centered approach to health communication is meant to centralize cultural voices in the articulation of health issues and potential solutions (Airhihenbuwa, 1995; Dutta-Bergman, 2005). To achieve this, Dutta (2007) notes, researchers must consider the key tenets that structure a culture-centered approach, i.e., recognize the linkages between structure and culture, agency, and voice, the notion of multiple and shifting contexts, and spaces of resistance. The culture-centered approach is geared towards examining how those cultural identities at the margins of a profit-driven health industry navigate the uneven distribution of resources.

A more culture-centered approach to this project would offer greater rhetorical benefits with regards to the reduction of stigma surrounding this population. In order to do this, the CDC would need to remove their voice from the message itself; this would create the space to listen to the stories and experiences of individuals without the interjection of an institutional voice. Removing the CDC from this message would re-centralize the voices of participants as the source of knowledge and experience – this is the main focus of the Culture-Centered Approach. Secondly, to make this campaign culture-centered, the CDC must also represent the voices of those who are living with HIV/AIDS who lack the type of resources that are available to more mainstream audiences. It is extremely important to highlight and expose how class status affects the way certain groups' health practices become stigmatized in a capitalist society.

This campaign needs to move away from focusing on PrEP as central to creating a post-AIDS society, which is positioned as a reason why de-stigmatization is possible (and needed) at this time, and instead move towards highlighting the array of lived experiences that show the complexities involved with living with HIV/AIDS from various class and cultural perspectives. Lastly, it is of utmost importance to manage the way representation unfolds in these types of campaign ads, as the current CDC ad places the burden of stigmatization on minority bodies. This does not help to reduce stigma regarding HIV/AIDS among these populations, instead it (re)positions these minority groups as the face of the disease. There needs to be an effort to show white, straight individuals as also dealing with this illness, as this is also part of the de-stigmatization process, to counter the historic rhetoric surrounding HIV/AIDS as being a Black, brown, and gay issue.

References

Airhihenbuwa, C. O. (1995). *Health and culture: Beyond the Western paradigm.* Thousand Oaks, CA: SAGE.

Atkin, C. K., & Rice, R. E. (Eds.). (2012). *Public communication campaigns* (4th ed.). Thousand Oaks, CA: SAGE.

Basu, A. (2011). HIV/AIDS and subaltern autonomous rationality: A call to recenter health communication in marginalized sex worker spaces. *Communication Monographs*, *78*(3), 391–408. doi:10.1080/03637751.2011.589457

Black, E. (1965). *Rhetorical criticism: A study in method*. New York: Macmillan.

Burke, K. (1937). *Attitudes toward history*. Berkeley; University of California Press.

Burke, K. (1945). *A grammar of motives*. Berkeley: University of California Press.

Burke, K. (1950). *A rhetoric of motives*. Berkeley: University of California Press.

Centers for Disease Control and Prevention. (2018, September). *National press conference kicks off 2018–2019 flu vaccination campaign*. Retrieved from https://www.cdc.gov/flu/spotlights/press-conference-2018-19.htm

Centers for Disease Control and Prevention. (2020). *Let's stop HIV together campaign at a glance*. Retrieved from https://www.cdc.gov/stophivtogether/pdf/preventionresources/cdc-lsht-factsheet-at-a-glance.pdf

Dillon, P. J., & Basu, A. (2014). HIV/AIDS and minority men who have sex with men: A meta-ethnographic synthesis of qualitative research. *Health Communication, 29*, 182–192. doi:10.1080/10410236.2012.732911

Dutta, M. J. (2008). *Communicating health: A culture-centered approach*. Malden, MA: Polity.

Dutta, M. J. (2017). Culture-centered communication and social change: Listening and participation to transform communication inequalities. In L. Chen (Ed.), *Intercultural Communication* (pp. 309–329). Berlin & New York: Mouton de Gruyter.

Dutta-Bergman, M. J. (2005). Theory and practice in health communication campaigns: A critical interrogation. *Health Communication, 18*, 103–122.

Farmer, P. (2003). *Pathologies of power: Health, human rights and the new war on the poor*. Berkeley: University of California Press.

Fishbein, M., & Cappella, J. N. (2006). The role of theory in developing effective health communications. *Journal of Communication, 56*, S1–S17.

Karim, Q. A., Karim, S. S., Soldan, K., & Zondi, M. (1995). Reducing the risk of HIV infection among South African sex workers: Socioeconomic and gender barriers. *American Journal of Public Health, 85*(11), 1521–1525. doi: 10.2105/AJPH.85.11.1521

Kreps, G. L., & Sparks, L. (2008). Meeting the health literacy needs of immigrant populations. *Patient Education and Counseling, 71*, 328–332.

Lundberg, C. O. (2013). Letting rhetoric be: On rhetoric and rhetoricity. *Philosophy & Rhetoric*, *46*(2), 247–255. doi: 10.5325/philrhet.46.2.0247

Lupton, D. (1994). Toward the development of critical health communication praxis. *Health Communication, 6*, 55–67. doi: 10.1207/s15327027hc0601_4

Malkowski, J. A., Scott, B., & Keränen, L. (2016). Rhetorical approaches to health and medicine. *Oxford Research Encyclopedia of Communication*. Retrieved from https://oxfordre.com/communication/view/10.1093/acrefore/9780190228613.001.0001/acrefore-9780190228613-e-180

Meloncon, L, & Frost, E. (2017). Special issue introduction: Charting an emerging field *Communication Design Quarterly, 3*, 7–14. doi:10.1145/2826972.2826973.

McGuire, W. J. (2013). McGuire's classic input-output framework for constructing persuasive messages. In R. E. Rice & C. K. Atkin (Eds.), *Public communication campaigns* (4th ed., pp. 133–146). Thousand Oaks, CA: SAGE.

Rogers, E. M., & Storey, J. D. (1987). Communication campaigns. In C. R. Berger & S. H. Chaffee (Eds.), *Handbook of communication science* (p. 817–846). Thousand Oaks, CA: SAGE.

Scott, J. B., Segal, J. Z., & Keränen, L. (2013). The rhetorics of health and medicine: Inventional possibilities for scholarship and engaged practice. *Poroi, 9*, 1–6. doi:10.13008/2151-2957.1157

Segal, J. Z. (2005). *Health and the rhetoric of medicine*. Carbondale: Southern Illinois University Press.

Silk, K. J., Atkin, C. K., & Salmon, C. T. (2011). Developing effective media campaigns for health promotion. In T. L. Thompson, R. Parrott, & J. F. Nussbaum (Eds.), *Routledge handbook of health communication* (2nd ed., pp. 203–219). New York: Routledge.

Viswanath, K., & Ackerson, L. K. (2011). Race, ethnicity, language, social class, and health communication inequalities: A nationally-representative cross-sectional study. *PLoS ONE, 6*, e14550. doi:10.1371/journal.pone.0014550

Wakefield, M. A., Loken, B., & Hornik, R. C. (2010). Use of mass media campaigns to change health behavior. *The Lancet, 376*, 1261–1271.

Zoller, H., & Dutta, M. (2008). Afterword: Emerging agendas in health communication and the challenge of multiple perspectives. In H. Zoller & M. Dutta (Eds.), *Emerging perspectives in health communication: Interpretive, critical and cultural approaches* (pp. 449–463). Mahwah, NJ: Lawrence Erlbaum Associates.

5 Indigenous HIV/AIDS in the Context of 'Post-AIDS' Discourse

A Meta-Synthesis of Qualitative Research

B. Liahnna Stanley, Nivethitha Ketheeswaran and Brianna R. Cusanno

The HIV/AIDS epidemic has had a pernicious global impact over the last 40 years, claiming more than 30 million lives since it began (UNAIDS, 2019). The World Health Organization (WHO, 2018) estimates that 38 million people are currently living with HIV/AIDS across the world. Although rates of HIV transmission and HIV/AIDS-related deaths have been decreasing in recent years (UNAIDS, 2019), enhancing treatment and prevention remains a dominant global health priority, with the goal of eliminating HIV as a public health threat by 2030 (UNAIDS, 2016). Political rhetoric of "zero new HIV infections, zero discrimination, and zero AIDS-related deaths (UNAIDS, 2010) supports goals of "an AIDS-free generation" and ultimately "ending the AIDS epidemic" (WHO, 2015). As alluring as the idea of "ending AIDS" may sound, it is far from being reality. Enduring biomedical innovations and health campaigns to reduce HIV/AIDS to non-epidemic levels may ease public anxieties about HIV/AIDS, but in doing so perpetuates a discourse of "post-AIDS" (O'Brien, 2013; Mazanderani & Paparini, 2015; Persson, 2013; Walker, 2017) that negates the embodied and structural experiences of individuals and communities living with HIV and/or AIDS.

In this chapter, we seek to highlight the ongoing complexities of experiences of living with HIV and/or AIDS among Indigenous Peoples by synthesizing qualitative literature on Indigenous People living with HIV and/or AIDS (IPHAs) in contemporary "post-AIDS" discourse. In what follows, we reflect on the meanings of "post-AIDS," provide a background of how HIV/AIDS affects Indigenous individuals and communities at large, and discuss the importance for understanding experiences of IPHAs in the context of "post-AIDS" before presenting our synthesis of qualitative research on IPHAs. We conclude with a theoretical discussion on "post-AIDS" as part of the larger colonial project that exploits and erases Indigenous lives. It is our hope that such interventions recognize the role of colonialism in health complexities that are neglected in "post-AIDS" discourse.

DOI: 10.4324/9781003000945-7

"Post-AIDS" and Indigenous Health

Despite the ongoing HIV/AIDS epidemic, HIV/AIDS is largely rendered as merely a manageable and treatable health issue in the public health sphere. Biomedical innovations and interventions have made possible the transformation of HIV, shifting it from a terminal disease to a manageable long-term condition in which people can continue to live with HIV as opposed to dying from AIDS. This shift is marked by the increasingly widespread availability and use of the HIV combination treatment medication, HAART (Highly Active Antiretroviral Therapy – commonly known as the "AIDS cocktail") to manage, control, and prevent opportunistic transmissions of HIV/AIDS (Gilbert & Walker, 2009; Whiteside, 2015; Whiteside & Strauss, 2014). Soon after the 1996 International AIDS conference in Vancouver, where the effectiveness of protease inhibitors – a classification of antiretroviral drugs – was officially announced, a myriad of popular and gay and lesbian news outlets signaled that we had reached "the ends of the AIDS epidemic" (Román, 2007, p. 372).

Western biomedical and developmental discourse of "positive progress" (Johnston et al., 2015) for HIV/AIDS has not only obscured the social, cultural, economic, and geopolitical underpinnings that shape HIV/AIDS as a structural health issue, but has also contributed to what O'Brien (2013) notes as "a 'post-AIDS' culture, whereby a discourse of crisis and death has evolved into one of survival and living" (p. 75). "Post-AIDS" discourse implies that we have "moved on" from and are "beyond" HIV/AIDS. For the millions of people currently living with HIV/AIDS, however, there is little that is "post" about HIV and AIDS. Thus, the concept of "post-AIDS" should not be embraced unproblematically – to assume that we are beyond HIV/AIDS and have made any meaningful momentum to "end AIDS" is distorted and dangerous. The monolithic discourse of "post-AIDS" oversimplifies the complexities of HIV/AIDS, erasing the sociocultural practices of health that play a fundamental role in shaping the experience of HIV/AIDS (Walker, 2017). National (U.S.-based) and global public health agencies such as UNAIDS, WHO, the Centers for Disease Control and Prevention (CDC), and National Institutes of Health (NIH) play a significant role in perpetuating a "post-AIDS" discourse by advancing vigorous biomedical research programs to develop and test new drugs and prevention measures. These approaches focus on HIV/AIDS as an isolated issue apart from social, economic, cultural, and political factors that structure health, risk, and disease.

The impact of HIV/AIDS has been particularly devastating among Indigenous Peoples (Negin et al., 2015). For the purposes of this chapter, we use *Indigenous Peoples* to describe the culturally and geographically diverse groups that share similarities based on common experiences of colonialism. For Indigenous Peoples, the legacies of colonialism result in a range of sociohealth disparities, including racism, depression, poverty, food insecurity, substance misuse, homelessness, stigma, discrimination in health services, and disproportionate mortality rates (Anderson et al., 2016; Jones, 2006; King et al., 2009). These proximal comorbidities extend the colonialism of genocide, forced relocation, forced assimilation, and dispossession from land, family, and resources (Brave Heart & DeBruyn, 1998; Evans-Campbell, 2008; Glenn, 2015). Impacts of colonization and concomitant detriments are highly complex intra- and intergenerational drivers for Indigenous health that contribute to the marginalization of Indigenous Peoples within the countries in which they live (Czyzewski, 2011; Negin et al., 2015; Paradies, 2016). For example, as reported by the U.S. Census Bureau (2017), Indigenous Peoples in the U.S. experience the highest rate of poverty among any racial group, with approximately 26% of Indigenous Peoples living in poverty, which is double the national average of 13%. Indigenous communities also experience geographical isolation, which means they are less able to access healthcare and are underreported by HIV testing and surveillance programs. Accordingly, very few countries have reliable national surveillance data to record factual levels of HIV among Indigenous Peoples (UNAIDS, 2006). The woefully inadequate – and in some cases, nonexistent – public health data creates unique challenges for addressing and understanding health for Indigenous Populations (Smylie & Firestone, 2015).

As previously mentioned, Indigenous Peoples bear a disproportionate burden of health inequities that intersect with and heighten risk for HIV/AIDS. "Post-AIDS" discourse muffles HIV/AIDS as a contemporary health crisis and stagnates possibilities for mobilizing transformative HIV/AIDS interventions, thus exacerbating HIV/AIDS and related health issues among Indigenous Peoples. Moreover, the notion of "post-AIDS" ignores the embodied, everyday experiences of HIV/AIDS, which are structured by colonization, particularly for those in the Global South (Auerbach et al., 2011). Under colonial rule, the popular imaginary perceives both colonialism and Indigenous Peoples to be relics of the past – analogous to assumptions that HIV/AIDS is no longer a problem because Western biomedical innovations have moved the world "beyond AIDS." Examining Indigenous experiences of HIV/AIDS locates HIV/AIDS in the context of colonialism and centralizes colonialism as a driving force of Indigenous health and life potentialities, thus generating insight for understanding "post-AIDS" as part of the colonial project. The purpose of this meta-synthesis is to bring the unique experiences of IPHAs into the forefront to discuss how to better understand and address IPHA health in a "post-AIDS" era. In the next section, we detail the literature search, data appraisal, and synthesis procedures used in this study.

Methods

The purpose of this project was to synthesize literature describing the social, structural, and cultural experiences of IPHAs to understand how these phenomena are connected to and communicated within larger discourses of "post-AIDS." To accomplish this, we employed a synthesis of qualitative research related to these topics. Meta-synthesis refers to a range of methodological approaches that involve comparing, translating, and analyzing original findings from which new interpretations are generated (Finfgeld, 2003). In this study, we used meta-ethnography, an interpretive approach involving inductive analysis of related themes and concepts identified in qualitative studies (Noblit & Hare, 1998). The meta-ethnographic process as first outlined by Noblit and Hare (1998) and elaborated by Atkins and colleagues (2008) involves several steps, including identifying key findings of each study, determining relationships among studies, and comparing and contrasting cross-case conclusions in order to synthesize the main findings.

We limited our analysis to qualitative research for several reasons. Central to qualitative research are methodologies that privilege the points of view of research participants (Lindlof & Taylor, 2019) which is important for understanding the experiences of health and illness by the people living with them (Bosma et al., 2010). Qualitative research offers rich forms of data and interpretation that account for the significance of "lay knowledge" and sociocultural influences on perspectives and behaviors related to health in everyday life (Grypdonck, 2006), which is particularly important for experiences of health and illness at the margins. Additionally, qualitative data are marked by complex detail that are often unable to be wholly represented through quantitative methods (Popay et al., 1998).

We would be remiss not to acknowledge the inherent risks of this analysis, namely the perils of essentializing Indigenous lives. How health factors play out in the lived realities of Indigenous Peoples varies greatly across cultures, communities, and countries, and even more so in the context of various, ever-evolving cultural, political, economic, geopolitical, and development health agendas. For these reasons, any discussion that groups together "Indigenous Peoples" and "Indigenous experiences" involves considerable generalization that discounts the myriad of particularities within Indigenous networks that are shaped by various colonial assemblages. General experiences can be drawn from their collective Indigeneity but not all issues discussed in this review will affect Indigenous Peoples in the same way. While we reject a singular notion of Indigeneity, we suggest that analyzing common themes in the experiences of several Indigenous groups in different geographical sectors can inform our understanding of IPHA experience in a "post-AIDS" era.

Search Strategies and Inclusion Criteria

Our analysis began with a systematic literature search to identify peer-reviewed literature published from 2000 to 2019 that focused on HIV/AIDS and Indigenous Populations in North, South, and Central America. We chose to focus on IPHAs in the Americas to broaden the scope beyond the U.S. but also to not essentialize global experiences of Indigeneity. We consulted seven electronic databases: Communication Abstracts, Anthrosource, Applied Social Science Index and Abstracts, Medline via Proquest, Social Science full text, Proquest International Bibliography of Social Sciences, and Web of Science Core Collection. Searches were conducted using various databases with combinations of keywords including: (a) HIV/AIDS, (b) Indigenous, (c) Native American, (d) American Indian, (e) First Nations, (f) Aboriginal, (g) health, and (h) qualitative. Additional articles were identified by searching the bibliographies from retrieved articles.

Our search protocol generated 441 abstracts for review. Inclusion criteria for this analysis were: (a) published in English language, (b) published between 2000 and 2019, (c) focused on perspectives of Indigenous adult populations in the Americas, (d) focused on HIV/AIDS, and (e) utilized qualitative methods. We applied the initial criteria to each abstract and reduced the sample to 25 abstracts for review. Next, we removed irrelevant papers from the sample using two screening questions as informed by Campbell and colleagues (2003): (a) "Does this paper report on [original] findings from research and involved qualitative methods of data collection and analysis?" and (b) "Is this research relevant to the synthesis topic?" During this stage, we decided to narrow our focus to studies that involved IPHAs as participants, excluding studies that only interviewed healthcare providers or family members of IPHAs and studies that focused on HIV/AIDS prevention in Indigenous communities. This allowed us to focus more closely on the lived experiences of IPHAs, centering their own articulations of health. After applying these screening questions, we reduced the final sample to 14 abstracts. We then retrieved the full text of these articles for review.

Next, we synthesized findings from the included articles to develop overarching themes. We created a table that indexed exemplar quotes of each study relative to participants' experiences and overall goals of the studies (e.g., first-order constructs) as well as interpretations of each study as articulated in the original manuscripts (e.g., second-order constructs) (Rutter et al., 2010). We then grouped together recurring themes across all first- and second-level constructs and notated relationships among the constructs. Finally, we practiced constant comparison (Lindlof & Taylor, 2019) and used analytic memos to generate initial categories and preliminary third-order constructs. This iterative process of allowed us to organize literature based on observed relationships, resulting in themes that were both grounded in the included literature and representative of the larger whole. Ultimatetly, we generated three broad themes related to the material and discursive health experiences of IPHAs – *structural and symbolic violence*; *(silently) making sense of HIV/AIDS and identity*; and *resilience, agency, and resistance.*

Results

Structural and Symbolic Violence

Many of the IPHA participants' articulations of health and HIV/AIDS were in connection to discriminatory attitudes associated with HIV stigma, racism, and homophobia. Participants commented on the multilayered stigma they endured as Indigenous, HIV-positive individuals based on their race, sexuality, intravenous drug use, and/or involvement in sex work (Mill et al., 2009).

One Aboriginal participant referred to living with HIV as "the stigma within the stigma" and recalled being labeled as "another drunken Indian … a faggot drunken Indian" (Mill et al., 2010, p. 1473). Other participants were also aware of the racial stereotypes about addiction and alcoholism of Indigenous Peoples. A participant detailed the following to Barlow and colleagues (2008) about perceptions of Indigeneity and racism in healthcare settings:

> I've been to clinics when I've had an injury, whether it was due to drinking or not even drinking, that I think I felt a prejudice where they just kind of came in and took a glance, and "Oh, yeah, you did something stupid when you were drunk. And it doesn't really matter because you're just an Indian, and you're probably going to just go get drunk and do it again."
>
> (p. 167)

In addition to the salience of racist stereotypes, a two-spirit participant in Argüello and Waters's (2018) study commented on the compounding oppressive forces of being queer and Indigenous: "[I]t's like … society's telling us that … 'we don't belong in the world'" (p. 115). Relatedly, an Aboriginal woman expressed how intersecting factors affect and complicate her HIV/AIDS stigma:

> Um, I get calls, um, people call me a "squaw [a racist and misogynistic slur historically used for Indigenous North American women] who has AIDS" and, you know, you probably deserve it because squaws deserved dying, you know, "Since we can't kill you off, you might as well die off by AIDS."
>
> (McCall et al., 2009, p. 1773)

In another case, an Indigenous woman in Ontario shared a story to Greene and colleagues (2015) of her and her partner getting tested for HIV:

> I told him [partner] … when he went to go get tested, that it's higher in Native women to have HIV and that he's best off just to leave me and to stay away from me … you know what my nurse said? … My nurse tells me that it's higher in black men from the islands and that I should stay away from them … when he asked them for condoms they wouldn't give him free condoms, they told him to go buy a box if he wanted to stay with me.
>
> (p. 12)

The marginalizing impact of racism, sexism, and homophobia significantly influenced Indigenous Peoples' experiences of health and descriptions of HIV/AIDS, resulting in IPHAs feeling alienated and without adequate healthcare.

Structural and symbolic violence toward IPHAs also manifested in a lack of accessible and supportive health resources. While there are similar rates of HIV/AIDS among Indigenous People living in both urban and rural settings (Negin et al., 2015), limited access and travel required to seek health services – especially specialized health services – was exacerbated for participants living in remote areas, including Indigenous reservations (McCall et al., 2009; McKay-McNabb, 2006; Woodgate et al., 2017a). When participants did find culturally grounded health and support services, they described these spaces as like "home" and a "second family" that alleviated feelings of exclusion and isolation (Barlow et al., 2008). Moreover, difficulties with healthcare dovetails with stigma, which, for many participants, engendered a fear of rejection or discrimination when seeking healthcare services (Hatala et al., 2018; McCall et al., 2009; McKeown et al., 2004; Woodgate et al., 2017a, 2017b). In a focus group interview with Đào and colleagues (2019), participants reflect on the mistreatment by healthcare professionals as barriers to care: "I had to use the health center only one time, I was treated badly and never went back again" (p. 39). In the same study, participants commented on their mistrust of healthcare providers, lack of education on HIV/AIDS, and limited communication with children about safe-sex practices on the behalf of participants (Đào et al., 2019). Similarly, Indigenous women in Woodgate and colleagues' (2017a, 2017b) studies discuss how the child welfare system conflated the stigma of their HIV status with being unfit mothers; children are taken into care at birth solely because the women were HIV positive, even when they abstain from illicit substances, seek treatment, and receive prenatal care.

The limited access to health resources and knowledge related to HIV/AIDS prevented many IPHAs from obtaining basic resources for their health – a barrier IPHAs already face as minorities (Greene et al., 2015; Hatala et al., 2018; McKay-McNabb, 2006). For example, women participants in Đào and colleagues' (2019) study reported that they only received information on HIV/AIDS if they were pregnant. Lack of knowledge about HIV/AIDS contributed to underutilization of existing healthcare services and an overall struggle to maintain IPHAs' well-being (McCall et al., 2009). The multiple, intersecting conditions with which many IPHAs live create a unique set of challenges for IPHAs prioritizing and addressing their health needs, particularly for HIV.

HIV was just one of several problems for IPHAs in studies we analyzed. Sociocultural and economic concerns about food security, safe housing, child and family care, and maintaining other comorbidities such as addiction often took precedence over HIV treatment (Cain et al., 2013; McCall et al., 2009; McKeown et al., 2004; Nowgesic et al., 2015). As one participant explained to McCall and colleagues (2009): "It's hard to get there [the clinic] when I'm on a [crack] run" (p. 1774). In a similar vein, a participant expressed to Cain and colleagues (2013) that she was more concerned with her "alcohol abuse, trying to sober … up and learning about [her] addictions" (p. 819) than she was about her HIV. Another participant explained the concurrent effect of HIV, depression, and substance misuse:

> I think what it is, is that I really didn't feel so good about myself and I just didn't care …. Because looking back, you say, okay, crystal meth [methamphetamine] and the raw sex and the HIV, it was like a slow kind of suicide for me. I just wanted to get it over with. This is one way of doing it … and it's all because of depression.
>
> (Cain et al., 2013, p. 820)

This participant narrative illustrates the deep connections among stigma, health, and identity. The second theme we developed relates to how participants made sense of these complications in terms of their HIV/AIDS and identity.

(Silently) Making Sense of HIV/AIDS and Identity

The simultaneously reinforcing stigma and silence that surrounds HIV/AIDS among Indigenous Peoples significantly influenced participants' sensemaking of HIV/AIDS and identity. Noted by Argüello and Waters (2018), the lack of attention, education, and health resources dedicated to HIV/AIDS contributes to silence HIV and HIV resources within Indigenous life. Indeed, HIV/AIDS has been suggested to be a "silent killer" among Indigenous communities (Vernon, 2001). Participants mentioned issues of anonymity when seeking health services and support groups based on the fear that community members would find out about their health status (Argüello & Waters, 2018; Cain et al., 2013; Hatala et al., 2018; McCall et al., 2009; Mill et al., 2009, 2010; Woodgate et al., 2017a, 2017b). Participants attribute their fear of judgment and ostracization from friends, family members, and community members to the compounding stigma of HIV and homophobic stereotypes that assume HIV to be synonymous with being gay (Argüello & Waters, 2018; Hatala et al., 2018; Mill et al., 2009, 2010). For example, a participant in Mill and colleagues' (2010) study recalled the following incident:

> I have Kaposi's [sarcoma] on my left foot, on my large toe and … it looks like a big, black bruise—and so she [nurse] asked me what it was, and I explained it to her, and she said, "Why are your toenails painted?" And I looked at her and I said, "Well, they're not. That's part of the illness." And she said, "What?" And I explained to her … I kept my voice down, and I said, "Well, I'm HIV positive," and she walked out to another nurse and she said, "Why didn't you tell me there's a fag in there that has AIDS?"
>
> (p. 1474)

As mentioned in the above section on structural and symbolic violence, HIV is often conceptualized as a "gay disease" that deemphasizes the complexities of race, ethnicity, class, gender, sexuality, and ability in HIV treatment, resulting in negative experiences for IPHAs.

Internalized stigma resulted in participants expressing fears of being perceived as "dirty," "disgusting," or being told to "get away" or "don't touch me" (Hatala et al., 2018, p. 1103). A participant discussed with Hatala and colleagues (2018) her decisions for social withdrawal: "I avoid going out in public. I don't like to be seen sick when out not being well" (p. 1104). Because participants feel unable to discuss their health with friends and family, IPHAs lack the social support necessary to have open relationships with regard to their health and well-being as well as feeling reluctant to disclose to others (Cain et al., 2013; Hatala et al., 2018; McCall et al., 2009; Mill et al., 2010; Nowgesic et al., 2015; Woodgate et al., 2017b). While many participants in Cain and colleagues' (2013) study had supportive family, friends, and communities, most frequently participants told stories of being barred from talking and interacting with people they loved: "I've met my half-brothers and -sisters, and none of them wanted anything to do with me ... ever since they found out I was HIV, anyway" (p. 820). Feelings of shame and hopelessness perpetuated silence and nondisclosure about HIV (Argüello & Waters, 2018; Cain et al., 2013; Hatala et al., 2018; Mill et al., 2009, 2010; Woodgate et al., 2017b). A participant in Woodgate and colleagues (2017b) study shared that she refused antiretroviral therapy while imprisoned because of her anxieties around disclosing her HIV status to her peers:

> I didn't want to take meds because I figured somebody's going to know that I'm HIV... because I was in jail too and then the medicine cart .... I just, I was scared, and I didn't want to take the medication because of that reason. (p. 20)

The lack of discretion of the jail medicine cart is not unlike the highly public waiting areas of other local healthcare facilities for IPHAs (Đào et al., 2019). Importantly, the notion of HIV/AIDS as both a ubiquitous and silenced phenomenon troubles participants' sensemaking practices. Even if HIV is silenced, its affective and material presence is embodied and implied. These stigmatizing practices makes participants conceal health conditions from other people (Argüello & Waters, 2018; Cain et al., 2013; Greene et al., 2015; McCall et al., 2009; Mill et al., 2009, 2010; Woodgate et al., 2017a, 2017b).

In studies we analyzed, it was common for IPHAs to articulate HIV as taking center stage for their identity. As described by a participant in Argüello and Waters's (2018) study, HIV is akin to a given identity rather than a social and medical problem: "But I think ... asking how important for you to find out [your status]—because some people don't want to know if they're HIV positive. They don't want to ... get tested because they don't want to face the truth" (p. 112). HIV functions as a "truth" from which to hide and not confront. When reacting to an HIV diagnosis, participants described to Cain and colleagues (2013) that the diagnosis resulted in them "shut[ting] down" and getting "tunnel vision," with one participant sharing the following example after learning about her HIV status when she was pregnant: "I just kept crying and I couldn't talk .... I cried all the way home [from the doctor's office]. Got home, my mom, she ... said, 'What's the matter?' And I just burst out ... 'I'm going to die.'" (p. 818). Similarly, a participant detailed the following about how the HIV diagnosis impacted how others perceived her and how this affected her own identity: "I had no clue what was good about me anymore. It's like if you, you say you love me, but yet I know everything you hate about me. What is there to love? I don't even love myself anymore" (Woodgate et al., 2017b, p. 20). Participants also reflected on the ways in which their HIV/AIDS experiences channeled resilience, agency, and community advocacy.

Resilience, Agency, and Advocacy

Despite the myriad challenges faced by Indigenous Peoples living with HIV and/or AIDS, several participants described senses of resilience, strength, and determination when facing the future. Kinship and community are core cultural values among Indigenous Peoples, and it is unsurprising that many participants attributed their ability to withstand the difficult conditions of HIV/AIDS to their collective communities. Indigenous mothers in McCall and colleagues' (2009) study spoke to this sentiment, commenting that in their children they find a reason to stay alive and focus on their well-being. Social support was also identified as crucial to the health of Indigenous Peoples – a participant noted to Hatala and colleagues (2018) that she was able to find solace by disclosing her HIV status to family and no longer "living a lie." She continued:

> So my whole family knows that I'm HIV. I disclosed to them. And they're actually very supportive. They didn't ostracize me and push me away. And they're not scared of me—not scared to touch me or hug me. Like we don't discuss it openly all the time. I've shared my info, it's out there. If I need them, I'll ask them [family].
>
> (p. 1105)

Similarly, a participant talked with Greene and colleagues (2015) about the ways that peer support impacts feelings of community engagement and connection:

> It's by that engagement and that involvement with other people ... they teach you so much .... that's been the best thing, was having that connection to peers and people that actually were the front liners rolling out with HIV and pregnancy stuff. Like if I didn't have that connection, I don't know if I would have been that confident going through my pregnancy at all.
>
> (p. 23)

Spirituality and ancestral connections were also a significant factor for maintaining resilience, as told by a mixed heritage Métis participant: "I just made sure I took care of me, my medicine world, my spiritual, my mental, my emotional .... It's important ... both sides of my heritage" (McCall et al., 2009, p. 1775). Recalling the prominence of IPHAs feeling shunned, shamed, and ostracized for their HIV, community, spirituality, and social support networks become a critical nexus for sustaining health among Indigenous Peoples (Argüello & Waters, 2018; Barlow et al., 2008; Hatala et al., 2018; McCall et al., 2009; Woodgate et al., 2017a).

Several participants engaged in agentic behaviors, such as resisting categorization and subverting HIV labeling as strategies to mitigate the stigmatization and social control they experienced as IPHAs. For example, a participant in Mill and colleagues' (2010) study described how he minimized discrimination from healthcare workers by altering his appearance and dressing more "presentable .... than somebody who has, you know, come from the street" (p. 1476). In other instances, participants decided to disclose other comorbidities instead of their HIV to manage their HIV stigma, often in collusion with healthcare professionals. A participant in Mill and colleagues' (2010) study shared that, on the advice of a healthcare provider, they sometimes disclose their hepatitis C diagnosis, to alleviate discrimination because of their HIV diagnosis. The participant explained:

> He [the doctor] told me if I ever go to the hospital or anything else just tell them I have hepatitis C, do not tell them I have HIV. But then when I tell them I have HIV they completely turn; they're not the same kind of people. They don't even want to touch you.
>
> (p. 1476)

At the same time, disclosing one's HIV status can also be a way of reclaiming power. A participant in Woodgate and colleagues' (2017b) study said: "Yeah, I told everybody because I didn't want people to have information and use it against me so I just put it out there" (p. 21). The strategy of HIV/AIDS is to perpetuate silence and stigma, but in this instance, the tactic for managing stigma is being straightforward about one's HIV status. Further, because of the lack of integrative and comprehensive healthcare for HIV/AIDS and related issues among Indigenous Peoples, several participants chose to engage in survival behaviors such as sex work and nurturing comorbidities, such as addiction, to maintain equilibrium and manage HIV in addition to other demands of childcare, food and housing security, and transportation costs (Cain et al., 2013; McCall et al., 2009).

Although most IPHAs are reluctant to involve themselves in HIV/AIDS community activism due to fears related to disclosing their HIV status (McCall et al., 2009), adopting advocate roles was a particularly salient theme across studies we analyzed. For example, participants in Hatala and colleagues' (2018) study discuss being and becoming a "helper":

> I learned that just because I'm sick [with HIV], doesn't mean my life's over. I can still live a full functioning life. You can walk around out there and help one person, then it makes you feel better. I know that an important part of my life is to start to learn to give and be a model for others, hey. To do—not to be done to, not to be given, but to give.
>
> (p. 1106)

For other IPHAs, sharing their and experiences with HIV facilitated them accepting their diagnosis, normalizing HIV, and building community with other Indigenous Peoples, especially those who are also HIV positive (Argüello & Walters, 2018; Hatala et al., 2018; McCall et al., 2009; McKay-McNabb, 2006). Participant accounts suggest that IPHAs' survival, resistance, and meaning-making in the face of stigma and oppression are deeply relational endeavors.

It is through their connections and interactions with others – including family, friends, and other IPHAs – that participants foster self-worth and purpose (Argüello & Walters, 2018; Greene et al., 2015; Hatala et al., 2018; McCall et al., 2009). Through significant relationships, IPHAs are able to transform from the "spoiled" self (Goffman, 1963) – constructed by mainstream discourse that stigmatizes HIV/AIDS – into the "helper" or moralized self. For some IPHAs, becoming a helper means, "sharing their story and journey with others to potentially help them along their own illness journeys" (Hatala et al., 2018, p. 1106). In oral societies, storying is a tradition of uplifting and nourishing sacred kinship and community, which is particularly important for IPHAs who experience various health perils.

Discussion

Our meta-synthesis of 14 qualitative, peer-reviewed research reports reveals that the experiences of IPHAs in the Americas are structured and constrained by systemic factors of colonized perceptions of health, sociocultural practices, and the (lack of) access to health resources. Participants described the silence surrounding HIV/AIDS among Indigenous Peoples, difficulties with health disclosure and social connection, multilayered discrimination, limited access to health services, and dehumanizing healthcare, resulting in participants feeling "dirty" and "disgusting." Participants' struggles with navigating HIV/AIDS are compounded by structural and cultural forces of marginalization and colonization, including stigma, isolation, and social inequity. Overall, health and HIV/AIDS resources for Indigenous individuals and communities are intimately anchored to deeper historical and structural roots of colonization, oppression, and trauma that impact and exacerbate Indigenous health in specific and contextually complex ways. Indigenous healing is embedded in Indigenous knowledges, spiritualities, and ecologies that are unintelligible to the dominant framework of Western health modalities, which engenders a poverty of both Indigenous health and spirit. Our discussion focuses on three main points: one, disentangling health apart from individualized Western perspectives of health that are incomprehensible to Indigenous health ecologies; two, grounding "post-AIDS" as a mechanism of the colonial project; and three; providing practical suggestions to better understand and address Indigenous health and healing.

Western notions of health are located within capitalistic neoliberal assumptions about health, illness, and recovery, which attribute health behavior to individual lifestyle choices without considering the roles of social structures in the manifestation of health and disease (Zoller, 2005). From our analysis it is clear that the dominant, biomedical model of healthcare for addressing HIV/AIDS among Indigenous Peoples is flawed and dismisses the embodied relationalities of health resulting from a long history of colonized erasures of Indigenous ontologies and epistemologies. In other words, dominant health frameworks cannot capture Indigenous knowledges of healing, relationalities, and embodiments because they are beyond Western taxonomies of health and individualism.

Our synthesis of previous research is consistent with Farmer's (2003) notion of structural violence, that is, the systematic ways in which the embedded social, cultural, and political organization of our social worlds make populations more vulnerable to illness and death by depriving them of their basic needs. Although all peoples living at the margins experience inequities, the severe violence, suffering, and marginalization experienced by Indigenous Peoples deserves particular attention.

Indigenous health disparities are embedded in continued colonial assemblages that superimpose Western rationalities onto Indigenous traditions of health and healing that accumulatively negate Indigenous well-being, values, and customs (Paradies, 2016). The violent synthesis of objective Western health modalities into Indigenous cultural healing involves modernizing and reconfiguring Indigenous traditions to classify Indigenous ways of knowing into Western epistemological and ontological catalogs that deny and disregard Indigenous traditions. Structural violence functions alongside colonialism and the "logic of elimination," which seeks the erasure of Indigenous Peoples to facilitate their replacement by white settlers and settler logics (Wolfe, 1999). Western (medical) biopower underpins the chronic and pervasive colonial impetus to displace, regulate, and undermine societies through an epistemological invasion that forces subjugated peoples and communities under colonial domination to assimilate to the values and belief systems of the colonizers (Hokowhitu, 2016). The seeming finality of Indigenous disappearance and settler replacement includes the replacement of traditional social and cultural practices of medicine and healing, such as healing circles, curing ceremonies, and mind–body–spirit connectivity, with mainstream models of healthcare that prioritize individual behavioral modifications. These models cannot comprehensively address the cultural context of health among Indigenous Peoples and, thus, constrain Indigenous agency insofar as health is scripted by the culturally incongruent structures that surround their lives.

To better understand IPHA experience and improve health outcomes for colonized subjugated populations, then, we must first recognize "post-AIDS" as a colonial capitalist logos to address the colonial implications of their HIV/AIDS status and health risks. Grounding "post-AIDS" steeped in colonial logics is critically important for addressing health and health structures through which Indigenous People live their lives. What is presented as a seemingly altruistic goal of "ending AIDS" via Western biomedical intervention, "post-AIDS" discourses permeate the historical and ongoing colonial project that have resulted in generations of subordination and elimination of Indigenous Peoples who face a multilayered reality of discrimination and disadvantage on macro, meso, and micro levels as demonstrated in our analysis. The notion of "post-AIDS" promotes colonial ideals that carve deep cognitive and cultural erasures of health and healing while simultaneously superimposing modalities of health that reduce health to an isolated biomedical issue. Though the biomedical model of health can aid individuals to overcome disease entirely through health treatment, "post-AIDS" discourses erase the complex realities of IPHAs for whom disease burden is amplified by colonialism. This erasure itself is a form of structural violence, for it fails to take into account the various social, cultural, and economic factors and consequences of health and illness. In a "post-AIDS" world, it is paramount to acknowledge the multiple co-occurring diseases that organize the social, cultural, and economic experience of health among colonized and subjugated populations in order to reduce HIV risk and improve health for IPHAs.

Current IPHA literature does not account for how "post-AIDS" as a contemporary colonial logic further suppresses Indigenous health potentialities. "Post-AIDS" weaponizes Western biomedical technologies – technologies that are antithetical to Indigenous practices – to perpetuate the myth that we are "beyond AIDS" (Gilbert & Walker, 2009; Whiteside & Strauss, 2014). "Post-AIDS" serves as yet another colonizing erasure of the complexities of health among Indigenous People. Instead of treating the various health-related challenges that Indigenous People experience, "post-AIDS" discourse utilizes techniques of biopower that exact on Indigenous Populations to discipline them to conform to a colonial society in which Indigenous individuals and communities are subject to colonized notions of health, gender, sexuality, and ways of living (Morgensen, 2011). For example, although poverty, substance misuse, shame, and loneliness are all contributing factors to HIV/AIDS, participants largely articulate these issues as an extension of HIV/AIDS rather than a contributing factor to HIV/AIDS. IPHAs are limited in health resources to remedy these problems and, thus, must become their own health advocates for resistance and survival. The ideological work of these discourses function to normalize a process of modernization that further disconnects Indigenous Populations from their traditional health and healing praxes.

The array of destructive and productive practices of health, including poverty, insecure housing, substance misuse, and trauma among Indigenous Peoples, forces IPHAs into particularly precarious positions and warrants an exigent understanding of contemporary Indigenous health. We suggest research addressing health among Indigenous People should take seriously the synergistic interaction of multiple adverse conditions that complicate health experiences among Indigenous Peoples. Syndemics theory is a valuable approach for understanding health as a holistic and interdependent entity. Syndemics, or the "aggregation of two or more diseases … that exacerbates the negative health effects of any or all of the diseases" (Singer et al., 2017, p. 941). In line with Jolivette's (2016) radical love framework, which offers a comprehensive model of healing that accounts for the cultural, economic, and spiritual traumas enveloping Indigenous life-worlds, a syndemic-informed approach to health defies colonial logics that assume health to be individual and disintegrated from social, economic, and cultural factors. Lastly, we suggest health practitioners and researchers create democratized spaces that acknowledge, honor, and listen to the voices and concerns of Indigenous Peoples to co-construct culturally relevant health interventions. Health reform alone will not suffice, which means radically transforming the organizational procedures of health services and delivery to heed Indigenous traditions and knowledges. While we cannot demolish colonial structures, current health practices for Indigenous Peoples are subpar at best. These practical steps of synergistic radical love and a colonial reckoning of "post-AIDS" are critical for interweaving Indigenous embodied knowledges of spiritual, relational, and ecological traditions to transform Indigenous health and healing in a "post-AIDS" era.

References

Anderson, I., Robson, B., Connolly, M., Al-Yaman, F., Bjertness, E., King, A., ... & Pesantes, M. A. (2016). Indigenous and tribal peoples' health (*The Lancet*-Lowitja Institute Global Collaboration): A population study. *Lancet*, *388*, 131–157. https://doi.org/10.1016/S0140-6736(16)00345-7

Argüello, T. M., & Walters, K. (2018). They tell us "we don't belong in the world and we shouldn't take up a place": HIV discourse within two-spirit communities. *Journal of Ethnic & Cultural Diversity in Social Work*, *27*, 107–123. https://doi.org/10.1080/15313204.2017.1362616

Atkins, S., Lewin, S., Smith, H., Engel, M., Fretheim, A., & Volmink, J. (2008). Conducting a meta-ethnography of qualitative literature: Lessons learnt. *BMC Medical Research Methodology*, *8*, 1–10. https://doi.org/10.1186/1471-2288-8-21

Auerbach, J. D., Parkhurtss, J., & Caceres, C. (2011). Addressing the social drivers of HIV/AIDS for the long-term response: Conceptual and methodological considerations. *Global Public Health*, *6*(Suppl 3), S239–S309. https://doi.org/10.1080/17441692.2011.594451

Barlow, K., Loppie, C., Jackson, R., Akan, M., MacLean, L., & Reimer, G. (2008). Culturally competent service provision issues experienced by aboriginal people living with HIV/AIDS. *Pimatisiwin*, *6*, 155–180.

Bosma, H., Apland, L., & Kazanjian, A. (2010). Review: Cultural conceptualizations of hospice palliative care: More similarities than differences. *Palliative Medicine*, *24*, 510–522. https://doi.org/10.1177/0269216309351380

Brave Heart, M. Y. H., & DeBruyn, L. M. (1998). The American Indian holocaust: Healing historical unresolved grief. *American Indian and Alaska Native Mental Health Research*, *8*, 60–82. https://doi.org/10.5820/aian.0802.1998.60

Cain, R., Jackson, R., Prentice, T., Collins, E., Mill, J., & Barlow, K. (2013). The experience of HIV diagnosis among Aboriginal people living with HIV/AIDS and depression. *Qualitative Health Research*, *23*, 815–824. https://doi.org/10.1177/1049732313482525

Campbell, R., Pound, P., Pope, C., Britten, N., Pill, R., Morgan, M., & Donovan, J. (2003). Evaluating meta-ethnography: A synthesis of qualitative research on lay experiences of diabetes and diabetes care. *Social Science & Medicine*, *56*, 671–684. https://doi.org/10.1016/s0277-9536(02)00064-3

Czyzewski, K. (2011). Colonialism as a broader social determinant of health. *International Indigenous Policy Journal*, *2*, 1–14. https://doi.org/10.18584/iipj.2011.2.1.5

Đào, L. U., Terán, E., Bejarano, S., Hernandez, I., Reina Ortiz, M., Chee, V., Flores, M., Izurieta, R., Baldwin, J., & Martinez Tyson, D. (2019). Risk and resiliency: The syndemic nature of HIV/AIDS in the indigenous highland communities of Ecuador. *Public Health*, *176*, 36–42. https://doi.org/10.1016/j.puhe.2019.02.021

Evans-Campbell, T. (2008). Historical trauma in American Indian/Native Alaska communities: A multilevel framework for exploring impacts on individuals, families, and communities. *Journal of Interpersonal Violence*, *23*, 316–338. https://doi.org/10.1177/0886260507312290

Farmer, P. (2003). *Pathologies of power: Health, human rights, and the new war on the poor.* Berkeley: University of California Press.

Finfgeld, D. L. (2003). Meta-synthesis: The state of the art – so far. *Qualitative Health Research, 7,* 893–904. https://doi.org/10.1177/1049732303253462

Gilbert, L., & Walker, L. (2009). "They (ARVs) are my life, without them I'm nothing"—experiences of patients attending a HIV/AIDS clinic in Johannesburg, South Africa. *Health & Place, 15,* 1123–1129. https://doi.org/10.1016/j.healthplace.2009.06.006

Glenn, E. N. (2015). Settler colonialism as structure: A framework for comparative studies of U.S. race and gender formation. *Sociology of Race and Ethnicity, 1,* 54–74. https://doi.org/10.1177/2332649214560440

Goffman, E. (1963). *Stigma: Notes on the management of spoiled identity.* New York: Penguin Books.

Greene, S., Ion, A., Nicholson, V. J., Beaver, K., Derry, R., & Loutfy, M. (2015). "Who is there to support our women?" Positive Aboriginal women (PAW) speak out about health and social experience and needs during pregnancy, birth and motherhood. *Canadian Journal of Aboriginal Community-Based HIV/AIDS Research, 7,* 1–32.

Grypdonck, M. (2006). Qualitative health research in the era of evidence-based practice. *Qualitative Health Research, 16,* 1371–1385. https://doi.org/10.1177/1049732306294089

Hatala, A. R., Bird-Naytowhow, K., Pearl, T., Peterson, J., del Canto, S., Rooke, E.,… Tait, P. (2018). Being and becoming a helper: Illness disclosure and identity transformations among indigenous people living with HIV or AIDS in Saskatoon, Saskatchewan. *Qualitative Health Research, 28,* 1099–1111. https://doi.org/10.1177/1049732318764394

Hokowhitu, B. (2016). Monster: Post-Indigenous studies. In A. Moreton-Robinson (Ed.), *Critical Indigenous studies: Engagements in first world locations.* (pp. 83–101). Tuscon, AZ: The University of Arizona Press.

Johnston, D., Dean, K., & Rizzo, M. (2015). The political economy of HIV. *Review of African Political Economy, 42,* 335–341. https://doi.org/10.1080/03056244.2015.1065603

Jolivette, A. J. (2016). *Indian blood: HIV and colonial trauma in San Francisco's two-spirit community.* Seattle: University of Washington Press.

Jones, D. S. (2006). The persistence of American Indian health disparities. *American Journal of Public Health, 96,* 2122–2134. https://doi.org/10.2105/AJPH.2004.054262

King, M., Smith, A., & Gracey, M. (2009). Indigenous health part 2: The underlying causes of the health gap. *Lancet, 374,* 76–85. https://doi.org/10.1016/S0140-6736(09)60827-8

Lindlof, T. R., & Taylor, B. C. (2019). *Qualitative communication research methods* (4th ed.). Thousand Oaks, CA: SAGE.

Mazanderani, F., & Paparini, S. (2015). The stories we tell: Qualitative research interviews, talking technologies and the 'normalisation' of life with HIV. *Social Science & Medicine, 131,* 66–73.

McCall, J., Browne, A. J., & Reimer-Kirkham, S. (2009). Struggling to survive: The difficult reality of Aboriginal women living with HIV/AIDS. *Qualitative Health Research, 19,* 1769–1782. https://doi.org/10.1177/1049732309353907

McKay-Mcnabb, K. (2006). Life experiences of Aboriginal women living with HIV/AIDS. *Canadian Journal of Aboriginal Community-Based HIV/AIDS Research, 1,* 5–19.

McKeown, I., Reid, S., & Orr, P. (2004). Experiences of sexual violence and relocation in the lives of HIV infected Canadian women. *International Journal of Circumpolar Health, 63,* 399–404. https://doi.org/10.3402/ijch.v63i0.17944

Mill, J., Edwards, N., Jackson, R., Austin, W., MacLean, L., & Reintjes, F. (2009). Accessing health services while living with HIV: Intersections of stigma. *Canadian Journal of Nursing Research*, *41*, 168–185.

Mill, J. E., Edwards, N., Jackson, R. C., MacLean, L., & Chaw-Kant, J. (2010). Stigmatization as social control mechanism for persons living with HIV and AIDS. *Qualitative Health Research*, *20*, 1469–1483. https://doi.org/10.1177/1049732310375436

Morgensen, S. L. (2011). *Spaces between us: Queer settler colonialism and Indigenous decolonization*. Minneapolis: University of Minnesota Press.

Negin, J., Aspin, C., Gadsden, T., & Reading, C. (2015). HIV among Indigenous peoples: A review of the literature on HIV-related behaviour since the beginning of the epidemic. *AIDS and Behavior*, *19*, 1720–1734. https://doi.org/10.1007/s10461-015-1023-0

Noblit, G., & Hare, R. (1998). *Meta-ethnography: Synthesizing qualitative studies*. Newbury Park, CA: SAGE.

Nowgesic, E., Meili, R., Stack, S., & Myers, T. (2015). The Indigenous Red Ribbon Storytelling Study: What does it mean for Indigenous peoples living with HIV and a substance use disorder to access antiretroviral therapy in Saskatchewan? *Canadian Journal of Aboriginal Community-Based HIV/AIDS Research*, *7*, 27–40.

O'Brien, C. (2013). Performing POZ: Irish theatre, HIV stigma, and "post-AIDS" identities. *Irish University Review*, *43*(1), 74–85. https://doi.org/10.3366/iur.2013.0056

Paradies, Y. (2016). Colonisation, racism, and Indigenous health. *Journal of Population Research*, *33*, 83–96. https://doi.org/10.1007/s12546-016-9159-y

Persson, A. (2013). Non/infectious corporealities: Tensions in the biomedical era of "HIV normalization." *Sociology of Health and Illness*, *35*, 1065–1079. https://doi.org/10.1111/1467-9566.12023

Popay, J., Rogers, A., & Williams, G. (1998). Rationale and standards for the systematic review of qualitative literature in health services research. *Qualitative Health Research*, *8*, 341–351. https://doi.org/10.1177/104973239800800305

Román, D. (2007). Not-about-AIDS. In J. G. Reinett & J. R. Roach (Eds.), *Critical theory and performance* (pp. 372–394). Ann Arbor: University of Michigan Press.

Rutter, D., Francis, J., Coren, E., & Fisher, M. (2010). *SCIE Systematic research reviews: Guidelines* (2nd ed.). London: Social Care Institute for Excellence.

Singer, M., Bulled, N., Ostrach, B., & Mendenhall, E. (2017). Syndemics and the biosocial conception of health. *The Lancet*, *389*, 941–950. https://doi.org/10.1016/S0140-6736(17)30003-X

Smylie, J., & Firestone, M. (2015). Back to the basics: Identifying and addressing underlying challenges in achieving high quality and relevant health statistics for Indigenous populations in Canada. *Statistical Journal of the IAOS*, *31*, 67–87. https://doi.org/10.3233/SJI-150864

UNAIDS. (2006). *Permanent forum on Indigenous issues: Fifth session*. Retrieved from https://www.unaids.org/sites/default/files/media_asset/unaidsindigenousissuespaper_en_0.pdf

UNAIDS. (2010). *UNAIDS strategy 2011–2015 Getting to Zero*. Retrieved from https://files.unaids.org/en/media/unaids/contentassets/documents/unaidspublication/2010/JC2034_UNAIDS_Strategy_en.pdf

UNAIDS. (2016). *Global AIDS update*. Retrieved from https://www.who.int/hiv/pub/arv/global-AIDS-update-2016_en.pdf?ua=1

UNAIDS. (2019). *Global HIV & AIDS statistics — 2019 fact sheet*. Retrieved from https://www.unaids.org/en/resources/fact-sheet

United States Census Bureau. (2017). *2017 American community survey 1-year estimates.* Retrieved from https://factfinder.census.gov/faces/tableservices/jsf/pages/productview.xhtml?src=bkmk#

Vernon, I. S. (2001). *Killing us quietly: Native Americans and HIV/AIDS.* Lincoln: University of Nebraska Press.

Walker, L. (2017). Problematising the discourse of "post-AIDS." *Journal of Medical Humanities, 41*, 95–105. https://doi.org/10.1007/s10912-017-9433-9

Whiteside, A. (2015). The key question in the AIDS epidemic in 2015. *Review of African Political Economy, 42*(145), 455–466. https://doi.org/10.1080/03056244.2015.1064371

Whiteside, A., & Strauss, M. (2014). The end of AIDS: Possibility or pipe dream? A tale of translations. *African Journal of AIDS Research, 13*(2), 101–108. https://doi.org/10.2989/16085906.2014.927780

Wolfe, P. (1999). *Settler colonialism and the transformatiton of anthropology.* London: Continuum Publishing Group.

Woodgate, R. L., Zurba, M., Tennent, P., Cochrane, C., Payne, M., & Migone, J. (2017a). A qualitative study on the intersectional social determinants for indigenous people who become infected with HIV in their youth. *International Journal for Equity in Health, 16*(1), 1–12. https://doi.org/10.1186/s12939-017-0625-8

Woodgate, R. L., Zurba, M., Tennent, P., Cochrane, C., Payne, M., & Migone, J. (2017b). "People try and label me as someone I'm not:" The social ecology of Indigenous people living with HIV, stigma, and discrimination in Manitoba, Canada. *Social Science & Medicine, 194*, 17–24. https://doi.org/10.1016/j.socscimed.2017.10.002

World Health Organization. (2015). *Guideline on when to start antiretroviral therapy and on pre-exposure prophylaxis for HIV.* Retrieved from https://www.who.int/hiv/pub/guidelines/earlyrelease-arv/en/

World Health Organization. (2018). *Global Health Observatory (GHO) data.* Retrieved from https://www.who.int/gho/hiv/en/

Zoller, H. M. (2005). Health activism: Communication theory and action for social change. *Communication Theory, 15*(4), 341–364. https://doi.org/10.1111/j.1468-2885.2005.tb00339.x

6 Neoliberal Hegemony and National HIV/AIDS Policy in India

Somrita Ganchoudhuri and Mohan Jyoti Dutta

The acquired immunodeficiency syndrome (AIDS) caused by the human immunodeficiency virus (HIV) is considered as a disease of inequality, distributing risks of infection and access to care along the lines of global–national–local inequalities in the distribution of resources (Acharya & Dutta, 2012; Dutta, 2008; Farmer, 1999). Global public health response (Lupton, 1995; Sastry & Dutta, 2011) to HIV/AIDS is framed within the neoliberal logic of market promotion, with privatization and economic growth often projected as solutions to HIV/AIDS. The global knowledge economy of HIV/AIDS response forms an industry of NGOs, academics, and enterprises, funded by international financial institutions (IFIs) and private foundations (such as the Bill and Melinda Gates Foundation), shaping the discursive and material terrains around HIV/AIDS prevention, treatment, and management (Dutta, 2008; Sastry & Dutta, 2011). The ideological construction of "post-AIDS," punctuating a narrative register for the end of HIV/AIDS, forms the basis for the neoliberal re-organizing of health care. The rhetoric of ending AIDS mobilizes instruments of privatization, delivered through the "rolling back" of the state as an infrastructure for public health to "roll out" a reworked state in collaboration with private capital, communication agencies, civil society, and foundations. "Post-AIDS," in other words, serves as the discursive canvas for the transformation of health care, holding up the material interests of private actors profiting from the mechanisms of the market.

Several scholars argue that articulation of health stems from neoliberalism, which propagates individual entrepreneurial freedom as the way to gain maximum benefit through liberalization and privatization (Dutta, 2016; Sastry & Dutta, 2013). The ideology of HIV/AIDS prevention and response is shaped by transnational corporations, private foundations, the World Bank (WB), the United States Agency for International Development (USAID), and the International Monetary Fund (IMF), generating knowledge claims about effective forms of response to HIV/AIDS. This ideology constructs health as an individual behavior, placing it in the realm of private responsibility, and foregrounding technological advancements such as antiretroviral treatment for HIV/AIDS patients that can be secured through participation in the global free

DOI: 10.4324/9781003000945-8

market (Dutta, 2016; Sastry & Dutta, 2011, 2013). Globally, the discourse of HIV/AIDS response links the success story to public–private partnerships (Dutta & Acharya, 2015; Sastry & Dutta, 2011, 2013). This chapter attempts to deconstruct the dominant discourse of HIV/AIDS in state response, by attending to the discursive formations in the National AIDS Control Organization (NACO) policy documents, situating these documents in relationship to the "post-AIDS" ideology. It is important to understand that the dominant discourse of HIV/AIDS in India did not happen in isolation; it impacted and informed the dominant discourse of health in general. Moreover, the discourse of "post-AIDS," setting specific targets to be met, forms the basis of introducing the logics of market, privatization, efficiency, and technology into the organizing of health in general. Through the framework of HIV/AIDS, the state–corporate nexus reworks the public health structure to serve the privatized logics of the market. In this chapter, we discuss how neoliberal narratives were weaved into the dominant discourse of HIV/AIDS, and how this became the pretext of dismantling public health program and the role of the state. The individualized conceptualization of health in the context of HIV/AIDS dictated the meanings of health in totality and the stress on public–private partnerships for efficient health solutions served the agendas of privatization of health structures, leading to the minimization of the role of the state.

NACO and HIV/AIDS Discourse in India

NACO, the nodal agency for policy formulation for HIV/AIDS in India, monitors India's HIV/AIDS control programme through the HIV/AIDS Prevention and Control Societies, which assist in instrumentation of one National Plan at state levels across the country (NACO, 2016). Within India's bicameral legislative system, the national plan lays out the conceptual framework for state and local level implementations, as well as controls the direction of state and local level HIV programs through the allocation of economic resources. In this chapter, we examine the policy discourse of NACO, attending to the ways in which NACO constructs HIV/AIDS, the risks attached to it, and the state response to it. We argue that the NACO policy framework for India's HIV/AIDS response reflects neocolonial hegemony, the hegemony of the Global North on the Global South through the ideological power held by global foundations. Worth noting here is the work performed by the "post-AIDS" ideology in securing the hegemony for private foundations. The neocolonial/neoliberal tropes shed light on how the discourse of HIV/AIDS surrounding individual health behavior and change primarily drives attention from the importance of public health programs, thus assigning much of the responsibility to individuals who are at risk of HIV/AIDS and gradually becoming the pretext for dismantling the public health ideology and practices.

Between 2002 and 2012, the Bill and Melinda Gates Foundation invested over $350 million in India for the development of an HIV/AIDS response framework, funding the Avahan program and directly injecting money into

NACO, with the goal of propping up the fight to end HIV/AIDS in India. The investment of the foundation in India's HIV/AIDS framework was to implement, scale up, and demonstrate the proof-of-concept for a business framework to HIV/AIDS response. We situate our analysis of the NACO documents in the backdrop of this powerful role of the foundation in shaping the Indian state's HIV/AIDS response strategy, guided by the partisan ideology of the foundation in reworking India's HIV/AIDS response as a business strategy. The nation-state, through the framework of influence, is reworked into an instrument of hegemonic transnational capital, redirecting public health toward serving private interests of profiteering, delivered through individualized models of prevention and care. The overarching ideology of individual behavior change forms the zeitgeist of the neoliberal ideology, actively working to dismantle the role of the state in developing structural solutions (Dutta, 2016). The NACO policy document, as a reflection of the ideological formation that constitutes HIV/AIDS state response, anchors the materiality of HIV/AIDS related practices among civil society organizations, state bodies, and public health infrastructures. What becomes apparent in the context of India is the powerful role played by the Bill and Melinda Gates Foundation in reformulating the Indian public health system more broadly, and the HIV/AIDS response system specifically, in the neoliberal ideology.

Neoliberal Governmentality and Healthcare

The underlying theoretical argument of neoliberalism is that human development is best achieved through higher economic growth with free functioning of the market; liberation of individual entrepreneurial freedom enables maximum utilization and allocation of resources, therefore leading to overall development (Dutta, 2008; McGregor, 2001). However, postcolonial scholarship highlights that, through the tropes of neoliberalism, a symbolic and material exploitation of the Third World even in the absence of the European imperialist continues (Dutta, 2016; Loomba, 1998; Said, 1978; Sastry & Dutta, 2011; Spivak, 1998). In the context of health, the symbolic representation of the Third World as primitive validates the hegemony of the West; for instance, the lack of knowledge of the Third World is posed as a justification of public health intervention programmes of the West. What remains hidden in the construction of disease is poverty, the root of increasing vulnerability of the poor to HIV/AIDS in the Global South, deepened by structural adjustment programs (SAPs) of World Bank (Escobar, 1995; Farmer, 1992). The powerful ideology of neoliberalism projects the role of state as inefficient while highlighting the need for privatization and free market as most beneficial for the development of the state (McGregor, 2001). This presence of SAPs and absence of government policies to ensure the fair redistribution of a nation's wealth widen the gap between haves and have-nots, and healthcare gap being one of them (Farmer, 1992; McGregor, 2001).

Global health inequities are perpetuated with global health policies that do not attempt to understand the cultural and historical context of the sites in which they intervene (Basu & Dutta, 2009; Dutta, 2008; Farmer, 1992; Sastry & Dutta, 2011). Several studies suggest the pressing need for drawing attention to the contextual specificity of the sites of interventions by drawing attention to the socio-cultural context in which health behaviour occurs (Basu & Dutta, 2009; Dutta, 2008; Lupton, 1995). The dominant understanding of HIV/AIDS based on a Western understanding of the disease lacks the subjectivity of the native body quintessentially undermining their meanings and understanding of the disease shaped in their cultural context (de Souza, 2007; Farmer, 1992). The neoliberal notion of HIV/AIDS constructs the disease at an individual level; the individualistic tenet of neoliberalism glorifies the effectiveness of individual responsibility of being healthy, and this sidelines the importance of public good and community (Campos & Farmer, 2003; Sastry & Dutta, 2013), solidifying the existing notion of people with health problems as being irresponsible without questioning the structural barriers such as access to hospitals that increases their vulnerability to diseases (Farmer, 1992; McGregor, 2001).

Diseased bodies become sites of intervention and markets for pharmaceutical companies keeping "humanitarian reasons" and greater "self-protection" in mind while facilitating the neoliberal agenda of free enterprise and private property (Sastry & Dutta, 2011). The logic of neoliberalism embedded in the construction of disease continues to dominate globally as "common sense," eradicating the scope of any other alternative discourse (Sastry & Dutta, 2013).

NACO Policy and HIV/AIDS

NACO, the nodal agency for policy formulation for HIV/AIDS in India, monitors the HIV/AIDS control programme through HIV/AIDS Prevention and Control Societies, which assist in instrumentation of one National Plan at State level (NACO, 2019). NACO, launched in 1992 to implement India's first National AIDS Control Programme (NACP), is a division of the Ministry of Health and Family Welfare (NACO, 2019). NACO holds a position of utmost importance since all HIV/AIDS programmes in India follow NACO's guidelines. The State AIDS Control Society of NACO monitors the non-governmental organizations that implement the programme at the state level.

In 1986, after the first cases of HIV/AIDS in the country were diagnosed, the Indian National AIDS Council monitored the HIV/AIDS programme along with support from local NGOs. In 1992, NACP was launched, with the end of Cold War and the advent of economic liberalization in India. NACO was formed as a "semi-autonomous temporary project management organization" to formulate a nationwide programme with US$84 million worth international development assistance credit from World Bank (Nambiar, 2012, p. 719). During this era of economic liberalization, the New Economic Policy of 1991 was adopted, and SAPs of the World Bank and the International Monetary Fund were implemented by opening domestic markets to the globalized economy, as India was facing severe fiscal and trade imbalances and huge inflation (Nambiar, 2012; Upadhyay, 2000). Under the purview of this policy, widespread disinvestment in health sector was initiated, along with an upsurge in foreign investment and privatization of industries like telecommunications and power generation (Nambiar, 2012; World Bank, 1999). This led to the NGO-isation of India (Roy, 2004) with accelerated growth of NGO-led projects of health development, funded by international donors (Nambiar, 2012).

Scholars argue that the neoliberal capitalist policies of SAPs to liberalize the Indian economy have increased poverty, inequality, and have led to poor(er) economic opportunities in the Global South (Upadhyay, 2000). The neoliberal policies of globalization, which result in the inequitable distribution of resources, is linked to the inequitable impact of HIV/AIDS on different segments of the population (Acharya & Dutta, 2012). The communities at risk of HIV/AIDS in India, as marked by NACO, are female sex workers (FSWs), men who have sex with men (MSM), injecting drug users (IDUs), and bridge populations (truckers and migrants).

Until now, NACP has been implemented in five phases, and each comprises of various objectives and missions. For example, NACP II (1999–2006) focused on Targeted Interventions on High Risk Groups (HRGs) viz. FSWs, MSM, IDUs, and bridge populations, while also decentralizing its implementation to the district level (NACO, 2016). NACP III (2206–2011) aimed at the general population – mostly youth, who are often referred to as the "workforce." The stress on "workforce" is important, as HIV/AIDS is often portrayed as a threat to global production because disease is viewed as a threat to the productive force (Farmer, 1999). Thus, the emergent need for dealing with HIV/AIDS is positioned within the paradigm of global production.

Impact of Neoliberal Policies on HIV/AIDS Campaigns

The neoliberal organizing of health is embedded in most of the solutions offered in the HIV/AIDS programmes, which are at an individual level and attempt to bring change in individual beliefs and attitude (Basu & Dutta, 2007; Dutta, 2007). What remains absent with dominant articulations of health as private and individual responsibility is the structural violence carried out by SAPs, imposed by IFIs such as the World Bank, which has led to deepening poverty and health disparities in the Global South (Basu & Dutta, 2007, 2009). The implementation of SAPs in low- and middle-income countries resulted in the privatization of various state-owned assets, free market, and foreign direct investment as per the conditions mandated by the World Bank. This also led to the weakening of investment in public healthcare programs and an increased role of NGOs in catering to the communities in the absence of public healthcare infrastructure (Pfeiffer & Chapman, 2010; Roy, 2004; Turshen, 1999;). Thus, the neoliberal articulation of HIV/AIDS as a private and individual responsibility ultimately serves the agendas of hegemonic structures.

NACO and its Discursive Articulations

NACO's annual reports provides a wide coverage of HIV/AIDS prevention programmes, care, support, and treatment, along with a detailed description of its success and future plans. They provide the most credible summary of state-driven responses to HIV/AIDS in India, along with a detailed overview of HIV/AIDS programmes. These reports, thus, serve as an entry point to make sense of the dominant discourse of HIV/AIDS in India.

We analyzed all of NACO's available annual reports from 2008–2009 to 2016–2017, paying particular attention to its preventive services and targeted interventions among HRGs. In the rest of this essay, we present our analysis. We highlight NACO's behavior change strategies, how NACO's discourse promotes condom use as business, the privatization of healthcare, and the co-optation of voices of the communities at risk.

Behavior Change

In case of HRGs, especially FSW, MSM, and the bridge population, behavior change and condom promotion are considered primary solutions. The depiction of decline in HIV prevalence among them is narrated as the result of successful interventions of campaigns on behavior change and condom promotion. Consider the following excerpt that explains the primary role played by campaigns designed for behavior change and condom promotion:

> Considerable decline in HIV prevalence has been recorded among Female Sex Workers at national level (5.06% in 2007 to 2.67% in 2011) and in most of the States where long standing targeted interventions have focused on behavior change and increasing condom use.
>
> (NACO, 2015, p. 404)

In this excerpt, we notice that the focused measures on behavioral change and condom promotion are highlighted as the reasons for the decline from 5.06% in 2007 to 2.67% in 2011. Here, the primary emphasis is on articulations such as individual behavior change, condom promotion, and improvement of technical efficiencies in the discursive space of HIV prevention.

What goes missing in the discourse are the structural inequities that, for example, FSWs are subjected to due to the nature of their job, which is considered clandestine (Basu, 2011). Several scholars suggest that the reason for HIV spread among this group is not a result of their unawareness and lack of knowledge of the spread of HIV/AIDS through unprotected sex (Basu & Dutta, 2011; Bowen et al., 2011). It is because of the lack of their power to negotiate with their clients who are not ready to use condoms (Basu, 2011; Carrasco et al., 2018). But the report does not highlight the structural inequities faced by FSWs; on the other hand, it showcases the increasing condom usage and behavior change among sex workers due to the successful interventions of NACO. This one-way flow of communication – from NACO to its stakeholders -- eliminates the possibility of dialogue with marginalized populations who are considered a part of HRGs, while putting an end to the possibility of listening to the voices of affected communities and discussing the problems they face. It essentially fails to create a space for discussing their everyday lived experiences that shapes their health. Therefore, possible stories of hunger, poverty, stigma, discrimination, physical and mental stress, alcohol consumption during sex, risk, and lack of family support remain subsumed by the celebratory discourse of condom-use-related individual behavior change.

Apart from HRGs – i.e., FSW, IDU, MSM, and transgender individuals/hijras – another group considered vulnerable to HIV is the bridge population that comprises long-distance truckers and migrant populations. As stated in NACO (2015) report, "These risk groups include long distance truckers and migrant workers and are commonly referred to as bridge populations owing to their perceived role in passing the HIV infection from the core groups to general population" (p. 405). This report explains the various targeted intervention projects for the bridge population along with the higher risk groups. Below is an excerpt:

> HIV testing and ART linkages among HRGs: NACO guidelines specify that all core HRGs should be tested for HIV once every six months …. Condom distribution among HRGs: As per NACP strategy, all sexual encounters of HRGs should be protected by consistent and correct usage of condoms.
>
> (p. 407)

The report stresses the compulsory and consistent usage of condoms during any sexual encounter of truckers but fails to question the deep-seated structural inequities that construct the trucker population's lived experiences. Here are excerpts that depict the discourse on the bridge population in the realm of HIV/AIDS:

> These populations, due to the nature of their work and mobility, are more likely to come in contact with HRGs and constitute a major proportion of the clients of sex workers …. In addition, long distance truckers also show high levels of vulnerability and thus form an important part of bridge population.
>
> (NACO, 2015, p. 405)

> [E]vidence indicates the possible role of bridge population including high-risk migrants and long-distance truckers in fuelling the HIV epidemic.
>
> (NACO, 2014, p. ix)

> Long-distance Truckers and Single Male Migrants constitute a significant proportion of clients of sex workers.
>
> (NACO, 2011b, p. 5)

These excerpts highlight the mobile nature of their job and how they contribute to the increasing vulnerability to HIV/AIDS among the general population by passing it on, but it essentially ignores the underlying reasons behind this mobile job. The mobility in their life exists because of the failure of structural configurations due to "liberalization, lack of belonging to a set social structure, a highly unorganized industry with no income or other safety nets, a transient livelihood and long absences from their families, communities, and social support systems" (Dutta & Acharya, 2015, p. 258). The dominant discourse of HIV/AIDS ignores the everyday struggles of the truckers/migrants, though it does narrate the role of migration behind the spread of HIV/AIDS among the migrant population such as truckers and their spouses. But it essentially ignores the underlying factors that contribute to the construction of their new identity – "the bridge population" – and only what remains discoursed is their role in spreading HIV/AIDS among the general population, and the need for behavior change among them. It ignores the deep-seated structural inequality that positions the lives of truckers at the margins and the conditions that are created at the margins. The lived experiences of truckers are constituted amid long work hours that impact their physical and mental health, longing for home, having long distances to cover, a lack of sleep and quality food, financial burden, exploitation by truck owners and agents, and lack of access to healthcare resources (Apostolopoulos & Sönmez, 2007; Apostolopoulos et al., 2013; Dutta & Acharya, 2015). The neoliberal logic of health takes for granted their hardships and health risks and portrays them as the ones responsible for carrying the disease from high-risk populations to the general population.

Condom Promotion as a Business

The NACO annual reports frame the "Targeted Condom Social Marketing Programme" as one of the most important initiatives under NACP-IV. The language of marketing is further highlighted in the following excerpt that outlines the agenda behind the social marketing programme:

> The thrust areas under the programme have been to expand social marketing programme to saturate coverage in districts characterized by high HIV prevalence and/or high family planning need and to increase the demand for condoms among high risk, bridge and general population.
>
> (NACO, 2015, p. 420)

The marketing strategy of expanding social marketing programmes to reach a wider population with high HIV/AIDS prevalence is highlighted with an emphasis on increasing the demand for condoms. The marketing logic embedded in this programme emphasizes increasing the demand of condoms among its customers (e.g., the truckers) and ensuring the availability of the product – condomw, in this case. The condom promotion programme resonates with a typical business model, often iterating the words "demand" and "supply."

Another excerpt that highlights the marketing strategies deployed for the success of "Targeted Condom Social Marketing Programme" (CSMP):

> NACO targeted Condom Social Marketing programme focuses on providing easy accessibility of condoms. The coverage and sustainability of non-traditional outlets is enhanced as they facilitate easy accessibility of condoms in rural and far flung areas. The programme also focus on saturation of high-risk areas i.e. truckers halt points .... All kinds of condom selling outlets located around these high risk areas are also covered in systematic approach under CSMP.
>
> (NACO, 2016, p. 351)

Increasing demand for condoms, which is then met by access to condoms with easy availability even in non-conventional outlets like petrol pumps stations, which are frequently visited by truckers, embodies the marketing logic of demands. Here is an articulation narrating the target groups as consumers: "Participants, as the most important consumer interface that facilitates condom purchase action were motivated to stock condoms and contribute in demand creation process by this means" (NACO, 2015, p. 421). The construction of identity of HRGs as consumers and facilitators of condom demand generation demonstrate the deep-seated marketing logic in such campaigns. Such articulation of health situates the health behavior in the realm of individual choice, thus ignoring the structural inequalities that constrain access to health resources, perpetuating the capitalist logic of considering community members as customers, and increasing demand among them while also involving them in the demand-generation process. The campaigns, designed by the marketing logic of contemporary global organizations, focus on diffusing their products by increasing the supply in various rural and urban areas, and its demand is increased by demand-generation programs across states (Dutta & Acharya, 2015). The marketing logic of demand and supply based on neoliberal ideologies of health erases the traditional view of health as a fundamental right and the need for public investment for good health (Sastry & Dutta, 2011).

Privatization of Healthcare

As a state entity involved in developing, implementing, and evaluating an overarching national level HIV/AIDS plan, NACO plays a key role in setting the agenda. An overarching theme in NACO's articulation of HIV prevention and management is privatization; the formulation of HIV/AIDS monitoring, prevention, and response as private functions are constructed in the realm of profits. Public–private partnerships have been mentioned as one of the successful new initiatives by NACO because of its reach with a vast number of people within limited amounts of time. This public–private partnership is considered the most efficient one in reaching people suffering from sexually transmitted infections (STIs) and reproductive tract infections (RTIs). Privatization is, thus, seen as a mechanism for extending the reach of interventions. Here is one articulation narrating the necessity of public–private partnership: "The involvement of private practitioners for providing STI services to HRG at such a large scale is one of the few successful initiatives globally" (NACO, 2016, p. 419). Although India has a state-driven public health system, the emphasis on private practitioners depicts simultaneously the backgrounding of public resources and public health infrastructures in addressing HIV/AIDS.

One of the new initiatives implemented by NACO is the Preferred Private Provider approach. Below is an excerpt that describes this approach:

> Preferred Private Provider approach has been rolled out to scale up STI/RTI services to HRG population under TI Projects. These providers are selected by the community members through group consultation. This approach has enhanced access to services for the HRG.
>
> (NACO, 2014, p. 35)

It is worth noting that, on one hand, the Preferred Private Provider approach is described as a participatory part of the HIV/AIDS campaign, where community members have the option to select providers of their own choice; on the other hand, these providers have to follow a standardized guideline provided by campaign planners and are trained according to that. Therefore, participation is built on the framework provided by the planners even though it portrays the community's authority in the selection process. The concept of privatization is framed in the form of participation as choice in the marketplace.

Here is another excerpt that brings forth the importance of privatization in dealing with HIV/AIDS:

> The major proportion of patients with STI/RTI seek services from the vast network of private health care delivery systems ranging from freelance private practitioners to large public hospitals ... It has been felt that reaching out to maximum numbers of people suffering from STI/RTI is not possible without partnership with private sector and organized public sectors.
>
> (NACO, 2015, pp. 419–420)

In NACO's report, the importance of tie ups with private organizations has been reiterated in order to increase its reach to this big population as well as to increase the efficiency of the proposed interventions. Partnerships with private healthcare are justified by stating how such partnerships have garnered success globally and how the majority of the population is dependent on the services provided by this enormous network of private healthcare providers. Here is another articulation of this need for public–private partnership: "The involvement of private practitioners for providing STI services to HRG at such a large scale is one of the few successful initiatives globally" (NACO, 2015, p. 419). Thus, in this campaign, the public–private partnership is justified, stating its efficiency, how people prefer their services, and how it has been a success globally. Also, it is evident that despite the depiction that the community members choose their preferred provider, ultimately the community members get co-opted to serve the planners' agendas. The privatization of health has raised concern among several scholars who argue that the basic idea underlying privatization overturns the traditional notion of health as a fundamental right and a public investment (Sastry & Dutta, 2013; Zoller, 2008). The promotion of privatization in NACO's report suggests the incorporation of neoliberal ideology that projects role of state as inefficient and the need for privatization and free market as effective solutions for development of state, and therefore in the context of health (McGregor, 2001).

Co-optation of Voice

Peer-led approaches are considered the key characteristic of Targeted Intervention (TI) projects aimed at HRGs. Once HRGs have been identified, targeted interventions draw upon characteristics of the targeted groups to offer persuasive interventions that deliver behavior change. In the articulations of HRGs, thus, exists the paradoxical framing of group participation as a channel of dissemination, situated in the backdrop of the framing of group members as passive recipients of the intervention designed by experts. Voice, thus, is situated amidst the overarching logic of fixing the agentic capacity of the group within the ambits of the intervention, as designed by experts and their overall managerial logics. The following excerpts are examples of the framing of participation within the managerial ontology of targeting:

> People from the high risk community are engaged to deliver services and act as agents of change, targeting high-risk behaviours and practices and not identities/individual choices, linking with services and commodities provision, dissociating risk from behaviours e.g. risk of STI and HIV infection from sex work, involving communities and their issues within the broader framework of interventions, adapting to the cultural and social milieu of the target audience. TI projects provide a package of prevention, support and linkage services to HRGs through an outreach-based service delivery model .... In addition, various organisations/institutions of repute have been engaged as State Training and Resource Centres (STRCs) to conduct capacity building activities for the TI programme.
>
> (NACO, 2015, p. 406)

> In order to ensure the quality of TI programme, capacity building and enhancing the technical skills of NGO/CBO staff is very important. Therefore, in order to provide uniform, quality training to different categories of staff working with NGOs/CBOs, viz., program managers, counsellors, finance accountants, outreach workers, peer educators and link workers, NACO has institutionalized the training and capacity building process with the establishment of the State Training and Resource Centres (STRC).
>
> (NACO, 2011a, p. 11)

The TI projects talk about including the voices of the community and adapt the social and cultural factors of the community, albeit within the umbrella logic of the intervention. Ironically, catering to the prescribed service model, which includes standardized services such as screening for and treatment of STIs, free condom and lubricant distribution among core groups, designed in a top-down framework by experts, is framed in the logic of participation. Participation and targeting exist side-by-side, with participation having been co-opted into the broader goals of targeting. The TI projects, even though are considered to have a peer-led approach, use participation as a channel to implement the agendas designed by the experts, with participation being configured as a channel for dissemination. Therefore, the peer-led approach utilizes community participants as agents to diffuse the dominant understanding of HIV/AIDS, exemplified in condom promotion and screening of STIs as solutions without really creating spaces for dialogue with the community on the nature of solutions. The possibility of open dialogue with community about its cultural and social contexts in which health behavior occurs is absent in the presence of a hegemonic prescribed service model. This one-way flow of communication – from expert to community – further solidifies the agendas of the campaign in the name of a peer-led approach.

Here is another articulation: "[V]arious organisations/institutions of repute have been engaged as State Training and Resource Centres (STRCs) to conduct capacity building activities for the TI programme" (NACO, 2015, p. 406). The community is provided with training by STRCs and, thus, they continue to serve the agendas of the campaign planners. The SRTCs are positioned as exemplars of participation, framed within the overarching logic of campaign promotion. The predetermined package of prevention, support and linkage services to HRGs leaves no space for an open dialogue with the community. The language of capacity building framed as part of participation pushes the agenda of the status quo in HIV prevention. Hence, TI programmes become tools to serve the hegemonic agendas of the campaigns and as means to co-opt the voices of the community while framing it as a peer-led approach.

Conclusion

The construction of HIV/AIDS by the state in India mirrors the neoliberal construction of the disease as an individualized behavior-based phenomenon to be managed through expert-driven, top-down interventions. The NACO annual reports, as reflections of the state's agenda and priorities, depict the symbolic and material interventions that are imagined and brought about by the state, and constructed in the service of global capital. The reports offer an inside view of the state's imagination of health and its management. As evidenced, at the peak of the funding flows from the Gates Foundation, and after the departure of the Foundation from India's HIV/AIDS program, the NACO policy framework mirrors the neoliberal ideology promoted by the Foundation (Dutta, 2016), replicating the Foundation's agenda of turning HIV/AIDS prevention and treatment into a business. The framing of the disease as an individual risk reproduces the framing put forth by the Foundation, serving the global hegemony of neoliberal governmentality of HIV/AIDS by turning health into an individual artifact, foregrounding individual-level behavioral choice, and constructing health interventions in the realm of individual behavioral decisions that express the agentic expressions of audience segments marked as "at risk" and/or "hard-to-reach." NACO, as a body of the Indian state created to tackle the disease, replicates the neo-colonial and neoliberal logics of individualist intervention, framing the risk agenda of national control around the high-risk individual, decontextualized from the structural contexts of HIV/AIDS. Principles of segmentation are drawn upon to mark high-risk segments of the population, formulated in the form of individual lifestyle behaviors and risky practices, simultaneously obfuscating the structural contexts of HIV/AIDS.

As we have argued in this chapter, HIV infections are constituted amid the precarity of lives at the margins of neoliberal governmentality that enable the unregulated flows of capital, material, and labor across sites of local-national-global profiteering. Salient in the discourse is the framing of at-risk groups that pose threats to the security of the nation state, and to the global status quo of the market. Behaviors then are constituted in relationship to these overarching power structures of risks, erasing simultaneously critical interrogations of the neoliberal local–national–global power structures that constitute the risks to health. For instance, the framing of sex workers as an at-risk group remains oblivious to the structural contexts of sex work, the displacement of poor women from their sources of livelihood in the Global South, migratory patterns brought about by accelerated transformations in economies, and the gendered precarities constituted amid economic displacement of the poor from their sources of livelihood. Similarly, the framing of truckers as "bridge population" remains oblivious to the risks, structural threats, and vulnerabilities that are borne by truckers amid rapidly transforming economies, with poor worker protections and weakening of worker collectivization processes through state-driven neoliberal interventions.

The emphasis on behavior change connects HIV/AIDS to solutions in/of the market, formulating the prevention of HIV/AIDS as social marketing. At-risk groups relate to the state's intervention programs as consumers in the market. Behaviors presented in the realm of participation in the market are tied to the global neoliberal apparatus of profiteering from health risks, marrying behavior-change solutions to market opportunities. Health is, thus, privatized, with public–private partnerships offered as solutions to the target audiences who are framed as consumers of the health products being sold. The behavior change industry that emerges through this discursive frame is tied to new market opportunities for introducing interventions, and intrinsically, therefore, tied to the creation of an at-risk market that can be targeted for individualist consumption. Within this framing of HIV/AIDS solutions as public–private partnerships, the participation is narrowly framed in the narrative of individual choice, attached to consumer engagement in the market. Citizens, framed as consumers, are connected to the logics of the market, turned into opportunities for private profit-making, and incorporated into hegemonic structures of participation. The language of capacity building is presented as a framework for disseminating the market-based logic of interventions and health services, with its goal being building the capacity of precarious communities identified as at-risk to be integrated with the market. Ironically then, participation is constituted within the dominant logics of the market and is constrained within the narrow agendas of profiteering through the promotion of products that are designed by experts in their managerial logics, devoid of opportunities for voices of community members to be heard. Infrastructures for participation are absent even as market friendly preconfigured structures are put forth as channels for engagement (Dutta, 2016). The voices of communities on the margins are raised in order to be co-opted into enhancing the efficiency and effectiveness of neoliberal HIV/AIDS interventions, tied to creating and promoting new markets, sold as behavior change.

Overall, this dominant discourse of HIV/AIDS has shaped the dominant discourse of health in general, thus limiting the plurality of ideas, questioning the structural violence leading to lack of access to health structures in certain communities, and providing meaningful solutions. The weakening of public health programs in a country leads to withdrawal of ideology that narrates health as a human right; instead, the individualized health discourse prevails, solidifying the notion that the responsibility of good health primarily lays with individuals. Paradoxically, this neoliberal ideology mobilized by the ideology of "ending AIDS" constitutes impossibilities of eliminating HIV/AIDS. Simultaneously, to prop up the "end of AIDS" discourse, a wide array of empirical accounts are strategically selected and propped up, while working through various techniques to erase articulations from the margins. As NACO's policy framework demonstrates, the rhetorical construction of the "end of AIDS" is deployed to fundamentally re-organize healthcare as a private commodity, dismantling the existing public health systems, and introducing large-scale precarities. Our analysis points toward the violence embedded in the ideology of "post-AIDS," colonizing spaces of community participation and state-driven public health systems to turn them into sites of transnational profiteering.

References

Acharya, L., & Dutta, M. (2012). Deconstructing the portrayals of HIV/AIDS among campaign planners targeting tribal populations in Koraput, India: A culture-centered interrogation. *Health Communication*, *27*, 629–640, doi: 10.1080/10410236.2011.622738

Apostolopoulos, Y., & Sönmez, S. (2007). Tracing the diffusion of infectious diseases in the transport sector. In Y. Apostolopoulos & S. Sönmez (Eds.), *Population mobility and infectious disease* (pp. 131–156). Boston, MA: Springer.

Apostolopoulos, Y., Sönmez, S., & Massengale, K. (2013). Sexual mixing, drug exchanges, and infection risk among long-haul truck drivers. *Journal of Community Health*, *38*(2), 385–391. doi:10.1007/s10900-012-9628-y

Basu, A. (2011). HIV/AIDS and subaltern autonomous rationality: A call to recenter health communication in marginalized sex worker spaces. *Communication Monographs*, *78*(3), 391–408. doi:10.1080/03637751.2011.589457

Basu, A., & Dutta, M. J. (2007). Centralizing context and culture in the co-construction of health: Localizing and vocalizing health meanings in rural India. *Health Communication, 21*, 187–196, doi: 10.1080/10410230701305182

Basu, A., & Dutta, M. J. (2009). Sex workers and HIV/AIDS: Analyzing participatory culture-centered health communication strategies. *Human Communication Research, 35*, 86–114. doi: 10.1111/j.1468-2958.2008.01339.x

Bowen, K. J., Dzuvichu, B., Rungsung, R., Devine, A. E., Hocking, J., & Kermode, M. (2011). Life circumstances of women entering sex work in Nagaland, India. *Asia-Pacific Journal of Public Health, 23*(6), 843–851. doi:10.1177/1010539509355190

Campos, N. G., & Farmer, P. (2003). Partners: Discernment and humanitarian efforts in settings of violence. *The Journal of Law, Medicine & Ethics, 31*(4), 506–514, doi: 10.1111/j.1748-720X.2003.tb00118.x

Carrasco, M. A., Nguyen, T. Q., Barrington, C., Perez, M., Donastorg, Y., & Kerrigan, D. (2018). HIV stigma mediates the association between social cohesion and consistent condom use among female sex workers living with HIV in the Dominican Republic. *Archives of Sexual Behavior, 47*(5), 1529–1539. doi:10.1007/s10508-018-1186-7

De Souza, R. T. (2007). *NGOs and empowerment: Creating communicative spaces in the realm of HIV/AIDS in India* (Doctoral dissertation). Purdue University, West Lafayette, IN. Available from ProQuest Dissertations & Theses Global. (UMI No. 304836288)

Dutta, M. J. (2007). Communicating about culture and health: Theorizing culture-centered and cultural sensitivity approaches. *Communication Theory, 17*, 304–328. doi: 10.1111/j.1468-2885.2007.00297.

Dutta, M. J. (2008). *Communicating health: A culture-centered approach.* Malden, MA: Polity.

Dutta, M. J. (2016). *Neoliberal health organizing: Communication, meaning, and politics* (Vol. 2). New York: Routledge.

Dutta, M. J., & Acharya, L. (2015). Power, control, and the margins in an HIV/AIDS intervention: A culture-centered interrogation of the "Avahan" campaign targeting indian truckers: Power, control, and the margins in HIV/AIDS. *Communication, Culture & Critique, 8*(2), 254–272. doi:10.1111/cccr.12078

Escobar, A. (1995). *Encountering development: The making and unmaking of the third world.* Princeton, NJ: Princeton University Press.

Farmer, P. (1992). *AIDS and accusation: Haiti and the geography of blame.* Berkeley: University of California Press.

Farmer, P. (1999). *Infections and inequalities: The modern plagues.* Berkeley: University of California Press.

Loomba, A. (1998). Situating colonial and postcolonial studies. In J. Rivkin & M. Ryan (Eds.), *Literary theory: An Anthology* (2nd edition; pp. 1100–1111). Maiden, MA: Blackwell Publishing.

Lupton, D. (1995). *The imperative of health: Public health and the regulated body.* Thousand Oaks, CA: Sage.

McGregor, S. (2001). Neoliberalism and health care. *International Journal of Consumer Studies, 25*(2), 82–89, doi: 10.1111/j.1470-6431.2001.00183.x

NACO. (2011a). *Annual report 2008–09.* Retrieved from http://naco.gov.in/sites/default/files/Annual_Report_NACO_2008-09.pdf

NACO. (2011b). *Annual report 2009–10.* Retrieved from http://naco.gov.in/sites/default/files/NACO_AR_English%202009-10_NEW.pdf

NACO. (2014). *Annual report 2013–14.* Retrieved from http://naco.gov.in/sites/default/files/NACO_English%202013-14.pdf

NACO. (2015). *Annual report 2014–15.* Retrieved from http://naco.gov.in/sites/default/files/annual_report%20_NACO_2014-15_0.pdf

NACO. (2016). *Annual report 2015–16.* Retrieved from http://naco.gov.in/sites/default/files/Annual%20Report%202015-16.pdf

NACO. (2019). *About us.* Retrieved from http://naco.gov.in/about-us

Nambiar, D. (2012). HIV-related stigma and NGO-isation in India: a historico-empirical analysis. *Sociology of Health & Illness*, 34(5), 714–729, doi: 10.1111/j.1467–9566.2011.01428.x

Pfeiffer, J., & Chapman, R. (2010). Anthropological perspectives on structural adjustment and public health. *Annual Review of Anthropology*, *39*, 149–165.

Roy, A. (2004, August). *Public power in the age of empire.* Speech at the American Sociological Association Conference, San Francisco, CA.

Said, E. W. (1978). *Orientalism.* New York: Pantheon Books.

Sastry, S. J., & Dutta, M. J. (2011). Postcolonial constructions of HIV/AIDS: Meaning, culture, structure. *Health Communication*, *26*, 437–449, doi: 10.1080/10410236.2011.554166

Sastry, S. J., & Dutta, M. J. (2013). Global health interventions and the "common sense" of neoliberalism: A dialectical analysis of PEPFAR. *Journal of International and Intercultural Communication*, *6*(1), 21–39, doi: 10.1080/17513057.2012.740682

Spivak, G. C. (1998). *A critique of postcolonial reason: Toward a history of the vanishing present.* Cambridge, MA: Harvard University Press.

Turshen, M. (1999). *Privatizing health services in Africa.* New Brunswick: Rutgers University Press.

Upadhyay, U. D. (2000). India's new economic policy of 1991 and its impact on women's poverty and AIDS. *Feminist Economics*, *6*(3), 105–22.

World Bank. (1999). *Project appraisal document on a proposed credit in the amount of USD 140.82 million to India for a second national HIV/AIDS control project* (No. 18918-IN). Washington, DC: World Bank Group.

Zoller, H. M. (2008). Technologies of neoliberal governmentality: The discursive influence of global economic policies on public health. In H. M. Zoller & M. J. Dutta (Eds.), *Emerging perspectives in health communication: Meaning, culture and power* (pp. 390–410). New York: Routledge.

Part II

Rhetorics and Relations

7 "I Might as Well Be Dead"

Aging with HIV in the "Post-AIDS" Era

Bernice McCoy and Nancy Romero-Daza

Death is a universal phenomenon. However, its definition and the exact event that marks its occurrence can differ depending on the context. Death has commonly been described in three categories: clinical, biological, and social. Biological and clinical death are declared when key vital functions (e.g., heartbeat, breathing) that keep a person's body alive cease to function. Social death occurs when an individual dies in a social sense and is treated as non-existent (Borgstrom, 2017). Thus, while clinical and biological death define the demise of the physical organism, social death marks the end of a human's social identity (Sweeting & Gilhooly, 1992). In most societies, social death is believed to always follow physical death. However, social death can precede physical death if people consider someone as "already dead" while their physical body is still alive (Mulkay, 1993). This paper outlines the concept of social death and its use in social science research by examining the experience of individuals who are living with a highly stigmatized and stigmatizing condition such as HIV/AIDS. We present a qualitative analysis of the lived experience of six African American men and their personal philosophies on negotiating their "social death" as they age with HIV in the "post-AIDS" era.

History and Definitions of Social Death

In reviewing social death, we must refer to the initial work of Goffman and his concept of mortification and "non-person" treatment (Goffman, 1961). Mortification was introduced in Goffman's description of institutions such as jails, prisons, boarding schools, and mental hospitals. Goffman states that the culture of these institutions is symbolic of isolation from the outside world and reinforced by physical barriers such as fences and locked doors. Upon admission, individuals undergo a process of "trimming" where they are stripped of personal possessions (e.g., clothes) and all attributes that individualize a person: autonomy, freedom, and self-determination. They are then lumped into the "largest and most abstract of social categories, that of human beings" (Goffman, 1961, p. 261; Sweeting & Gilhooly, 1992). Here, all aspects of life (e.g., work, sleep, and play) are shared with others in the same locale, which is often controlled by a higher authority. Thus, individuals entering these settings undergo a process

DOI: 10.4324/9781003000945-10

of "mortification" where they are "dispossessed of roles they held in the outside world" (Goffman, 1963, p. 253). Goffman (1961, 1963) also notes how staff often create a social distance between themselves and these individuals so as to safeguard themselves from the treatment occurring inside these institutions. This distancing leads to what Goffman terms "non-person treatment," where staff in fact acts as if the person does not exist (Goffman, 1961, p. 352).

Goffman's work served as a foundation for the fields of ethnography, anthropology, and medical-thanatology – the scientific study of death – in their production of the definitions of "social death." The first definition can be traced back to 1907, where Hertz noted how death meant not only the end of life, but also the destruction of the "social being grafted upon the individual" (Hertz, 1960, p. 77). Based on data of nineteenth-century anthropologists, Hertz contrasted the then-held belief by most Western societies that death was immediate with those of non-Western societies, as reflected in their temporary burial rituals (Hertz, 1960). These societies believed that the deceased soul lingered and therefore the individual was still a "partial member of society" and in need of food and company (Nzioka, 2010). Mandelbaum (1958) illustrates such a case among the Kota of South India, who observe two funeral ceremonies – a Green Funeral and a Dry Funeral. The Green Funeral is held to observe the cremation of the individual's body and the Dry Funeral – lasting 11 days – is held in remembrance of the individual's life. The Kota believe that a person is not socially dead until the conclusion of the Dry Funeral.

In addition, Hertz illustrated that individuals who are in mourning are also considered "people of death" (Hertz, 1960). The scholar provides the example of the Hupa People who, while in mourning, are viewed as one and the same with the corpse of the deceased. As the scholar states, "[T]hey [Hupas in mourning] live in darkness, dead themselves from a social point of view, because any active participation on their part in collective life would only spread abroad the curse they carry in them" (Hertz, 1960, p. 52). Another example of this is burial rituals of the Orthodox Jews. Their bereavement process lasts for approximately a year, during which recreational activities are prohibited, mourning garments are worn, and the bereaved are visited by family and friends. At year's end, the tombstone is dedicated during an unveiling ceremony, and the formal mourning process concludes.

Among medical-thanatologists, Sudnow (1967) was the first to recognize that social death can precede biological death (Sweeting & Gilhooly, 1997). Sudnow defines social death as: "[T]hat point at which socially relevant attributes of the patient begin permanently to cease to be operative as conditions for treating him, and when he is essentially already dead" (Sudnow, 1967, p. 74; Sweeting & Gilhooly, 1991). Though he acknowledges Goffman's argument that social death is the asocial treatment of a person (i.e., "non-person treatment"), Sudnow believes that this argument is ambiguous and prefers to limit the term to the literal sense of "death" (Sweeting & Gilhooly, 1991). Sudnow cites several examples of social death based on his observations from two U.S. hospitals, where he described how the social value of the patients near death determined the level and effort of treatment provided by medical personnel. Sudnow observed a nurse forcing a dying woman's eyelids shut due to the fact that it would have been more difficult to close them upon actual death; the completion of autopsy permits for the dying; familial arrangements for burial of the not-yet deceased; and the disposal and compartmentalization of personal belongings of the dying prior to death (Sudnow, 1967).

Similar to Sudnow, Kastenbaum (1969) defined social death as: "[A] situation in which there is absence of those behaviors which we would expect to be directed towards a living person and the presence of behaviors we would expect when dealing with a deceased or non-existent person" (Kastenbaum, 1969, p. 309, 1977). The researcher points out that "a significant aspect of being a person is being a person in the eyes of others" (Kastenbaum, 1977, p. 311; Sweeting & Gilhooly, 1991). He further extends his definition of social death to include the status of individuals who have transgressed societal norms. This includes individuals who have violated a taboo, those living with a stigmatized disease (e.g., HIV/AIDS), and those who are seen to lose "live person status" (e.g., the elderly or terminally ill) (Sweeting & Gilhooly, 1991). An elderly individual abandoned in a nursing home where family members cease to visit him, yet where they still make decisions about his life, exemplifies the situation described by Kastenbaum.

Kalish (1968), delves further into the notion of social death and sub-divides the concept into two main categories: self-perceived and other-perceived. Self-perceived social death is when an individual presumes that they are "as good as dead" and that their social role in life has terminated. Other-perceived social death is when society concludes that an individual, who people once knew and acknowledged as alive, is now thought to be dead (Kalish, 1968). Kalish also examines the impact of social death on living family and friends as members of the departed. He discusses that families and friends may parallel much of what Sudnow observed in U.S. hospitals – that families will make burial and cremation arrangements and give away the deceased's belongings before actual physical death occurs (Kalish, 1968). However, he also points out that families and friends become impatient if the occurrence of the physical death takes too long.

Use of the Social Death Construct

The concept of social death has been used in a wide variety of disciplines. Králová (2015) highlights how this concept has been broadly applied to explore empirical topics including genocide, displacement, slavery, and dementia. However, she states that the wide use of the term within numerous disciplines has created ambiguity surrounding its application and that there is a need for conceptual clarity

Králová (2015) conducts a systemic review to highlight the applicability of this conceptual framework. She identified three central tenets mentioned by scholars in the social death literature: loss of social identity, loss of social connectedness, and loss associated with the disintegration of the body. Social identity is one's sense of self as a member of a social group (or groups). Králová states that an individual's social identity is lost when they are viewed as inadequate in the eyes of others. The reasons for this loss can be varied and may include personality traits, embodied characteristics, value systems, and low social, economic, or cultural capital. The loss of social identity results in social abandonment of which social death is a consequence. Second, regarding the loss of social connectedness, Králová points out that since human beings are inherently social, we suffer profound loss when our social connections and roles in society are severed. An extreme example of such loss is that associated with solitary confinement, a mechanism commonly instituted in prisons. As Guenther (2013) writes, "There are many ways to destroy a person, but one of the simplest and most devastating is through solitary confinement" (p. xi). From this example, Králová emphasizes that the loss of multiple social roles or identities is a likely cause of social death. Third, Králová details the role of the body in social death. She states that our social identity is inevitably connected to our bodies (Hockey & Draper, 2005). Hence, when our body shows visible signs of deterioration – whether due to illness or old age – our social identities and interactions become undermined and disrupted. Thus, in dying, the physical body's profound deterioration is viewed as "disgusting" and something unworthy of social connection. Kellehear (2007) states that the individual experiences "shameful dying."

Social Death and HIV

Understanding the notion of social death is important as we enter the "post-AIDS" era and witness the greying of the epidemic. In 2016, nearly half of the people living with HIV in the U.S. were aged 50 years or older (CDC, 2019). Significant advancements in HIV treatment regimens have transformed HIV from a death sentence to a chronic, manageable condition. However, there are positives and negatives associated with this new reality of aging with the virus. While life expectancy has improved, older adults aging with HIV/AIDS still face numerous unique obstacles not encountered by their younger counterparts. These obstacles include multiple stigmas associated with their age (i.e., ageism) and sero-status, and a greater likelihood for isolation and loneliness, all of which can contribute to their social demise.

For aging individuals, death is perceived as "natural" or "appropriate" and is viewed as the gradual relinquishment of life "which has reached its allotted span" (Kastenbaum, 1972; Raphael, 1984; Sweeting & Gilhooly, 1997, p. 96). This view is historically premised on the assumption that the "prerogative" of older individuals in society was to die (Sweeting & Gilhooly, 1997; Williamson, 1979). Due to nineteenth-century improvements in nutrition, sanitation, and social conditions, there was a dramatic drop in mortality rates and an increase in the number of individuals who were surviving beyond the age in which they could either be contributing members of society or provide for themselves (Sweeting & Gilhooly, 1997).

Today, survival into old age is no longer unusual with many individuals living into late retirement (Sweeting & Gilhooly, 1997). However, in most industrial societies there is a strong emphasis on the productivity of adults and on their economic worth (i.e., contribution and value). Thus, a working adult is worth more than an elderly adult in terms of human capital. An elderly person's value in society is seen as rapidly depreciating. As a result, society may stereotype and exclude elderly individuals as they are considered not to be of much value. Interestingly, this notion of age-based worth can continue even after an elderly individual has passed. Prior (1989) illustrates this notion in the autopsies of elderly individuals where medical examiners paid greater importance to autopsies of the "economically active age groups" rather than to those of the elderly (Sweeting & Gilhooly, 1997, p. 97).

Furthermore, aging individuals are also most likely to face social seclusion. Many suffer a reduction in their social support networks due to family and friends living far away, having predeceased them, or being emotionally distant. Aging individuals are least likely to travel, their engagement in social activities is diminished, and many actually live in isolation. Combined with the expectancy of death, this "reality" of the life of the elderly leads society to think of them as having no future worth – that they might as well be dead. As Kastenbaum states, "[A] person may come to be classified as socially dead precisely because he has not died ... but has instead outlived his social context" (Kastenbaum, 1969, p. 17). This perception may be further enhanced if the elderly individual is placed in an institution such as a nursing home. As Kastenbaum emphasizes, "admission to an age-segregated institution suggests or confirms to many people the idea that 'it is all over but the dying'".

As a condition that affects not only the physical, but also the social wellbeing of individuals, HIV/AIDS plays an important role in the experience of social death. Due to its primary transmission through sexual contact and intravenous drug use, HIV/AIDS has become a metaphor for moral and physical contamination. It is through this moralization of HIV/AIDS that HIV positive individuals are viewed as having a "spoiled identity, which may result in prejudice, stigma, and the loss of social identity" (Nzioka, 2010, p. 14). The disclosure of a "spoiled identity" often equals social death. To avoid a "spoiled identity," HIV positive individuals will often conceal their status and normalize their HIV positivity. They avoid disclosure to family and friends for fear of rejection and to physicians who may express negative attitudes towards them due to their being infected with HIV. In addition, they refrain from activities that signal their diagnosis, such as seeking appropriate health care (e.g., receiving HAART) or participating in HIV support groups.

However, the concealment of one's HIV status and avoidance of social death can only occur for so long, particularly for individuals who did not receive medical treatment when the epidemic started. When the immune system continues to deteriorate and the disease manifests in the individual's body, AIDS-related conditions will become visible and much harder to hide than in the initial stages of infection. In the absence of treatment, bodily expressions such as HIV wasting syndrome (i.e., severe weight loss) and Kaposi's sarcoma (patch stage lesions that eventually form into nodular tumors) will appear (Alonzo & Reynolds, 1995). This has the greatest implications for progression towards social death, and loss of personhood as stigma, the biophysical disease process, and social identity issues are now intensified. Colman notes that this "often results in a special kind of downward mobility" as affected individuals "lose their place in the social hierarchy" (Coleman, 1988, p. 100).

While most individuals who are presently aging with HIV/AIDS are likely undergoing medical treatment that considerably decreases the outward manifestations of infection, their condition interplays with the general aging process to magnify the impact of "social death." Understanding the occurrence of social death among older people living with HIV and/or AIDS (PLHIV) is particularly salient in the "post-AIDS" era, when advances in medicine are increasing the period between diagnosis and physical death. Although numerous studies have captured the long-term effects of HIV medications on the aging body, few have examined the lived experience of those who are facing social death in the context of aging bodies and HIV/AIDS. This paper contributes to fill this gap in the literature by presenting the results of an exploratory study conducted among men who are currently aging with HIV/AIDS and experiencing social death.

Study Participants and Methods

The six participants whose stories are highlighted in this paper are a sub-sample of those who took part in a larger study exploring the current health status and life-experiences of African American men (N=35) who are aging with HIV in Hillsborough County, Florida. Purposive sampling was used to recruit participants who previously completed the Antiretroviral Treatment and Access to Services (ARTAS) program at a local community-based organization. The ARTAS program – an individual-level intervention – links individuals recently diagnosed or previously diagnosed with HIV and without care for six months to medical and social services. The larger study sought to address HIV disparities in access to care among African Americans. Further inclusion criteria for participants in the larger research study was to identify as a male (transgender female-to-male included), be 50 years of age or older, and reside within Hillsborough County.

The larger research study consisted of two main phases. The goal of Phase I was to create a profile and obtain general knowledge of the state of health of the 35 participants. Phase I consisted of an open-ended questionnaire in which data were obtained on self-reported socio-demographic information including age, sexual orientation, educational attainment, employment status, household income, and health insurance status, among others. Additionally, the date and location of the participants' HIV and/or AIDS diagnosis, current medical issues, functioning status, medication/treatment regimens, social support network(s), and current receipt of social (e.g., case management) and mental health services were also collected. In addition, participants were asked to free-list and pile-sort their health care concerns, barriers, and facilitators. Participants' Health

Related Quality of Life (HRQoL) – a multi-dimensional concept utilized to assess the impact of one's health status on overall life satisfaction (Healthy People.gov 2020, 2019), was also assessed through the Medical Outcomes Study HIV Health Survey (MOS-HIV). The tool is comprised of 34 items that include six scale scores (i.e., mental health, physical function, role function, general health perceptions, social functioning, and pain) derived from the MOS-20-Item Short Form Health Survey (SF-20) and components believed to be substantial in HIV disease (e.g., health distress, QoL, energy/fatigue levels, cognitive functioning, etc.) (Delate & Coons, 2001).

The goal of Phase II was to capture the life course perspective (life experience) of older African Americans who are aging with HIV. A person's life history, timing of their diagnosis, and length of time living with HIV can have an effect on life pathways, expectations, and overall illness experience. Of primary interest exploring the differences and similarities of the life course perspectives of individuals who were diagnosed prior to the introduction and availability of Highly Active Antiretroviral Therapy (HAART) (i.e., prior to 1995, pre-HAART era) and those individuals diagnosed during the post-HAART era (after 1996). Of secondary interest was documenting the participants' reflections on life and death as well as their definition, experience, and mechanisms of coping with social death. Research participants were separated into their respective eras based on their date of diagnosis. A subsample of six research participants – three from each era – was then selected at random and contacted to participate in two subsequent open-ended interviews. The first interview was used to capture details of participants' life course, while the second interview aimed at capturing the participants' viewpoints on life, death, and social death. The rich qualitative data obtained from these six individual interviews are presented and discussed in the sections below.

The first author first began taking an interest in the topic in 2014 while she was working as a Prevention Specialist at a local substance abuse agency within their HIV Services Department. While in this position, she facilitated the implementation of a state-funded High Impact Prevention Program (HIP), which targeted the Black/African American community in Hillsborough County, Florida. The program was comprised of several individual, group, and community-level interventions to address the needs of individuals who were HIV-negative, whose HIV-status was unknown, and PLHIV. A key intervention within this program was that of "Antiretroviral Treatment and Access to Services" (ARTAS). This intervention serves to link newly diagnosed individuals into services and medical care and to re-engage PLHIV who had fallen out of care for six months or more.

As the researcher enrolled individuals into the ARTAS program, it became increasingly evident that older clients living with the virus faced social challenges different from those of younger cohorts of PLHIV. Differences were even evident between aging individuals who had lived with the virus for a while and older individuals recently diagnosed with the virus. The first author found that her older clients – particularly men – experienced a greater lack of social support, increased stigma, and increased stereotypes due to their older age, their HIV status, and, for some, their sexual orientation. These challenges were further compounded by the lack of senior-specific services, end-of-life planning services, support for companions caring for individuals LHIV, housing support, and income support within the Hillsborough County area. This spurred the author to begin to research and assesses the current state of health of the aging, Black/African American male population LHIV so as to begin to identify gaps in AIDS Service Organizations' (ASO) current programming towards addressing these unique challenges.

Data Collection

Data were collected through an open-ended interview guide developed by the first author, based on the "Life Story Interview" model, Life Course Theory, and previous research on social death. The interview guide was designed with assistance from key informants who had extensive knowledge and experience working with both aging populations and HIV-positive individuals. The key informants involved in this development process included a healthcare professional, two individuals from a local AIDS service organization, and an expert in the field of aging. The research project was approved by the University of South Florida Institutional Review Board. With consent of research participants, all interviews were audio-recorded.

All audiotapes of interviews were transcribed verbatim. In addition, each transcription was simultaneously reviewed with participant audio recordings and researcher notes to ensure thoroughness and accuracy. Next, the first author, alongside a colleague, undertook a process of open coding for two interview transcripts, one from the pre-HAART era and one from the post-HAART era. Utilizing an inductive approach, the transcripts were analyzed for salient themes and used to develop a preliminary codebook. The parent and sub-parent codes found throughout the transcripts were compared between the two coders and used to create and define specific codes. Any emergent themes found throughout the transcripts were also coded and included in the preliminary codebook. Afterwards, reviewed transcripts were imported into AtlasTi software where the first author further assessed inter-coder reliability along with other concordances and discrepancies. Codes that were agreed upon and missing/not matched were noted with '1' and '0' respectively. Cohen's Kappa, which measures inter-rater agreement for qualitative items, was applied to find substantial agreement until all coding discrepancies were reconciled throughout the transcripts. Thematic and content analyses were then completed until saturation was reached. This procedure was then used to assess, analyze, and code the remaining four transcripts.

The Participants

In order to contextualize the findings of this research, it is necessary to offer a detailed background of the individuals who participated in the study. The following biographical sketches of the six participants offer a glimpse into their stories as PLHIV who are experiencing the aging process and facing social death. All the names used are pseudonyms.

Edward (Post-HAART Era)

Born in 1969, Edward was enlisted in the Army in 1988 at 19 years of age. He was discharged in 1991 when, as he shared, "my partyin' years began." He was diagnosed with HIV in 1998 at the age of 29, following a "casual hookup" with a male. Edward knew of the man's HIV status but stated, "[I] was out there drinkin' and druggin' and didn't care." Edward did not find out he was positive until he was arrested for possession of paraphernalia and was sent to county jail where he received HIV testing. Edward shared that after his diagnosis he simply shut down. He interacted with no one. Although he was offered the opportunity to begin a medication regime while in jail, Edward decided against it: "Back then, the HIV clinic was separated from everything else. People started asking questions as to why I was called to see a doctor in that [HIV clinic] area." Edward was released from jail in 1999 and enrolled in a drug-treatment program. It was then that he decided he needed to not only control his drug addiction, but also to manage his life living with HIV. In 2013, Edward began getting involved in local organizations and governing boards, and educating others about HIV. However, the desire to be so forthcoming about his life and living with HIV was not always there: "I was really nervous, but I saw that I had to educate folks." Today, Edward is happily married to his sero-discordant partner of five years, and his viral load is undetectable. He continues to be an HIV advocate in his community.

William (Pre-HAART Era)

Born in 1957, William was raised in South Florida. He had a religious upbringing with his father being a Methodist minister. He was heavily involved in the church, was part of his prayer group, and helped serve food in the church kitchen. William was diagnosed with HIV in 1990 at the age of 33, after having "the worst hook-up of my life" with a female friend. Upon confirmation of his diagnosis, he began making funeral arrangements and assigning beneficiaries. For a year, he was deeply depressed and full of anxiousness, regret, and guilt. However, William stated, "I woke up one day realizing that I can't stay stuck on stupid for the rest of my life … I have too much to live for." William shared being inspired by other long-term survivors and seeing how they were taking HIV medicines everyday and fighting the virus. This served as a motivator for William – "It showed me that I could do that too!" Disclosure was the greatest obstacle for William in living with HIV. Though most of his family and friends became aware of his diagnosis after several years, he did not disclose his status to his mother until 2013. Due to her being in a fragile state of health, William thought disclosure of his status would have "sent my mother to her grave." Even so, William shared that his mother had a keen sense that something was different.

Once, during a visit, she asked William, "Are you sick? You look like you may be sick." Today, William is in good health and his viral load is stabilized. He stays busy attending support groups and being involved in the church, singing in its choir, and serving as a trustee.

Tony (Pre-HAART Era)

Born in 1958, Tony comes from a long line of family members employed in the healthcare industry. His mother is a healthcare administrator, while his sister is a registered nurse at a local hospital. Tony himself once attended school to be a nurse practitioner. When the HIV epidemic first emerged in the 1980s, both Tony's mother and sister were among the first cadre of AIDS caretakers to work in the hospitals' AIDS wards. Tony volunteered daily alongside his sister and recalled helping to care for and provide comfort for the individuals hospitalized in the ward. As he states, "[W]hen I was diagnosed in 1984, I really wasn't in shock … I was already pretty familiar with HIV. I knew what the disease did." Tony's partner passed away from AIDS-related complications in 1984. Tony admits knowing that his partner had HIV. However, little was known regarding the etiology of the disease and how it was contracted. When news regarding the sexual transmission of the virus came to light, Tony and his partner began using protection. However, by then, it was too late. After his partner passed, Tony was in no rush to get tested. It was not until one and a half years later that he received a positive test result.

Darnell (Pre-HAART Era)

Darnell, 59-years-old, was diagnosed with HIV in 1992 while incarcerated. He was 25 years old and, as he stated, "[i]n jail, the disease was out of sight out of mind. Also, I just thought it was one of those things that could never happen to me." Darnell went against his better judgment and became involved with a man during his incarceration. When other inmates found out whom he was involved with, they told him, "Oh damn son … that guy's got it." Even then, he did not rush to get checked. It was not until he felt a knot in the back of his neck that he decided to get tested. Darnell shared that his test result came back indefinite and further tests had to be done. However, he had an inkling that he was positive. He felt the disease manifesting quickly in his body. Darnell detailed how his body began "wasting away"; he weighed a measly 110 pounds at the time of diagnosis. Doctors placed him on several vitamins and Ensure shakes to improve nutritional and weight levels. It was not until two weeks following his HIV test that he received confirmation of a positive test result. Darnell shared, "[W]hen I received, my diagnosis my mind went blank. At that time, I didn't know much about the disease. But what I did know was that it was taking people away real fast. I wasn't ready to accept that; I wasn't ready to die." Darnell shared that he did not come to terms with his diagnosis until five years post-incarceration, in 1997. "It wasn't until after I got out of jail that reality hit. My count while in jail was 2000, but when I got out it was 350 … that's when I knew that I had to get on medication."

Roger (Post-HAART Era)

Born in Miami, Florida, Roger was enlisted in the United States Army from 1978 to 1984. He was honorably discharged and decided to move to Hillsborough County, Florida. "Being that I did my time in the Army, I thought I could just wild out ... didn't know that having some fun was going to lead to this [HIV]." Roger shared that the thought of having HIV never crossed his mind: "If it weren't for my friend who dragged me to the Miami Dade Health Department in 1997, I don't know what would have happened." In detailing the day he received his diagnosis, Roger said: "They [nurses] were making such a huge commotion over me and beating around the bush with giving me the news. When they told me, I said, 'I'm positive? That's it? I thought you told me I was going to be dying tomorrow!' I let out a sigh of relief. Honestly, I began laughin'!" The nurse practitioner kept asking Roger if he was alright as laughter was not a usual reaction on receiving a positive diagnosis. However, Roger shared that he had an "optimistic spirit about the disease." He further shared, "I didn't think that being [HIV] positive was a negative thing. I knew I could get on the meds ... there were some good new ones rollin' out at the time and things were lookin' up for those who had it [HIV]." Several years following his diagnosis, Roger received further news that he had prostate cancer. "Now the cancer... that knocked me down. That's when thoughts of death crossed my mind." However, Roger shared that he "buckled down" and focused on taking care of himself. He maintained his medication regime and cancer treatment. Twenty-eight years later, Roger is happily cancer free and has an undetectable viral load.

Clint (Post-HAART Era)

Born in 1973, Clint was the youngest participant at diagnosis (25 years old). He detailed being very much in the know regarding HIV and how to prevent transmission. He shared that he had attended educational seminars where individuals living with AIDS would speak about their experiences and their fight to stay alive. "I knew protection was everything. I was very much into using condoms. I even had my own condoms because I didn't trust anyone else with their condoms. I had friends in the 1980s. I saw what HIV did to them. I wasn't going to let THAT be me." However, Clint never knew that his ability to negotiate condom use would be stripped away from him. In 1998, while serving time in prison, Clint was beaten and raped by four men, one of whom was HIV positive but did not know it at the time. Clint described the horrific pain he endured following the incident, sharing, "I woke up in the infirmary ... didn't even know that had happened until I went to the bathroom and s*&t was just not right ... the nurses there had to stitch me up. My jaw was broken." Shortly following the incident, Clint was transferred to a local county jail to serve the remainder of his sentence. It was there that Clint received word that one of the men that raped him had tested positive for HIV. Clint immediately requested testing. His results were negative initially, but Clint has an inkling that his status would change. Subsequent testing six months later showed not only a positive result, but that he had acquired three different strains of the virus and had "full-blown AIDS." Clint shared, "I remember thinking, 'NO NO NO.' … Why me? What did I do to deserve this? Please Lord, just kill me now. I don't want to live this life." Following the diagnosis, Clint fell into a deep depression and attempted suicide three times. It took a "jet black queen" (a woman of trans experience), who was also living with HIV and who was admitted to the prison, to convince him to live. Today, Clint shares that he lives with an undetectable viral load and is "healthy as an ox." He serves as a condom ambassador for a local AIDS Service organization and is also certified to provide rapid HIV testing throughout Hillsborough County.

Salient Themes

The thematic analysis of the six in-depth interviews conducted with the participants described above revealed several salient themes that highlight their journeys from exposure to diagnoses, treatment, and present-day status. Central to these themes is the issue of social death, manifested in different degrees and at different points in time.

Being Left Behind

All participants diagnosed during the pre-HAART and early post-HAART eras felt as though they are being socially excluded due to being left behind in current HIV initiatives. Though their lives have been saved with life-altering HIV medications, they still face unique challenges, which, they feel, are not being recognized by HIV organizations and policy makers. As Darnell stated:

> HIV is so mainstreamed now … so much is focused on prevention and so that those of us who've been living with it for so long are sort of being forgotten. Which don't get me wrong, [prevention] is good, but don't forget about us! A lot of programs that were once available back in the day have kind of fallen to the wayside. We [individuals living with HIV] are all lumped together now, but we aren't all the same."

Pre-HAART participants stated that their being "lumped together" gives them the feeling that their personal histories and experiences are not distinguished but, rather, considered the same as the experience of older individuals diagnosed with HIV today. As William stated, "*There is a big difference between a 50-year-old person who has HIV and a 75-year-old person who has HIV. We were diagnosed in two different worlds.*" Pre-HAART individuals detailed how they struggled with uncertainty and tried to assert control over their lives. Participants detailed having symptoms comparable to post-traumatic stress disorder (PTSD), where they are consistently anxious, nervous, and "on guard." Many participants described experiencing reccurring depression, anger, and fear. Even after many years, survivor's guilt is also prominent among the pre-HAART participants. As William further shared, *"Why me? Why am I still here and my friends are gone?"*

The feeling of being hidden is particularly evident among gay, bisexual, and other men-who have sex with men (MSM) and who are aging with HIV. Several participants shared experiencing a "triple stigma" associated with public misconceptions regarding HIV, ageism, and homophobia. Some shared how social programming is primarily focused on young adults, because HIV is not seen as something that affects the elderly population. Four participants also detailed that, of the existing LGBT social services and programs, few address the impacts of living with HIV, the process of aging, and other syndemic factors – substance use, mental health, and poverty – that are prominent among these aging men. Adding some context to the multiple psychosocial burdens that this population faces, Darnell shared:

> I am one of those older adults that I'm always dealing with [things] like keeping a roof on my head and a stomach full of food, not to forget staying sober. I don't really focus on the fact that I have HIV. It's just one of many things that is part of my life.

Furthermore, participants iterated that there is already a shortage of healthcare providers who are trained to provide culturally competent HIV health care. With the greying of the epidemic has come the greying of the HIV healthcare field. They fear this shortage will result in regression in the quality of care they receive. As William stated,

> Early on when this [HIV epidemic] first came out and I'd see my doc, I was simply defined by my numbers. Didn't really matter what my name was. It was … what is your [CD4] count? How much of the virus do you have in you? What can we do to raise your numbers? Didn't matter what my name was or where I came from. It's like I was a specimen or something. But, you know, things change. Today, my doc spends a lot of time with me, going through all my issues, side effect of the meds and whatnot.

This further extends to the provision of culturally competent LGBT care. As Tony iterated:

> I'm so worried as my doc retired this past year and the nurse practitioner, I have will be retiring soon too. These are my people … my family really. They've practically been with me from the beginning [of the epidemic]. I'm so open with them … probably way too open with them [laughs] … about everything … my partners, sex …. But the thing about them is that they don't see me for being POZ but as someone who is living it up. I'm afraid that these new docs won't really SEE me. They are just going to treat me like any other patient, collect my numbers [CD4 and viral load] and send me on my way."

As the excerpts presented above suggest, the participants expressed a real concern about the potential loss of the relationships they have been able to cultivate throughout the years with their doctors and nurses. This sense of loss is further exacerbated by considerations about their future, which leads them to ponder their long-term plans.

Long-Term Planning

End-of-life planning is now considered an empowering process when, earlier in the HIV epidemic, there was not much time or space to be thoughtful about such plans. Now, that the prospect of old age is more real, participants are worried about how they will be taken care of, living with HIV as aging individuals. As William stated:

> How will we be treated as elders in our twilight years? It's coming, for so many of us who were told we had four or five months to live. Now it's 25 years later and I am left to wonder, ponder and worry about the people who will tend to our needs as we start losing the ability to tend to them ourselves.

Several participants also mentioned that since the introduction of anti-retroviral therapies, end-of-life issues have ceased to be of great concern. When discussions regarding end-of-life planning occur, physicians are hard-pressed to recommend resources for hospice and palliative care. In addition, numerous participants discussed their concerns about needing to move into assisted care facilities as they age. These participants expressed fear that such places will not have the expertise in dealing with their disease, and that they will face covert discrimination and be deemed "unworthy" of care due to being HIV positive. As Roger shared:

> I wonder ... when I make it to one of those places what people will think of me? Will they sit with me when I'm at the dining hall? Want to interact with me? What about the staff there? Will they answer my calls in the middle of the night if I'm in pain? How quickly will they respond to me?

Furthermore, MSM participants' fear of entering a nursing home is twofold, as they feel they will not only be discriminated against based on their HIV status, but also on the basis of their identifying as MSM.

For the participants, worries about inadequate care and potential isolation/discrimination in facilities where they will need to reside when they are no longer able to care for themselves may also relate to overall loss of social connections in other areas of their lives, as discussed below.

Loss of Social Connections

All participants detailed an impending social death due to the "chipping way of connections" and difficulty in replenishing these severed relations. Several Pre-HAART participants detailed initially surrounding themselves with other

PLHIV, creating informal networks upon diagnosis due to lack of support from friends and family. However, for many of these participants, the HIV-positive peers who survived the initial years of the epidemic are beginning to pass away due to old age and non-related HIV health issues. Often, the few family members that knew about their diagnosis and accepted them have relocated and no longer live within close proximity to them. For some, some familial relationships just never recovered. Such is the case for Clint, who shared:

> For me, many of these people [friends diagnosed with HIV] are gone now. Nobody else has gone through it … lost the number of friends that I have. And nobody will be able to understand it really … I always thought that these men that I made friends with would be around for me when I grew old. Now, I'm the only one of my friends that hasn't died. I have this picture of all of us together at home. I'm the only one still alive. THAT was my family. My blood family that I thought that was going to be … supposed to be … around for me … they ain't there.

Due to continued vigilance regarding disclosure of their status, many participants described hesitation in establishing new connections for fear that people will be uncomfortable being around them due to their HIV status. As Clint continues:

> I've had people say: go out and mingle … make new friends … but go out and mingle with who? I'm so afraid of what people will think. Also, I don't want to go through the whole rigmarole of having to disclose again. What if they accept me? What if they don't? I'm just too old for that … I'll just keep to myself.

Alongside the hesitation in establishing new friendships is the hesitation to engage in intimate relations. Three participants detailed how the current laws criminalizing HIV – the punishment of exposing another person to HIV – have caused them to think twice before engaging in sexual relationships or completely forgo entering these relationships altogether. Thus, they are driven into further isolation. As Roger shared:

> Let me start with saying, I. LOVE. Sex. But, you hear of this criminalization thing? I don't understand it. If I am always taking my meds like the doc says and if I use a condom that makes the chances for someone else to get it so, so low. So why do we have these laws in place? What if that person has 'the clap' or herpes? Do they get arrested for giving me that? I feel that those [STDs] things are worse because there isn't any meds to take to block you from getting that. You just find out you got it AFTER the fact. At least with HIV I'm taking my meds and I'm preventing it from the get-go. But hey, all I know is I don't need to be arrested. I've already gone to jail and I certainly don't need this nonsense [the criminalization of HIV] to send me back.

Even when there is the motivation to go out and make new connections and disclose their status, participants from both pre- and post-HAART eras shared that they consistently bounce between social acceptance and social exclusion. It is a repetitive, rollercoaster of emotions that is debilitating and exhausting. As Edward shared:

> It fluctuates daily. One day I might get shunned … talk about 'this ol' dirty man got that virus … don't give him your hand.' Some other days, I'm looked at like a hero … an inspiration … talk like, "You have lived this long with it [HIV] … that is unbelievable!' You learn how to tolerate it but, damn, it's tiring.

However, despite it being exhausting, two participants stated that the roller-coaster of emotions has allowed them to build resiliency and has even motivated further advocacy. As Roger notes:

> There are certain individuals that have just crossed me off their social list. There ain't nothin' I can do to change that … so to them I may no longer exist, but I continue on my way. I know who I am, and I continue to live my best life without 'em. If anything, I'm stronger without 'em! Their opinions of me don't affect me and the impact I'm trying to make in my community.

The comments presented here highlight the loss that the participants have experienced as their social networks erode for a variety of reasons, including the death of peers. Such loss presents challenges for the men's physical and emotional wellbeing, and underscore their vulnerability in their (actual or imagined) attempts to create new relations as they age with HIV. The resulting feelings of isolation and "social death" are further compounded by those who also experience a major shift in their productive capacity as they age with the disease, as described below.

Loss of Productive Capacity

For many participants, working prior to their diagnosis with HIV was a central part of who they were – a contributing member of society. As Darnell described, "I really liked my line of work. I worked with my hands and fixed up houses. My work kept my mind in a good place … kept me going and kept me alive." However, upon receiving a positive diagnosis, the pre-HAART participants quit their jobs, spent their retirement accounts and savings, and cashed in their insurance policies based on the assumption that their life was coming to an end. Similarly, those diagnosed in the early post-HAART era quit their jobs due to the unpredictable nature of the disease. Many of these participants detailed being limited by their occupational functioning due to fatigue, physical and cognitive limitations, medication side effects, and frequent medical appointments. However, with revolutionized HIV treatment and breakthroughs (e.g., one-pill-a-day drugs), living life with HIV has dramatically improved – so much so that it has caused participants to consider returning to the workforce. Yet a return to the workforce is lined with its own stressors. One issue is that of continuation of benefits. Most participants reported being on long-term disability or public assistance benefits (e.g., housing support, social support services, food assistance), which, due to eligibility requirements, force them to keep their income low. These benefits provide stability that many participants do not want to discontinue for the sake of employment. As Edward stated in discussing the idea of returning to work, "I haven't really had to give it [work] much thought. It's black and white for me. I just can't go back – not the way I want to anyways." Although programs such as the Ticket to Work and Work Incentive Improvement Act of 1999 (TWWIIA) provide opportunities for those receiving benefits to supplement their earnings through work, the anxiety regarding health insurance and medication coverage remains. A majority of participants receive assistance with premiums and with out-of-pocket costs for prescription drugs through programs such as AIDS Drug Assistance Program (ADAP) and Medicaid. This prescription coverage is essential, particularly for PLHIV who are not only aging with the virus but are dealing with non-infectious comorbidities – like cardiovascular disease, hypertension, and type 2 diabetes – with high drug costs. Edward continues, "I fought hard … it took time to get on this [ADAP] program … and Medicaid helps me out a lot for my other meds … I can't lose that help. I want to work, but just can't risk it." Thus, participants described being forced into a socially gray area, where they want to avoid social death by re-entering the workforce, but run the risk of physical death, should they lose the benefits that are extending their physical life.

The question of identity derived from participating in the workforce is also important to consider and can further make it difficult to combat social death. Participants may have left the workforce with a specific set of skills and sense of self that is now currently out of date or no longer relevant. Aging PLHIV may find that they physically cannot do the type of work they previously did. Participants like Darnell, who enjoyed hands-on work, shared, "This work [construction] is all I know. Even when I was in jail, I kept myself busy doing hands-on stuff. But the HIV caused me to get arthritis real bad in my hands now and I just can't do that type of work no more. Sure, I do odd-end things for people … even did some small painting work on my neighbor's house. But nothin' like I used to do before. So, if I could go back to work, what would I do? I'd be lost. I don't know anything else than what I know."

Returning to work additionally poses serious challenges related to the many stigmas that are associated with PLHIV. The process of obtaining employment may involve disclosure of sero-status, particularly given the fact that there may be large gaps in employment history. In addition, the need for accommodations (e.g., extended or more frequent breaks) may also cause PLHIV to have to disclose their status to employers, thus making themselves vulnerable to potential discrimination. As Williams described, "Disclosure to my family was bad enough for me. Heck, took me up until 2013 to tell my mom. I'm in a good state now. And those that know [about HIV status], know. I don't need to open up another can of worms. I'm too old for that."

Discussion

The six individuals whose stories are recounted here have benefitted from medical advances that allow them to live much longer lives than they had originally expected when they were each first diagnosed with HIV. However, while they have, so far, avoided physical demise, they experience social death on a regular basis. The disappearance of personal social networks through the death of HIV-positive peers, the loss of socially productive roles, and the realities of the natural aging process, among other factors, combine to create a sense of isolation, invisibility, and abandonment permeating their daily lives. These feelings are magnified by the all-too-common discrimination based on HIV status, sexual identity/orientation, race, and age to which the participants are subjected. Altogether, social death adds an additional layer of exclusion to a population already plagued by multiple social inequalities. Thus, in order to address the phenomenon of social death experienced by aging individuals living with HIV, there is a need to create strategies that respond to their lived experience.

HIV programming needs to account for the voice and perspective of older adults, especially those from underserved groups, such as the African American men included in this study. Current HIV/AIDS education and programming are primarily tailored to a younger population and most of the information/material provided does not address the numerous challenges specific to individuals who are aging with HIV (Roger, Migone & Kirkland, 2013). Particular efforts should focus on reducing HIV-related stigma, which often leads to social isolation and self-exclusion – two big contributors to social death. On a related note, there needs to be an increase in training for current and incoming HIV medical and other social service providers in meeting the unique needs for older adults living with HIV. For example, physicians may inadvertently play a role in maintaining stigma related to both HIV and aging as they may not consistently collect comprehensive sexual history and may not feel comfortable discussing sexuality with older adults. Research has shown that older adults may not be forthcoming with sexual health information or behaviors, particularly if they believe it will be perceived as inappropriate by their social circles, culture, and physicians. Healthcare providers can play a pivotal role in promoting the overall health and wellness of older persons aging with HIV. Central to this endeavor are efforts to address the biological as well as the psychosocial challenges salient to this population and to promote positive coping strategies to build resilience.

Further research should be conducted to study the experiences of elderly PLHIV and older gay or bisexual men who are living in congregate living facilities such as nursing homes and long-term care facilities. The few studies conducted on this issue have touched on how gay elderly persons residing within these settings are often assumed to be heterosexual and feel the need to hide their sexual orientation from residents and staff (Cahill & Valadez, 2013; Herdt & de Vries, 2004; Johnson, Arnette, & Koffman, 2005). This is problematic and causes long-term relationships with partners of the same sex to be devalued. Those that are "outed" as being gay may experience neglect, abuse, and discrimination by facility employees and healthcare personnel. Furthermore, there needs to be shift in how healthcare practitioners approach advanced-care planning and/or end-of-life care with individuals with advancing age and long-standing HIV infections. Currently, there appears to be more emphasis placed on the management of physical death, emphasizing medical and palliative care models, rather than on the lived experience of an individual dying with HIV (Kellehear, 2009). Such an approach can cause a premature "social death," as it denies PLHIV the opportunity to be active agents (e.g., express preferences for care, openly discuss end-of-life) within the context of their dying. Data have shown that since the arrival of HAART the practice of advanced care planning and/or end-of-life care has dwindled substantially. Fewer than half of PLHIV aged 50 and older report having had such discussions with a medical provider (Erlandson, et al., 2012; Sangarlangkarn & Appelbaum, 2016; Wenger et al., 2001). Even fewer discussions are likely among certain patient groups such as ethnic minorities, intravenous drug users, and those with lower education levels (Wenger et al., 2001). Discrepancies regarding what constitutes end-of-life discussions between patients and providers have also been captured (Selwyn & Rivard, 2003). With the increased longevity of PLHIV who are also suffering from multiple, complex chronic conditions related to aging, having these discussions now is more important than ever.

In order to address the physical and social isolation that increases the risk of social death among aging PLHIV, there needs to be greater funding to support better access to public transportation and for social-support programming. Social relationships and networks have been proven to play a pivotal role for older persons and PLHIV (Roger et al., 2012; Sankar et al., 2011). Numerous studies have illustrated that health is tied to a sense of connection with one's social environment (Loxterkamp, 2013). Rebuilding a connection between an individual and their community may play an important role in improving self-worth, strengthening a sense of belonging and purpose, and enhancing quality of life (Molassiotis et al, 2002; Simoni et al, 2011). This will allow a person to remain "socially alive" and pertinent within their society. Further, to address social death that results from the loss of employment, efforts need to be invested in initiatives to provide support for individuals who are looking to become economically productive.

A return to employment may offer individuals the ability to experience a "social re-birth." McReynolds (2001) found that PLHIV viewed employment as an activity that meant there was a future. Having a job offered a shift from being viewed as a person with a life-threatening illness to being viewed as someone who is healthy and a contributing member of society (Goldblum & Kohlenberg, 2005; McReynolds, 2001). Furthermore, being gainfully employed offers

PLHIV the ability to feel greater connectedness to others. Research has found that the social network of the workplace allows for the maintenance of a communal network and continual societal connections that PLHIV would otherwise not have access to (Conyers, 2004; Trujillo, 2010). Researchers have also found that employment provides a distraction from negative feelings and low self-esteem resulting from feeling like a burden on society due to long periods of unemployment (Brooks & Klosinski, 1999; Conyers, 2004). This facet of employment is important given past research demonstrating that unemployed individuals generally have higher rates of depression, anxiety, social isolation, and low self-esteem (Blalock & Mcdaniel, 2002). Such factors can be detrimental to older PLHIV. Currently, the HIV service community lacks the resources and knowledge to assist people in considering, starting, or seeking further training to re-enter the workforce. A coordinated effort is needed to raise awareness and educate HIV service providers about employment and economic opportunities for those aging with HIV. Education and inclusion of local vocational rehabilitation offices may assist in bolstering these efforts.

The implementation of strategies such as those described above can significantly increase the physical, mental, and social wellbeing of individuals who are facing both the natural progression of HIV disease, and the physical and mental changes of the normal aging process. More importantly, it can begin to address, and potentially reverse, the experience of social death that robs individuals of their place in society, and that slowly erodes their agency and their identity as they approach physical death. Programming directed at African Americans aging with HIV must be designed in ways that directly respond to their lived experiences as minorities whose everyday life is shaped by the pervasive racial disparities that still exist in the United States. The HIV experience for the Black community remains qualitatively different from that of individuals of other races/ethnicities. Black Americans remain one of the most economically disadvantaged demographic groups in the U.S. and are more likely to reside in neighborhoods with concentrated poverty, high rates of violence, poor infrastructure, and higher levels of incarceration than other racial and ethnic groups (Taylor, 2020). For Black PLHIV, poverty exacerbates the challenges of living and aging successfully with the virus. Unstable housing, inadequate transportation, and food insecurity are all factors that have been inextricably linked to poor outcomes along the HIV Care Continuum for Black Americans (Furlotte, Schwartz, Koornstra, & Naster, 2012; Himmelgreen, Romero-Daza, Turkon, Watson, & Sellen, 2009; Leaver, Bargh, Dunn, & Hwang, 2007; Tuller et al., 2010). The inability to meet basic health and nutritional needs worsens HIV, increases the risk for contracting other infections, and hastens the onset of AIDS. Further exacerbating poor outcomes is the lack of consistent access to quality health care. Many Black Americans are uninsured or underinsured and rely on public assistance and governmental programs, such as Medicaid, for healthcare coverage. However, despite approval for Medicaid expansion, 14 states, primarily in the South, rejected this expansion, leaving nearly 40% of Black PLHIV without medical coverage (The AIDS Institute, 2020). This is detrimental to individuals who are in their 50s and 60s, aging with HIV, and not yet eligible for Medicare. Given the fact that viral loads can increase from lack of access to care, the risk of infection to sexual partners increases, thereby fueling the epidemic.

The research described in this chapter is an initial attempt to shed some light on this important issue, one that needs to be fully explored if we are to enhance HIV-related services for individuals such as the men whose stories are portrayed here.

References

The AIDS Institute. (2020, May). Florida policy. *Florida AIDS Drug Assistance Program (ADAP): Facts, Problem, Solution, Action*. Retrieved from http://www.theaidsinstitute.org/florida-policy/adap/florida-aids-drug-assistance-program-adap-facts-problem-solution-action

Alonzo, A., & Reynolds, N. (1995). Stigma, HIV and AIDS: An exploration and elaboration of a stigma trajectory. *Social Science and Medicine, 41*, 303–315. doi:10.1016/0277-9536(94)00384-6

Blalock, A., & Mcdaniel, S. F. (2002). Effect of employment on quality of life and pscyhological functioning in patients with HIV/AIDS. *Psychosomatics, 43*(5), 400–404.

Borgstrom, E. (2017). Social death. *QJM: An Iternational Journal of Medicine, 110*, 5–7. doi:https://doi.org/10.1093/qjmed/hcw183

Brooks, R., & Klosinski, L. (1999). Assisting persons living with HIV/AIDS return to work: Programmatic steps for AIDS service organizations. *AIDS Education and Prevention, 11*, 212–223.

Cahill, S., & Valadez, R. (2013). Growing older with HIV/AIDS: New public health challenges. *American Journal of Public Health, 103*, e7–e15. doi:10.2105/AJPH.2012.301161

Centers for Disease Control and Prevention. (2019). *HIV and older Americans*. Retrieved from https://www.cdc.gov/hiv/group/age/olderamericans/index.html

Coleman, J. (1988). Social capital in the creation of human capital. *American Journal of Sociology, 94*, 95–120.

Conyers, L. (2004). Expanding understanding of HIV/AIDS and employment: Perspective of focus groups. *Rehabilitation Counseling Bulletin, 48*, 5–18.

Delate, T., & Coons, S. (2001). The use of 2 health-related quality-of-life measures in a sample of persons infected with human immunodeficiency virus. *Clinical Infectious Diseases, 32*, e47–e52. doi:10.1086/318492

Erlandson, K., Allshouse, A., Duong, S., MaWhinney, S., Kohrt, W., & Campbell, T. (2012). HIV, aging, and advanced care planning: Are we successfully planning for the future? *Journal of Palliative Medicine, 15*, 1124–1129.

Furlotte, C., Schwartz, K., Koornstra, J., & Naster, R. (2012). "Got a room for me?" Housing experiences of older adults living with HIV/AIDS in Ottawa. *Canadian Journal on Aging, 31*, 37–48.

Goffman, E. (1961). *Asylums: Essays on the social situation of mental patients and other inmates*. Garden City: Anchor Books.

Goffman, E. (1963). *Stigma*. New York: Simon & Schuster, Inc.

Goldblum, P., & Kohlenberg, B. (2005). Vocational counseling for people with HIV: The client-focused considering work model. *Journal of Vocational Rehabilitation, 22*, 115–124.

Guenther, L. (2013). *Solitary confinement: Social death and its afterlives.* Minneapolis: University of Minnesota Press.

Herdt, G., & de Vries, B. (2004). *Gay and lesbian aging: Resarch and future directions.* New York: Springer.

Hertz, R. (1960). *Death and the right hand.* New York: Routledge.

Himmelgreen, D. A., Romero-Daza, N., Turkon, D., Watson, S., Okello-Uma, I., & Sellen, D. (2009). Addressing the HIV/AIDS-food insecurity syndemic in sub-Saharan Africa. *African Journal of AIDS Research, 8*, 401–412.

Hockey, J., & Draper, J. (2005). Beyond the womb and the tomb: Identity, (dis)embodiement and the life course. *Body and Society, 11*, 41–58.

Johnson, M., Arnette, J., & Koffman, S. (2005). Gay and lesbian perceptions of discrimination in retirement care facilities. *Journal of Homosexuality, 49*, 83–102.

Kalish, R. (1968). Life and death-dividing the invisible. *Social Science and Medicine, 2*, 249–259.

Kastenbaum, R. (1969). Psychological death. In L. Pearson (Ed.), *Death and dying: Current issues in treatment of the dying person* (pp. 255–249). Cleveland, OH: Case Western Reserve University Press.

Kastenbaum, R. (1972). While the old man dies: Our conflicting attitudes towards the elderly. In B. Schoenberg, A. C. Carr, D. Peretz, & A. H. Kutscher (Eds.), *Psychosocial aspects of terminal care* (pp. 116–125). New York-London: Columbia University Press.

Kastenbaum, R. (1977). *Death, society and human experience.* St. Louis: Mosby Co.

Kellehear, A. (2007). *A social history of dying.* Cambridge: Cambridge University Press.

Kellehear, A. (2009). On dying and human suffering. *Palliative Medicine, 23*, 388–397.

Králová, J. (2015). What is social death? *Contemporary Social Science, 10*(3), 235–248.

Leaver, C., Bargh, G., Dunn, J., & Hwang, S. (2007). The effects of housing status on health-related outcomes in people living with HIV: A systematic review of the literature. *AIDS and Behavior, 11*(2), 85–100.

Loxterkamp, D. (2013). Humanism in the time of metrics. *British Medical Journal, 347*(4), f5539.

Mandelbaum, D. G. (1958). Social uses of funeral rites. *Eastern Anthropologist: A Quarterly Record of Ethnography and Folk Culture, 12*, 5–24.

McReynolds, C. (2001). The meaning of work in the lives of people living with HIV disease and AIDS. *Rehabilitation Counseling Bulletin, 44(2)*, 104–115.

Molassiotis, A., Callaghan, P., Twinn, S. F., Lam, S. W., Chung, W. Y., & Li, C. K. (2002). A pilot study of the effects of cognitive-behavioral group therapy and peer support/counseling in decreasing psychologic distress and improving quality of life in Chinese patients with symptomatic HIV disease. *AIDS Patient Care and STDs, 16*(2), 83–96.

Mulkay, M. (1993). Social death in Britain. In D. Clark (Ed.), *The sociology of death: theory, culture, practice* (pp. 31–55). Blackwell: Oxford.

Nzioka, C. (2010). The social meanings of death from HIV/AIDS: An African interpretative view. *Culture Health & Sexuality, 2*(1), 1–14. doi: 10.1080/136910500300831

Prior, L. (1989). *The social organisation of death: Medical discourse and social practices in Belfast.* Basingstoke: Macmillian.

Raphael, B. (1984). *The anatomy of bereavement: A handbook for the caring professions.* London: Hutchison.

Roger, K., Migliardi, P., & Mignone, J. (2012). HIV, social support, and care among vulnerable women. *Journal of Community Psychology, 40*(5), 487–500.

Sangarlangkarn, A., & Appelbaum, J. S. (2016). Caring for older adults with the human immunodeficiency virus. *Journal of the American Geriatrics Society, 64*, 2322–2329.

Sankar, A., Nevedal, A., Neufeld, S., Luborsky, R., & Luborsky, M. (2011). What do we know about older adults and HIV? A review of social and behavioral literature. *AIDS Care, 23*, 1187–1207. doi:10.1080/09540121.2011.564115

Selwyn, P., & Rivard, M. (2003). Palliative care for AIDS: Challenges and opportunities in the era of highly active anti-retroviral therapy. *Journal of Palliative Medicine, 6*, 475–487.

Simoni, J. M., Chen, W. T., Huh, D., Fredriksen-Goldsen, K. I., Pearson, C., Zhao, H. … Zhang, F. (2011). A preliminary randomized controlled trial of a nurse-delivered medication adherence intervention among HIV-positive outpatients initiating antiretroviral therapy in Beijing, China. *AIDS and Behavior, 15*(5), 919–929.

Sudnow, D. (1967). *The social organization of dying*. Englewood Cliffs, NJ: Prentice-Hall.

Sweeting, H. N., & Gilhooly, M. L. (1992). Doctor, am I dead? A review of social death in modern societies. *OMEGA—Journal of Death and Dying, 24*(4), 251–269.

Taylor, J. (2020, May). Racism, inequality and health care for African Americans. *The Century Foundation*. Retrieved from https://tcf.org/content/report/racism-inequality-health-care-african-americans/?session=1

Trujillo, M. (2010). Persons living with HIV/AIDS contemplating a return to work: A social cognitive career theory and constructivist theory perspective. *Journal of Rehabilitation, 76*, 51–56.

Tuller, D. M., Bangsberg, D. R., Senkungu, J., Ware, N. C., Emenyonu, N., & Weiser, S. D. (2010). Transportation costs impede sustained adherence and access to HAART in a clinic population in southwestern Uganda: A qualitative study. *AIDS and Behavior, 14*(4), 778–784.

Wenger, N. S., Kanouse, D. E., Collins, R. L., Liu, H., Schuster, M. A., Gifford, A. L., Bozzette, S. A., & Shapiro, M. F. (2001). End-of-life discussions and preferences among persons with HIV. *Journal of the American Medical Association, 285*(22), 2880–2887. https://doi. org/10.1001/jama.285.22.2880

Williamson, J. (1979). The challenge. In D. Doyle (Ed.), *Terminal care* (pp. 15–19). Edinburgh: Churchill Livingstone.

8 African American Mothers Living with HIV in the "Post-AIDS" Era

A Meta-Ethnographic Synthesis

Patrick J. Dillon and Satish K. Kedia

In March 2019, Dr. Robert Redfield – the former Director of the United States (U.S.) Centers for Disease Control and Prevention (CDC) – opened the National HIV Prevention Conference by appealing to audience members that "now is the time ... to put an end to the HIV epidemic once and for all" (Department of Health and Human Services, 2019a, para. 6). He then outlined the key strategies identified within the nation's *Ending the HIV Epidemic* (EHE) plan, which targets a 90% reduction in the number of new HIV infections by 2030 through expanded diagnostic, prevention, and treatment services (Department of Health and Human Services, 2020). This plan largely mirrors global HIV prevention efforts aimed at similar outcomes (Bekker et al., 2019; Joint United Nations Programme on HIV/AIDS, 2017; United Nations, 2015).

A few days later, the same conference closed with a session reminding attendees that addressing the continued impact of HIV on American society would require more than reducing the rate of new diagnoses; it would also require concerted efforts to assuage the inordinate effects of poverty, discrimination, and stigma on people living with HIV, particularly within communities of color (Department of Health and Human Services, 2019b). As part of this final session, Dr. Gail King, Professor and Director of the UCLA Sexual Health Program, highlighted the continued need to understand and attend to the unique HIV-related challenges of African American women, especially those with children or in need of reproductive health services (National Prevention Information Network, 2019).

Recent surveillance data support Dr. King's call for a greater focus on this subgroup, as African American women continue to bear an inequitable burden of new HIV diagnoses, those living with HIV, and HIV/AIDS-related deaths (Kaiser Family Foundation, 2020). In 2018, an estimated 4,114 African American women were newly diagnosed with HIV; this figure is more than twice the number of newly diagnosed Hispanic/Latina women (1,269) and non-Hispanic white women (1,491) combined (CDC, 2020). These new diagnoses are consistent with an overarching trend wherein African American women are significantly more likely to be diagnosed with HIV in their lifetime (1 in 56) than both Hispanic/Latina women (1 in 256) and non-Hispanic white women (1 in 941) (Hess et al., 2017). African American women also account for the highest percentage of HIV/AIDS-related deaths (58%) among women each

DOI: 10.4324/9781003000945-11

year – with HIV being the seventh leading cause of death for African American women between ages 25 and 44 (CDC, 2017, 2018a).

Despite being disproportionately affected by HIV/AIDS, African American women are less likely than women from other racial and ethnic populations to be linked to appropriate HIV services within a month of their diagnosis or to receive ongoing care (Cohen et al., 2004; Dasgupta et al., 2016; Lillie-Blanton et al., 2010; Lipira et al., 2019; Losina et al., 2009). African American women living with HIV frequently encounter multiple forms of disease-related stigma – which, in turn, is associated with a number of negative health outcomes such as depressive symptoms, reduced medication adherence, social isolation, and substance dependency (Grodensky et al., 2015; Lipira et al., 2019, 2020; Reif et al., 2019). Furthermore, when considering these HIV-specific issues combined with various markers of inequality, including racial/sexual discrimination, poverty, and infant/maternal health disparities among African Americans (DeNavas-Walt & Proctor, 2014; Geronimus, 1996; Robinson et al., 2019), it is apparent why Dr. King and other scholars believe that this population warrants further attention (Kapadia & Landers, 2019; National Prevention Information Network, 2019; Okoro & Odedina, 2017).

In particular, an increasing number of scholars have, in recent years, called for research that explores how living with HIV impacts African American women's experiences of motherhood and their reproductive health decisions (see, e.g., Fletcher et al., 2016; Kedia et al., 2019; Muze & Onsomu, 2017). These calls come as national survey data indicate that the majority of African American women living with HIV are of typical childbearing age (i.e., aged 18–44 years; CDC, 2018c; Fletcher et al., 2016). A number of recent studies also suggest that – similar to women of other races/ethnicities – a significant percentage of African American women living with HIV report the intention to give birth (Barnes & Murphy, 2009; Finocchario-Kessler et al., 2012; Fletcher et al., 2016; Kennedy et al., 2014).

Pregnancy intentions were widely discouraged in the early days of the epidemic due to the risk of perinatal transmission (often referred to as "vertical" or "mother-to-child" transmission); more recently, however, medical advancements – including widespread HIV testing, the proliferation of antiretroviral therapies, and safe breastfeeding protocols – have made motherhood a viable option for many women living with HIV in the U.S. and beyond (Blanche, 2020; CDC, 2018b). For example, despite an estimated 5,000 women living with HIV giving birth each year (Nesheim et al., 2018), the CDC notes that the annual number of HIV diagnoses attributed to perinatal transmission in the U.S. has declined over 95% during the past three decades, with a 41% reduction in such cases observed between 2012 and 2016.

With similar declines in perinatal transmission observed across the world, progress towards preventing mother-to-child transmission of HIV is considered to be one of the great accomplishments of the global effort to address this epidemic (Blanche, 2020; Joint United Nations Programme on HIV/AIDS, 2017; United Nations Children's Fund, 2019). Blanche (2020) argues, for instance, that "[w] ith continued efforts in screening and the organization of care and treatment of pregnant women, it is not unreasonable to expect that pediatric AIDS may virtually disappear and that children will only become infected in rare cases" (p. 20).

Despite this noteworthy progress, a closer look at perinatal transmission rates in the U.S. reveals that it is yet another marker of HIV-related disparity between African American women and those of other races/ethnicities. Children born to African American women accounted for 64% of pediatric HIV diagnoses attributed to perinatal transmission in 2017; the perinatal transmission rate per 100,000 live births is also five times higher among African American mothers than Hispanic/Latina and white women (CDC, 2018b). Additionally, while the virtual elimination of perinatal HIV transmission is by itself a laudable and important goal, achieving it would do little to address the aforementioned hardships experienced by African American mothers living with HIV. There is ample evidence that medical advancements can allow African American women living with HIV to have children with minimal risk of those children become HIV-positive; there is, however, little evidence to suggest that the U.S. healthcare system, or society as a whole, is doing enough to put these women (and their children) in a position to thrive (Fletcher et al., 2016; Kedia et al., 2019; Muze & Onsomu, 2017).

In this way, experiences of motherhood among African American women living with HIV embody many of the contradictions that have been identified within contemporary "post-AIDS" discourse (Mazanderani & Paparini, 2015; Persson, 2013; Walker, 2020). As Walker (2020) notes, the biotechnically informed logic of the "post-AIDS" era has the potential to overlook or negate the daily challenges associated with living with a stigmatized illness that has no cure –experiences that are "characterized by uncertainty, anxiety, [and] ongoing negotiation (emotional, social and economic)" (p. 96). Aligned with this critique, there is a vital need for scholarship that documents how present-day experiences of living with HIV, particularly among populations who encounter intersectional vulnerabilities, can inform practices and policies beyond biotechnical intervention aimed at improving the lives of those impacted by HIV (Mazanderani & Paparini, 2015; Persson, 2013). As Caiola and colleagues (2014) argue, such intersectional vulnerabilities are perhaps best exemplified by African American women; they further note that "[b]eing a mother adds an extra layer of complexity to the lives of women living with HIV" – as they experience increased stress associated with simultaneously managing their own and their children's needs while attempting to protect their children from HIV-related stigma (p. 292). These unique factors make African American mothers living with HIV a population that warrants specific scholarly attention. To this end, this chapter reports the findings of a meta-ethnographic synthesis (Atkins et al., 2008; Noblit & Hare, 1988) of qualitative studies focusing on African American mothers living with HIV, published between 2010 and 2020.

In the following section, we describe our methodological approach, which was informed by the practices of meta-ethnography (Borgnakke & Hillyard, 2020; Dillon & Basu, 2014; Noblit & Hare, 1988). Building from this approach, we then present our analytic framework – which draws upon the socioecological model (Auerbach et al., 2011; Baral et al., 2013) to organize the findings reported in the synthesized articles. Finally, we discuss how our analysis relates to contemporary "post-AIDS" discourse and how it can inform efforts to address the needs of African American mothers living with HIV.

Method

Methodological Approach

The present study was guided by the principles of meta-ethnography. Originally developed by Noblit and Hare (1988) and updated by Atkins et al. (2008), meta-ethnography provides a systematic method for synthesizing qualitative research studies. As Borgnakke and Hillyard (2020) note, meta-ethnography "preserves the particularities of the original studies while comparing and contrasting them to explore similarities and differences" (para. 1). Furthermore, consistent with the aims of this study – i.e., to better understand the lived experiences of African American mothers living with HIV – Dillon and Basu (2014) argue that meta-ethnography is well-suited to understanding how "lay knowledge" and socio-structural factors influence people's perspectives and experiences related to health and illness across studies (see also, Bosma et al., 2010; Dillon et al., 2012; Popay et al., 1998); it also well-suited for identifying the practical implications of qualitative research (Borgnakke & Hillyard, 2020; Dillon & Basu, 2014).

Search Strategies

We began our analysis by conducting a systematic literature search to identify peer-reviewed qualitative studies focusing on African American mothers living with HIV. More specifically, we searched seven electronic databases: (1) CINAHL, (2) PubMed, (3) PsychInfo, (4) Science Direct, (5) Web of Science, (6) ComAbstracts, and (7) Communication and Mass Media Complete. Each database was searched for relevant articles using the following key terms: [HIV OR AIDS OR HIV/AIDS] AND [Black OR African American OR African-American] AND [Women OR Female] AND [Mother OR Motherhood OR Maternal] AND [Qualitative OR Ethnographic OR Interpretive OR Interview]. We limited our search to articles published in English between 2010 and 2020. In addition to searching within the databases, we also checked the reference list of each retrieved article (Atkins et al., 2008). We used PubMed's "Related Searches" function to identify other potentially relevant publications.

Our initial search identified 1,846 manuscripts for this review (Figure 8.1). As a first step in the data extraction process, we created a spreadsheet listing citation information for each article; we used this spreadsheet to eliminate duplicate records (n = 27). We then evaluated each remaining record (n = 1,819) for inclusion, using two broad screening questions: (1) Does this article report on findings from research that involved qualitative methods of data collection

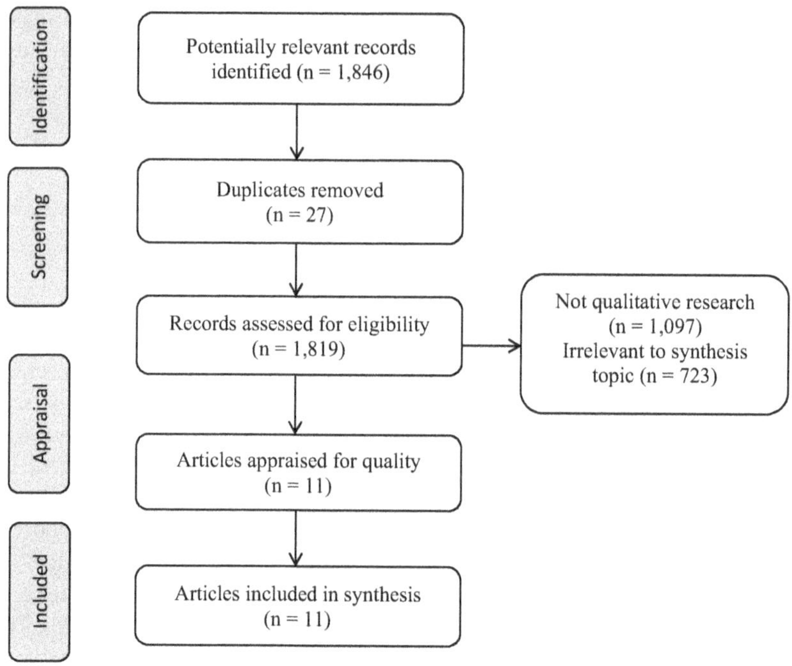

Figure 8.1 Literature search flowchart.

and analysis? and (2) Is this research relevant to the synthesis topic? (Campbell et al., 2003; Dillon & Basu, 2014). We ultimately retained 11 articles for data extraction and quality appraisal.[1]

Data Extraction and Quality Appraisal

The next step in the analysis process was to extract information from the retrieved articles to assess their methodological quality. Although there is little consensus regarding the role of the quality assessment in meta-ethnographic analysis, we followed previous researchers in using the assessment process as a means of eliminating potentially "poor" studies and to begin familiarizing ourselves with the individual articles (see, e.g., Atkins et al., 2008; Dillon & Basu, 2014; Sleijpen et al., 2016). We carefully read each manuscript and extracted information that was necessary for quality appraisal (e.g., research purpose, participant characteristics, data collection procedures, etc.). We then used the criteria established by Atkins et al. (2008) to evaluate the reported studies' methodological quality (see Table 8.1). The quality appraisal process revealed that all 11 studies met at least 80% of the Atkins et al. (2008) criteria; hence, we determined that all 11 articles were of sufficient quality to be included in the synthesis (see also Bosma et al., 2010; Dillon & Basu, 2014).

Table 8.1 Quality Appraisal Criteria (adapted from Atkins et al., 2008) and Results

Criteria	Yes	No	Unclear
1 Is this study qualitative research?	11	0	0
2 Are the research questions clearly stated?	5	6	0
3 Is the qualitative approach clearly justified?	11	0	0
4 Is the approach appropriate for the research question?	5	0	6
5 Is the study context clearly described?	11	0	0
6 Is the role of the researcher clearly described?	8	3	0
7 Is the sampling method clearly described?	10	1	0
8 Is the sampling strategy appropriate for the research question?	5	0	6
9 Is the method of data collection clearly described?	11	0	0
10 Is the data collection method appropriate to the research question?	5	0	6
11 Is the method of analysis clearly described?	8	3	0
12 Is the analysis appropriate for the research question?	5	0	6
13. Are the claims made supported by sufficient evidence?	11	0	0

Synthesis Procedures

The final step in the analysis process was to synthesize the data from each article. We began by reviewing each study's findings to identify primary themes and concepts; we then organized them into first-order (i.e., quotations attributed to study participants) and second-order (interpretations of the empirical data found in the original manuscripts) constructs (Bosma et al., 2010; Schutz, 1962). The first- and second-order constructs, taken verbatim from the original articles, were subsequently uploaded to *Dedoose,* a web-based qualitative analysis application (*Dedoose*, 2015).

We analyzed the extracted data using a three-stage process akin to the one described by Thomas and Harden (2008; see also Matthews et al., 2019). In the first stage, we read through each line of text, assigning initial codes to each one; we then began organizing these "free" codes (Thomas & Harden, 2008) into a rough framework that served as a starting point for synthesizing the studies. The second stage involved developing "descriptive" themes by comparing our initial codes (based on similarities and differences) and refining the framework we created in the first stage (Thomas & Harden, 2008). During the third and final stage, we developed a set of "analytical themes" (Thomas & Harden, 2008), which Matthews et al. (2019) describe as a process of inferring meanings "from the descriptive themes to go beyond the findings of the primary studies and address the aims of the review" (Matthews et al., 2019, p. 2289). In doing so, we developed a third-order analytical framework that was grounded in the accumulated body of evidence and formed a coherent interpretation of the whole (Bosma et al., 2010; Dillon & Basu, 2014).

Furthermore, to provide additional coherence to our interpretations and enhance the practical utility of our analysis, we followed other recent meta-ethnographies (see, e.g., Edeza et al., 2020) in organizing our findings within the structure of the socioecological model (Auerbach et al., 2011; Baral et al., 2013). More specifically, drawing on the selected manuscripts, we describe how the experiences of African American mothers living with HIV are impacted by structural/societal, interpersonal/social, and individual/personal factors in the U.S. (Baral et al., 2013; Edeza et al., 2020).

Results

Study Characteristics

As noted above, our final synthesis included 11 articles (representing 10 unique studies) that were published between 2010 and 2019 (Amutah et al., 2016; Amutah-Onukagha et al., 2018; Boehme et al., 2014; Caiola et al., 2017, 2018; Fletcher et al., 2016; Murphy et al., 2011; Muze & Onsomu, 2017; Peltzer et al., 2017; Tufts et al., 2010; Webel & Higgins, 2012). The articles primarily reported findings based on data collected via in-depth interviews (n = 8) and analyzed using various forms of content analysis (n = 7). Study samples ranged from a minimum of eight (Muze & Onsomu, 2017) to a maximum of 42 African American women living with HIV (Fletcher et al., 2016); the average sample included approximately 21 participants. In total, the 11 articles ostensibly reflect the perspectives of 207 unique participants drawn from various U.S. regions, including the Midwest (Peltzer et al., 2017; Webel & Higgins, 2012), the Northeast (Amutah et al., 2016; Amutah-Onukagha et al., 2018), the South (Boehme et al., 2014; Caiola et al., 2017, 2018; Fletcher et al., 2016; Muze & Onsomu, 2017; Tufts et al., 2010), and the West Coast (Murphy et al., 2011). See Table 8.2 for descriptive summaries of the included articles.

Consistent with Edeza et al. (2020), we organized the key themes identified during our analysis into three socioecological categories: (a) structural/societal, (b) interpersonal/social, and (c) individual/personal. Seven of the reviewed articles (63%) explicitly referenced structural/societal factors that impacted participants' experiences of motherhood while living with HIV. All 11 articles (100%) discussed interpersonal/social and individual/personal factors that impacted these experiences. In the remainder of this section, we discuss the themes we identified within each socioecological category, using relevant participant quotes (taken verbatim from the reviewed articles) to support our assertions.

Structural/Societal-Level Factors

Structural/societal-level factors relevant to African American mothers' experiences of living with HIV included the continued impact of societal stigma pertaining to HIV, intersectional (i.e., gender-, race-, and class-based) inequality, and barriers/facilitators to HIV-related care.

Societal HIV stigma. A number of the reviewed studies highlighted participants' perceptions regarding the continued impact of HIV-related stigma in American society (Caiola et al., 2017, 2018; Murphy et al., 2011; Muze & Onsomu, 2017; Peltzer et al., 2017; Tufts et al., 2010; Webel & Higgins, 2012) – noting, in particular, how this stigma impacted their relationships, health

Table 8.2 Brief Details about the Reviewed Studies

Author(s), year	*Title*	*Aim/focus*	*Participants/setting*	*Methodology*
Amutah et al. (2016)	Shaping the conversation: A secondary analysis of reproductive decision-making among Black mothers with HIV	Examines major influencers on mothers with HIV in their childbearing decisions, as well as how those influencers shape conversations with clinicians and healthcare providers regarding HIV treatment and prevention	Mothers living with HIV (N = 15); the majority of participants (n = 13) were African American Recruited from a single pediatric clinic located in New Jersey	Secondary analysis of in-depth interviews Thematic analysis
Amutah-Onukagha et al. (2018)	Missed opportunities for HIV prevention: Results of a qualitative study on mother-daughter communication	Examines the role of communication among African American mothers living with HIV and their daughters in HIV prevention	African American mothers living with HIV (N = 15) and their daughters (N = 15) Recruited from multiple HIV/AIDS clinics in Newark, New Jersey	Semi-structured interviews informed by Unified Theory of Behavior Change and the Normative Interpersonal Communication Theory Thematic analysis
Boehme et al. (2014)	A qualitative study on factors impacting HIV care adherence among postpartum HIV-infected women in the rural southeastern USA	Explores barriers and facilitators to HIV care experienced by postpartum women living with HIV	Mothers living with HIV (N = 18); majority of participants (n = 15) were African American Recruited from multiple HIV/AIDS clinics located in Alabama	Focus groups and Nominal Group Technique interviews (also included a survey component) Content analysis
Caiola et al. (2017)	Capturing the social location of African American mothers living with HIV: An inquiry into how social determinants of health are framed	Explores the social determinants of health for African American mothers living with HIV by examining how mothers describe their social location at the intersection of gender-, race-, and class inequality; HIV-related stigma; and motherhood	African American mothers living with HIV (N =18) Recruitment strategies included posting flyers at infectious disease clinics in North Carolina and mailing a study invitation	Three in-depth interviews over an eight-week period; second interview was conducted using a photo elicitation technique Content Analysis

(*Continued*)

Author(s), year	*Title*	*Aim/focus*	*Participants/setting*	*Methodology*
Caiola et al. (2018)	Black mothers living with HIV picture the social determinants of health	Explores the social determinants of health for Black mothers living with HIV in the southeastern region of the United States using a photo elicitation technique	African American mothers living with HIV (N =18) Recruitment strategies included posting flyers at infectious disease clinics in North Carolina and mailing a study invitation	Three in-depth interviews over an eight-week period; second interview was conducted using a photo elicitation technique Content Analysis
Fletcher et al. (2016)	"Out of all of this mess, I got a blessing':' perceptions and experiences of reproduction and motherhood in African American women living with HIV	Explores perspectives related to reproduction and motherhood in HIV-infected African American women of child- bearing capacity	African American women living with HIV who had children or were of childbearing age (N = 42) Recruited from five healthcare clinics and AIDS service organizations in South Carolina	Semi-structured interviews Thematic Analysis
Murphy et al. (2011)	HIV disease impact on mothers: What they miss during their children's developmental years	Explores whether or not mothers living with HIV felt that HIV had caused them to miss activities with their children while the children were growing up, what types of activities they had missed, the age of the child for each example, and how HIV had led to missing these activities	Mothers living with HIV (N = 57); approximately 35% of participants (n = 20) were African American Random sample of participants drawn from the Parents and Adolescents Coping Together III study (PACT III) who were originally recruited from Los Angeles, CA	In-depth interviews Grounded theory analysis
Muze & Onsomu (2017)	Our children, our hope: Voices of African American mothers living with HIV and rearing uninfected children	Focuses on the day-to-day experiences of African American mothers living with HIV who were caring for "uninfected" children	African American mothers living with HIV (N = 8) Recruited from a single community-based wellness agency in North Carolina	In-depth interviews Phenomenology; content analysis

Peltzer et al. (2017)	A qualitative description of HIV-infected African American women's experiences of psychological distress and their coping strategies	Examines experiences of psychological distress and use of coping strategies among African American women living with HIV	African American women living with HIV (N = 22) who reported psychological distress; 21 of the women had at least one child (M = 2) and one was pregnant Recruited from an internal medicine clinic in Kansas and an infectious disease clinic in Missouri	In-depth interviews Inductive content analysis
Tufts et al. (2010)	Self-care behaviors of African American women living with HIV: A qualitative perspective	Focuses on how African American women living with HIV women define self-care and what facilitates and hinders SC behaviors among these women	African American women living with HIV (N = 21); approximately 81% of the women (n = 17) had at least one child Recruited from a clinical practice that provided HIV care and treatment, two local AIDS service organizations, and community settings (i.e., beauty shops, laundromats, and takeout restaurants) in the southeastern US	Focus groups Content analysis
Webel & Higgins (2012)	The relationship between social roles and self-management behavior in women living with HIV/AIDS	Examines the main social roles of women living with HIV and explores how these roles relate to their self-management of HIV	Women living with HIV (N = 42); approximately 69% (n = 33) were African American and approximately 94% (n = 45) had at least one child or were pregnant Recruited through flyers posted at infectious disease clinics and AIDS service organizations located around Cleveland, OH	Focus groups Content Analysis

behaviors, and mental health status (see following sections for details). In many cases, study participants explained that the continued presence of societal-level stigma was linked to insufficient information about HIV and the tendency to equate it with irresponsible or immoral behavior. For instance, a participant in the Peltzer et al. (2017) study stated, "I'm not open with my diagnosis due to stigma and the ignorance" (p. 232); another participant in the same study offered the following example to illustrate the latter point:

> I don't get the stigma ... it's the same thing as cancer .... If I came and tell you I have leukemia, first thing you're going to say is, 'How can I help you? What do you need?' But I come and say I have HIV and the first thing you ask is, 'How'd you get it? What did you do?'
>
> (Peltzer et al., 2017, p. 231)

Intersectional discrimination and inequality. A few of the studies also described how experiences of HIV-related stigma were compounded by wider forms of intersectional (i.e., gender, race-, and class-based) discrimination and inequality (Boehme et al., 2014; Caiola et al., 2017, 2018; Murphy et al., 2011; Muze & Onsomu, 2017; Peltzer et al., 2017). This finding was most prominent in the Caiola et al. (2017) study, where the authors shared examples of participants explicitly identifying "the multidimensional and negative intersection of race, gender and HIV-related stigma" (p. 214); one participant, for example, stated:

> I don't know, it's like a lot of people ... for a Black woman, to me, they find out you're HIV or AIDS, you've got to be, you've got to have been a prostitute. Or you had to sell your body or you're considered a little bit like nasty ... you just can't let everybody know, it's not that I'm ashamed of this but there's a lot of cruelty out there you know?
>
> (Caiola et al., 2017, p. 214)

Other studies noted how structural inequalities driven by sexism and racism impacted participants' ability to access gainful employment or to secure safe, affordable housing, which in turn affected participants ability to pay for their antiretroviral medication and provide material resources for their children (Boehme et al., 2014; Caiola et al., 2018; Murphy et al., 2011; Muze & Onsomu, 2017; Peltzer et al., 2017).

Structural barriers and facilitators to HIV-related care. Participants in some of the reviewed studies also identified structural-level factors that served as barriers or facilitators to accessing HIV-related care. For example, participants in two studies identified unreliable mass transit systems and a lack of personal transportation as barriers to attending clinic visits (Boehme et al., 2014; Caiola et al., 2018). At an organizational level, participants in the Boehme et al. (2014) study identified scheduling conflicts (i.e., clinic office hours only being during typical working hours) and the lack of childcare services at healthcare facilities as barriers to scheduling and attending medical appointments; participants in the same study noted that this barrier could be offset to some extent by providers being available via telephone outside of typical clinic hours, which helped facilitate access to information, advice or both regarding their medication or other forms of self-care (Boehme et al., 2014).

Interpersonal/Social-Level Factors

Participants across the reviewed studies identified several salient interpersonal factors that impacted their experiences; these included encountering stigma in their social network, the dialectical nature of motherhood while living with HIV, the importance of social support, and varied perceptions of healthcare providers.

Enacted and anticipated HIV stigma. Although a number of studies addressed HIV-related stigma as a societal-level issue (see above), it was most often identified within interpersonal contexts – as study participants reported experiences with enacted stigma, anticipated stigma or both (see Earnshaw & Chaudoir, 2009) in their personal and professional relationships (Amutah et al., 2016; Caiola et al., 2017, 2018; Fletcher et al., 2016; Murphy et al., 2011; Muze & Onsomu, 2017; Peltzer et al., 2017; Tufts et al., 2010; Webel & Higgins, 2012). For example, participants in the Peltzer et al. (2017) study stated that they had friends and family members "turn on them" after disclosing their HIV diagnosis; likewise, a participant in the Tufts et al. (2010) study described encountering HIV-related stigma in the workplace, her faith community, and her own family: "I work with children, and my coworkers at the daycare say stupid things. At church they say stupid things. I want to blurt it out. I was scared. Even family will look at you like the ground" (p. 45). Some studies also reported that women felt stigmatized when interacting with healthcare providers (Amutah et al., 2016; Fletcher et al., 2016; Tufts et al., 2010; Webel & Higgins, 2012), with one participant telling Fletcher et al. (2016), "[T]here's still a lot of healthcare providers that live with [HIV-related] stigma" (p. 385).

These experiences made participants across several of the reviewed studies leery of disclosing their HIV status to others, even those closest to them (Amutah et al., 2016; Caiola et al., 2017; Murphy et al., 2011; Muze & Onsomu, 2017; Peltzer et al., 2017; Tufts et al., 2010; Webel & Higgins, 2012). A participant in the Amutah et al. (2016) study, for example, described her decision to withhold the information from her husband:

> I have this greatest fear. That's why I haven't told my husband. I have this greatest fear that he's just gonna disown me and the children. He loves me but this is a thing where it would really put this love to the test. Does he love me enough to understand?
>
> (p. S6)

Participants in some studies also worried about indirect disclosures – going as far as to avoid social situations, including their children's activities and events (Murphy et al., 2011; Peltzer et al., 2017), or refusing to take their antiretroviral medication in public spaces (Boehme et al., 2014) so as not to raise questions about their HIV status.

The dialectical nature of motherhood while living with HIV. Several studies also highlighted the dialectical nature of motherhood while living with HIV (Amutah et al., 2016; Amutah-Onukagha et al., 2018; Boehme et al., 2014; Caiola et al., 2017; Fletcher et al., 2016; Murphy et al., 2011; Muze & Onsomu, 2017; Tufts et al., 2010; Webel & Higgins, 2012). This idea is captured by a participant in Muze and Onsomu's (2017) study who stated:

> Sometimes, I just break down and cry, just seeing everything falling-down on me, but when I look at them, I say it's because of my children .... Taking care of them removes all worry about my situation from my mind. Sometimes I just wish that somebody would call and try to rescue me or something .... Of course, taking care of my child throws off my whole day because the focus is on my child.
>
> (p. 164)

As the participant cited above explained, women across the reviewed studies described their children as sources of "inspiration," "motivation," and "support," frequently identifying their maternal responsibilities as a reason to be more proactive about their HIV care and general health (Amutah et al., 2016; Boehme et al., 2014; Caiola et al., 2017; Fletcher et al., 2016; Muze & Onsomu, 2017; Tufts et al., 2010; Webel & Higgins, 2012). At the same time, however, participants also discussed the challenges they faced in attempting to care for their children while navigating the physical and emotional difficulties associated with HIV, most notably the side effects of their antiretroviral medication. More specifically, study participants recounted having trouble completing household tasks and not being able to engage in active playtimes; they also recalled missing out on their children's school and extracurricular activities because they did not feel well enough to attend (Caiola et al., 2017; Murphy et al., 2011; Muze & Onsomu, 2017; Tufts et al., 2010). Furthermore, a few studies also noted that attempting to prioritize their children's needs negatively impacted participants' HIV-related behaviors, such as by disrupting their medication-intake schedule or leading them to miss medical appointments (Boehme et al., 2014; Caiola et al., 2017; Murphy et al., 2011; Webel & Higgins, 2012). For instance, a postpartum participant in the Boehme et al. (2014) study explained how caring for her children led her to simply forget to take her medication: "When you got a child, you have to feed right at that moment, you can't stop [and it disrupts your schedule and you forget]" (p. 578).

The importance of social support. Considering the unique challenges associated with motherhood while living with HIV, participants in several of the reviewed studies emphasized the importance of receiving social support (Amutah et al., 2016; Boehme et al., 2014; Caiola et al., 2018; Muze & Onsomu, 2017; Peltzer et al., 2017; Tufts et al., 2010; Webel & Higgins, 2012). For example, women in the Boehme et al. (2014) study noted that family members (i.e., intimate partners, parents, and uncles) helped facilitate their attendance at clinical appointments as well as remind them to consistently take their antiretroviral medication; one participant, for instance, stated, "My old man. He reminds me a lot. Did you take your medicine today? You know, and he gets it for me" (Boehme et al., 2014, p. 579). For other women, it was their children who served as a primary source of support. A participant in the Tufts et al. study (2010), for example, described being supported by her daughter after being diagnosed; she recounted:

> When I first find out that I had the virus, I was so sad. I didn't want to come out. At the time I had this really supportive daughter that supported me all the way. She would say, 'Ma, that don't mean because you got that that people won't love you.' She the one that really brought me out.
>
> (Tufts et al., 2010, p. 44)

Participants in some of the reviewed studies also highlighted the HIV-related support they received from their religious communities (Caiola et al., 2018; Peltzer et al., 2017; Tufts et al., 2010).

In addition to the reviewed articles that highlighted how participants benefitted from social support, some studies identified the hardships that African American mothers living with HIV faced in its absence – with study participants in this situation reporting that they felt "isolated," "lonely," and "overwhelmed" without others to support them (Muze & Onsomu, 2017; Peltzer et al., 2017; Tufts et al., 2010; Webel & Higgins, 2012). In one study (Muze & Onsomu, 2017), participants also noted how the absence of supportive relationships made them fearful of what would happen to their children if they were to die or become incapacitated; one participant, for example, said, "Because I don't have any family to help me, sometimes I get scared thinking that about my child having to be raised by some stranger if something happens to me" (Muze & Onsomu, 2017, p. 165). Despite recognizing that they could benefit from social support, some participants in these studies were often reluctant to ask for it from their family and friends due to past negative experiences (Muze & Onsomu, 2017; Webel & Higgins, 2012) or to seek it from formal sources, such as support groups, due to confidentiality concerns (Peltzer et al., 2017; Tufts et al., 2010).

Another way that participants emphasized the importance of social support (or its absence) was related to reproductive health decisions. More specifically, participants in the Amutah et al. (2016) study revealed that their decisions about future pregnancies and their contraceptive options were mainly influenced by family members (specifically mothers and grandmothers) rather than healthcare providers. Similarly, the mothers in the Amutah-Onukagha et al. (2018) study described themselves as their daughters' primary resource for matters pertaining to HIV and reproductive health.

Varied perceptions of healthcare providers. Participants in the reviewed studies varied in their perceptions of relationships with healthcare providers. While, in some cases, women described feeling stigmatized by healthcare providers (Webel & Higgins, 2012) or avoiding discussing important topics with them (Amutah et al., 2016), participants' experiences in other studies were more mixed (Boehme et al., 2014; Fletcher et al., 2016; Tufts et al., 2010). This variability was particularly evident in the Fletcher et al. (2016) study, which focused largely on experiences pertaining to conception and pregnancy. For example, one participant expressed frustration that her providers frequently encouraged her to undergo a tubal ligation to avoid future pregnancies; she recalled, "Every visit they [healthcare providers] wanted to know whether I was gonna get my tubes tied. That [my status] shouldn't deter me whether I'm gonna have my tubes tied after having this baby" (Fletcher et al., 2016, p. 385). Alternatively, a participant in the same study described her healthcare providers as being supportive and providing her with advice to make an informed decision about getting pregnant:

> They [health care providers] got the same idea I have … just because you're positive … as long as you take your medicine and do what you're supposed to do, they don't see why a pregnancy is not something that you can do.
> (Fletcher et al., 2016, p. 385)

Individual/Personal-Level Factors

Individual/personal-level factors that impacted African American mothers' experiences of living with HIV included orienting to their identity as mothers, identifying the impact of HIV on their physical and mental health status, and personal feelings about reproductive health.

Orienting to their identity as mothers. Consistent with what past studies have described as a "mother-first" orientation (Basu & Dutta, 2011; Kedia et al., 2019), participants in the reviewed articles largely preferred to identify with and prioritize their role as mothers (Boehme et al., 2014; Caiola et al., 2017; Fletcher et al., 2016; Murphy et al., 2011; Muze & Onsomu, 2017; Tufts et al., 2010; Webel & Higgins, 2012). For example, when asked to choose the identity that most defined them and their experiences, the majority of women living with HIV who participated in Webel and Higgins' (2012) study chose a maternal one – with one participant stating that, above all else, "I'm the mom and I'm the grandma and I'm the auntie that likes to kick it with the young crowd" (p. e29). Likewise, Caiola et al. (2017) noted that for the majority of women who participated in their study, orienting towards motherhood acted as "an opposing health determinant" in their lives "against the HIV-related stigma and racism" they experienced (p. 214). One participant, for instance, described how motherhood "buffered" the negative effects of living with HIV while noting that her diagnosis simultaneously enhanced her maternal identity; she said, "So you know just being a mom and trying to be here for my children makes it [living with HIV] better for me" (Caiola et al., 2017, p. 216).

The physical and mental impacts of living with HIV. Several of the reviewed studies also highlighted various impacts that living with HIV had on participants' physical and mental health status (Caiola et al., 2017; Murphy et al., 2011; Muze & Onsomu, 2017; Peltzer et al., 2017; Tufts et al., 2010; Webel & Higgins, 2012). The most commonly cited physical symptoms were overwhelming fatigue and digestive issues – which, as noted in the previous section, were often associated with taking antiretroviral medication. For instance, when asked about her physical symptoms, a participant in the Murphy et al. (2011) study replied, "Fatigue ... I feel like I get tired—it will come like you can't control it .... It's not tired whereby I will try and force myself. No—it's that and that's it" (p. 365). Similarly, a woman in Muze and Onsomu's (2017) study stated:

> Some days, I don't feel like getting out of bed when I'm having nausea because of my HIV medicine, but because of my son, I force myself to. Sometimes, I don't even have enough energy to take care of myself on days that I fall sick.
>
> (p. 165)

As noted in the previous section and the quote cited above, participants often felt compelled to "power through" (Murphy et al., 2011) their physical symptoms to fulfill their caregiving responsibilities.

In addition to the physical impacts of HIV, some of the reviewed articles also reported that study participants experienced mental health conditions, such as depression, anxiety, and extreme stress. Peltzer et al. (2017) used the term *psychoemotional suffering* to denote the "significant distress experienced by all of the participants following the diagnosis of HIV infection" (p. 230); they also reported that suicidality was common among their participants, with one woman telling them that she had tried to end her life at least six times: "I tried to run out in the street and get hit by a car ... I tried three times to slit my wrists" (Peltzer et al., 2017, p. 230). In some cases, participants reported that their mental health status was negatively impacted by the perception that living with HIV (and its associated challenges) diminished their ability to care for their children (Caiola et al., 2017; Murphy et al., 2011; Peltzer et al., 2017). In other instances, study participants attributed their mental health challenges to internalizing the stigma they encountered – i.e., feeling as if it was somehow deserved or justified (Caiola et al., 2017; Murphy et al., 2011; Peltzer et al., 2017; Webel & Higgins, 2012). For example, African American mothers in the Murphy et al. (2011) study alternately described living with HIV as making them feel "ashamed" or that they had been "defiled."

Feelings about reproductive health. The final individual-level theme identified in the reviewed studies reflected participants' personal feelings regarding issues pertaining to reproductive health (Amutah et al., 2016; Amutah-Onukagha et al., 2018; Fletcher et al., 2016). The Amutah-Onukagha et al. (2018) study focused on how African American women living with HIV communicated with their daughters about reproductive health and HIV; their findings suggested that participants viewed communicating about reproductive health – especially the risks associated with HIV and other sexually transmitted infections – to be highly important and generally expressed a great deal of confidence in their ability to discuss such matters effectively.

Two other studies focused on how African American mothers living with HIV perceived the risks associated with future pregnancies. Participants in the Amutah et al. (2016) study generally expressed negative attitudes towards future pregnancies, frequently identifying the risk of perinatal transmission as a key factor. One participant, for example, explained that her desire to have multiple children shifted after being diagnosed with HIV during her first pregnancy:

> Well I did want to have at least two children …. But now that I know I'm HIV-positive I know that I shouldn't, it's not wise for me to have another child because that child could come out infected. I was blessed with my son but I don't know the chances of my next child being infected and I wouldn't want to subject them to that.
>
> (Amutah et al., 2016, p. S5)

The women who participated in the Fletcher et al. (2016) study were more varied in their feelings about future pregnancies; however, as with participants in the Amutah et al. (2016) study, the driving factor appeared to be their perception regarding the risk of perinatal transmission. For instance, a participant who felt positively about future pregnancies emphasized that she viewed the risk of perinatal transmission as minimal for women who consistently took their antiretroviral medication; she said, "Make sure that you take your medication so you'll be undetected like myself and because there's a 1% chance that your child could have it" (Fletcher et al., 2016, p. 385).

Discussion

This meta-ethnography identified critical themes pertaining to the experiences of African American mothers living with HIV in the United States. The reviewed articles represent the lived experiences of 207 participants across 11 articles residing in diverse U.S. regions. Our analysis of these articles extracted a number of salient factors that impact participants' day-to-day lives at the structural/societal level (i.e., societal-level stigma; intersectional discrimination and inequality; structural barriers and facilitators to HIV-related care), the interpersonal/social level (i.e., anticipated and enacted stigma; the dialectical nature of motherhood; the importance of social support; varied perceptions of healthcare providers), and the personal/individual level (orienting to the identity of motherhood; physical and mental health status; reproductive health perceptions).

The socioecological themes identified across the reviewed articles offer insight into the disconnect between "post-AIDS" discourse and the day-to-day realities of living with HIV – particularly for marginalized populations such as African American mothers. The success of biotechnical innovations such as antiretroviral therapies (and, more recently, pre-exposure prophylaxis) have undoubtedly transformed the experience of living with HIV and emboldened policymakers to cast an optimistic vision of a "post-AIDs" world. However, suggesting that the proliferation of these technologies signals that society has moved beyond HIV is a misplaced notion that, as Walker (2020) argues, negates "the embodied and structural experience of living with HIV and AIDS" in contemporary society (p. 95).

Consistent with Walker's (2020) argument, the best evidence that society has not moved beyond HIV is the enduring reality of HIV-related stigma. As recounted by the African American mothers in the studies reviewed here, HIV is far from transforming into an "ordinary illness" (Sontag, 1989); instead, living with HIV continues to serve as a deeply discrediting attribute (Goffman, 1963) that permeates every area of their lives, contributing to negative health outcomes, limiting their ability/willingness to seek needed social support, and compromising their ability to care for themselves and their children. The impact of HIV-related stigma on participants' social support is particularly important. Consistent with a number of extant studies indicating a positive link between social support and HIV-related outcomes, including antiretroviral adherence and improved mental health (DiMatteo, 2004; Edwards, 2006; Knowlton et al., 2007; Turan et al., 2016; Vyavaharkar et al., 2011), participants in the reviewed studies frequently highlighted the various ways they benefited from the support they received from family members, friends, and members of their faith communities. Alternatively, when the women's loved ones "turned on" them (Peltzer et al., 2017) or it was perceived that they would (Amutah et al., 2016) due to HIV-related stigma, the women were left on their own.

According to the reviewed studies, HIV-related stigma also appears, in some cases, to compel them to prioritize their identity as mothers – an orientation that has been described elsewhere as "mother-first identity" (Basu & Dutta, 2011; Kedia et al., 2019). While this orientation can serve a symbolic and motivational function, there is evidence that prioritizing motherhood in this way can produce negative consequences for mothers living with HIV if they begin to feel as though their physical limitations (or other factors) are preventing them from living up to the maternal caregiving standards they have set for themselves or have internalized from external sources. More specifically, this perception can lead to depressive symptoms and internalized stigma, which in turn are associated with reduced antiretroviral therapy adherence (see, e.g., Kedia et al., 2019; Turan et al., 2016).

In addition to the enduring presence of HIV-related stigma, Walker (2020) further argues that "post-AIDS" discourse has traditionally overlooked the ways that "intersectional vulnerabilities" (e.g., those associated with race, class, and sexuality) impact the experience of living with HIV and vice versa. Likewise, participants in the reviewed studies noted how varied forms of discrimination and economic insecurity exacerbated the challenges of living with HIV, noting, in particular, how their limited access to economic resources and the lack of flexibility in their employment arrangements compromised their HIV-related care and the ability to care for their children. Participants also described the difficulties associated with securing safe, affordable housing and being forced to use unreliable mass transit systems because they did not have access to personal transportation.

Although HIV-related stigma and intersectional vulnerability have frequently been overlooked in contemporary "post-AIDS" discourse (Walker, 2020), there is some evidence that this trend may be shifting. For example, in a recent article published in *Lancet HIV*, Andersson et al. (2020) highlighted the growing movement to account for the concurrent challenges facing "people living and aging with HIV who still have suboptimal [health-related quality of life],

with regards to their mental, sexual, and physical wellbeing" (p. e129; see also Lazarus et al., 2016). In particular, they highlighted the need for increased efforts to understand how HIV-related stigma occurs at various socioecological levels within specific populations and to develop stigma-reduction interventions that address the needs of people who experience intersectional inequality (Andersson et al., 2020). Although there are, to our knowledge, currently no stigma-reduction interventions that have been designed specifically for African American mothers living with HIV, there are at least two reported interventions that could potentially be adapted to their needs. Rao et al. (2012) reported that a workshop intervention designed for African American women living with HIV resulted in a statistically significant reduction in self-reported internalized stigma; likewise, Barroso et al. (2014) reported similar results in participants' response to a digital stigma-reduction intervention designed for women living with HIV in the American South. Ideally, any stigma-reduction efforts targeted to African American mothers living with HIV would also be coupled with resource-based interventions, such as those described by Webel et al. (2013) – i.e., those that provide access to material resources and instrumental support in the form of childcare, financial assistance, and stable housing.

Limitations

The review presented in this chapter should be considered in light of some potential limitations. First, despite a thorough and meticulous literature search, it is possible that we may have overlooked potentially relevant research reports. In the same vein, we restricted our searches to only peer-reviewed journal articles to limit the scope of this synthesis to manuscripts with well-defined goals that align with the primary focus of this review. Second, while we believe our analysis is representative of the experiences of the African American mothers living with HIV who participated in the reviewed studies, it is important to note that the themes and (especially) the quotations were already selections from large data sets that the respective authors already selected to support a particular line of argument in the original articles (Atkins et al., 2008; Dillon & Basu, 2014). Finally, it should be noted that, as others have argued (see, e.g., France et al., 2014), synthesizing previous findings in the manner prescribed by meta-ethnography sacrifices some of the contextual nuance that is a hallmark of qualitative scholarship; ultimately, however, we align with those who argue that, despite its limitations, synthesizing qualitative health research in this manner "facilitates a broader impact and interpretability for individual qualitative works, and is critical to advancing the state of this literature" (Edeza et al., 2020, p. 7) on a specific research topic.

Conclusion

Shortly after Dr. Robert Redfield finished his opening remarks at the HIV Prevention Conference, Dr. Anthony Fauci, Director of the National Institute of Health's National Institute of Allergy and Infectious Diseases, stepped to the microphone to share his thoughts on the ambitious plan outlined in *Ending the Epidemic*. As he concluded, Dr. Fauci spoke of the "highly effective" tools developed to eliminate new HIV transmissions and the ethical and moral responsibility that the nation has to implement them (Department of Health and Human Services 2019a).

There is no debate that reducing the number of people living with HIV is an important and laudable goal. However, harkening back to Dr. Gail King's words and the words of the African American mothers living with HIV who took part in the studies reviewed as part of this synthesis, it is equally important to remember the ethical and moral responsibility that the country has to those already living with HIV, especially within communities of color. As our analysis suggests, focusing on addressing the enduring presence of HIV-related stigma and the intersectional vulnerabilities that characterize their experiences is an excellent place to begin.

Note

1 Consistent with previous meta-ethnographies (see, e.g., Dillon & Basu, 2014), we chose to integrate studies that included participants outside of our population of focus (i.e., participants who did not identify as African American or who did not have children) as long as the articles clearly attributed specific ideas/experiences to African American mothers living with HIV (see Table 8.2 for study details)

References

Amutah, N. N., Gifuni, J., & Wesley, Y. (2016). Shaping the conversation: A secondary analysis of reproductive decision-making among Black mothers with HIV. *Clinical Medicine Insights: Women's Health*, 9s1. https://doi.org/10.4137/CMWH.S34671

Amutah-Onukagha, N. N., Opara, I., Hammonds, R., & Guthrie, B. (2018). Missed opportunities for HIV prevention: Results of a qualitative study on mother-daughter communication. *Journal of HIV/AIDS & Social Services, 17*(4), 384–401. https://doi.org/10.1080/15381501.2018.1502708

Andersson, G. Z., Reinius, M., Eriksson, L. E., Svedhem, V., Esfahani, F. M., Deuba, K., ... Ekström, A. M. (2020). Stigma reduction interventions in people living with HIV to improve health-related quality of life. *The Lancet HIV, 7*(2), e129–e140. https://doi.org/10.1016/S2352-3018(19)30343-1

Atkins, S., Lewin, S., Smith, H., Engel, M., Fretheim, A., & Volmink, J. (2008). Conducting a meta-ethnography of qualitative literature: Lessons learnt. *BMC Medical Research Methodology, 8*(1), 21. https://doi.org/10.1186/1471-2288-8-21

Auerbach, J. D., Parkhurst, J. O., & Cáceres, C. F. (2011). Addressing social drivers of HIV/AIDS for the long-term response: Conceptual and methodological considerations. *Global Public Health, 6*(sup3), S293–S309. https://doi.org/10.1080/17441692.2011.594451

Baral, S., Logie, C. H., Grosso, A., Wirtz, A. L., & Beyrer, C. (2013). Modified social ecological model: A tool to guide the assessment of the risks and risk contexts of HIV epidemics. *BMC Public Health, 13*(1), 482. https://doi.org/10.1186/1471-2458-13-482

Barnes, D. B., & Murphy, S. (2009). Reproductive decisions for women with HIV: Motherhood's role in envisioning a future. *Qualitative Health Research, 19*(4), 481–491. https://doi.org/10.1177/1049732309332835

Barroso, J., Relf, M. V., Williams, M. S., Arscott, J., Moore, E. D., Caiola, C., & Silva, S. G. (2014). A randomized controlled trial of the efficacy of a stigma reduction intervention for HIV-infected women in the Deep South. *AIDS Patient Care and STDs, 28*(9), 489–498. https://doi.org/10.1089/apc.2014.0014

Basu, A., & Dutta, M. J. (2011). 'We are mothers first': Localocentric articulation of sex worker identity as a key in HIV/AIDS communication. *Women & Health, 51*(2), 106–123. https://doi.org/10.1080/03630242.2010.550992

Bekker, L.-G., Ratevosian, J., Spencer, J., Piot, P., & Beyrer, C. (2019). Governance for health: The HIV response and general global health. *Bulletin of the World Health Organization, 97*(3), 170–170A. https://doi.org/10.2471/BLT.19.230417

Blanche, S. (2020). Mini review: Prevention of mother–child transmission of HIV: 25 years of continuous progress toward the eradication of pediatric AIDS? *Virulence, 11*(1), 14–22. https://doi.org/10.1080/21505594.2019.1697136

Boehme, A. K., Davies, S. L., Moneyham, L., Shrestha, S., Schumacher, J., & Kempf, M. C. (2014). A qualitative study on factors impacting HIV care adherence among postpartum HIV-infected women in the rural southeastern USA. *AIDS Care, 26*(5), 574–581. https://doi.org/10.1080/09540121.2013.844759

Borgnakke, K., & Hillyard, S. (2020). Meta-Ethnography. *SAGE Research Methods Foundations.* Retrieved from https://doi.org/10.4135/9781526421036857960

Bosma, H., Apland, L., & Kazanjian, A. (2010). Review: Cultural conceptualizations of hospice palliative care: more similarities than differences. *Palliative Medicine, 24*(5), 510–522. https://doi.org/10.1177/0269216309351380

Caiola, C., Barroso, J., & Docherty, S. L. (2017). Capturing the social location of African American mothers living with HIV: An inquiry into how social determinants of health are framed. *Nursing Research, 66*(3), 209–221. https://doi.org/10.1097/NNR.0000000000000213

Caiola, C., Barroso, J., & Docherty, S. L. (2018). Black mothers living with HIV picture the social determinants of health. *Journal of the Association of Nurses in AIDS Care, 29*(2), 204–219. https://doi.org/10.1016/j.jana.2017.09.011

Caiola, C., Docherty, S. L., Relf, M., & Barroso, J. (2014). using an intersectional approach to study the impact of social determinants of health for African American mothers living with HIV. *Advances in Nursing Science, 37*(4), 287–298. https://doi.org/10.1097/ANS.0000000000000046

Campbell, R., Pound, P., Pope, C., Britten, N., Pill, R., Morgan, M., & Donovan, J. (2003). Evaluating meta-ethnography: A synthesis of qualitative research on lay experiences of diabetes and diabetes care. *Social Science & Medicine, 56*(4), 671–684. https://doi.org/10.1016/S0277-9536(02)00064-3

Centers for Disease Control and Prevention. (2017). *HIV Mortality 2017.* Retrieved from https://www.cdc.gov/hiv/pdf/library/slidesets/cdc-hiv-surveillance-mortality-2017.pdf

Centers for Disease Control and Prevention. (2018a). *HIV surveillance in women 2018 (preliminary).* Retrieved from https://www.cdc.gov/hiv/pdf/library/slidesets/cdc-hiv-surveillance-women-2018.pdf

Centers for Disease Control and Prevention. (2018b). *HIV by group: Pregnant women, infants, and children.* Retrieved from https://www.cdc.gov/hiv/group/gender/pregnantwomen/index.html

Centers for Disease Control and Prevention. (2018c). *HIV by group: Women.* Retrieved from https://www.cdc.gov/hiv/group/gender/women/index.html

Centers for Disease Control and Prevention. (2020). *HIV surveillance report 2018 (updated).* Retrieved from https://www.cdc.gov/hiv/pdf/library/reports/surveillance/cdc-hiv-surveillance-report-2018-updated-vol-31.pdf

Cohen, M. H., Cook, J. A., Grey, D., Young, M., Hanau, L. H., Tien, P., … Wilson, T. E. (2004). Medically eligible women who do not use HAART: The importance of abuse, drug use, and race. *American Journal of Public Health, 94*(7), 1147–1151. https://doi.org/10.2105/AJPH.94.7.1147

Dasgupta, S., Oster, A. M., Li, J., & Hall, H. I. (2016). Disparities in consistent retention in HIV care—11 states and the District of Columbia, 2011–2013. *Morbidity and Mortality Weekly Report, 65.* https://doi.org/10.15585/mmwr.mm6504a2

Dedoose (6.1.18). (2015). [Computer software]. SocioCultural Research Consultants. www.dedoose.com

DeNavas-Walt, C., & Proctor, B. D. (2014). *Income and poverty in the United States: 2013.* U.S. Department of Commerce, Economics and Statistics Administration, U.S. Census Bureau: Washington, DC.

Department of Health and Human Services. (2019a, March 19). *CDC National HIV Prevention Conference opens with focus on ending the HIV epidemic.* Retrieved from https://www.hiv.gov/blog/cdc-national-hiv-prevention-conference-opens-focus-ending-hiv-epidemic

Department of Health and Human Services. (2019b, March 25). *HIV stigma in focus at closing session of CDC's National HIV Prevention Conference.* Retrieved from https://www.hiv.gov/blog/hiv-stigma-focus-closing-session-cdc-s-national-hiv-prevention-conference

Department of Health and Human Services. (2020, May 8). *What is ending the HIV epidemic: A plan for America?* Retrieved from https://www.hiv.gov/federal-response/ending-the-hiv-epidemic/overview

Dillon, P. J., & Basu, A. (2014). HIV/AIDS and minority men who have sex with men: A meta-ethnographic synthesis of qualitative research. *Health Communication, 29*(2), 182–192. https://doi.org/10.1080/10410236.2012.732911

Dillon, P. J., Roscoe, L. A., & Jenkins, J. J. (2012). African Americans and decisions about hospice care: Implications for health message design. *Howard Journal of Communications, 23*(2), 175–193. https://doi.org/10.1080/10646175.2012.667724

DiMatteo, M. R. (2004). Social support and patient adherence to medical treatment: A meta-analysis. *Health Psychology, 23*(2), 207–218. https://doi.org/10.1037/0278-6133.23.2.207

Earnshaw, V. A., & Chaudoir, S. R. (2009). From conceptualizing to measuring HIV stigma: A review of HIV stigma mechanism measures. *AIDS and Behavior, 13*(6), 1160. https://doi.org/10.1007/s10461-009-9593-3

Edeza, A., Karina Santamaria, E., Valente, P. K., Gomez, A., Ogunbajo, A., & Biello, K. (2020). Experienced barriers to adherence to pre-exposure prophylaxis for HIV prevention among MSM: A systematic review and meta-ethnography of qualitative studies. *AIDS Care,* 1–9. https://doi.org/10.1080/09540121.2020.1778628

Edwards, L. V. (2006). Perceived social support and HIV/AIDS medication adherence among African American women. *Qualitative Health Research, 16*(5), 679–691. https://doi.org/10.1177/1049732305281597

Finocchario-Kessler, S., Sweat, M. D., Dariotis, J. K., Anderson, J. R., Jennings, J. M., Keller, J. M., … Trent, M. E. (2012). Childbearing motivations, pregnancy desires, and perceived partner response to a pregnancy among urban female youth: Does HIV-infection status make a difference? *AIDS Care, 24*(1), 1–11. https://doi.org/10.1080/09540121.2011.596514

Fletcher, F., Ingram, L. A., Kerr, J., Buchberg, M., Richter, D. L., & Sowell, R. (2016). "Out of all of this mess, I got a blessing": Perceptions and experiences of reproduction and motherhood in African American women living with HIV. *Journal of the Association of Nurses in AIDS Care, 27*(4), 381–391. https://doi.org/10.1016/j.jana.2015.12.003

France, E. F., Ring, N., Thomas, R., Noyes, J., Maxwell, M., & Jepson, R. (2014). A methodological systematic review of what's wrong with meta-ethnography reporting. *BMC Medical Research Methodology, 14*(1), 119. https://doi.org/10.1186/1471-2288-14-119

Geronimus, A. T. (1996). Black/white differences in the relationship of maternal age to birthweight: A population-based test of the weathering hypothesis. *Social Science & Medicine, 42*(4), 589–597. https://doi.org/10.1016/0277-9536(95)00159-X

Goffman, E. (1963). *Stigma: Notes on the management of spoiled identity.* New York: Simon & Schuster.

Grodensky, C. A., Golin, C. E., Jones, C., Mamo, M., Dennis, A. C., Abernethy, M. G., & Patterson, K. B. (2015). "I should know better": The roles of relationships, spirituality, disclosure, stigma, and shame for older women living with HIV seeking support in the South. *Journal of the Association of Nurses in AIDS Care, 26*(1), 12–23. https://doi.org/10.1016/j.jana.2014.01.005

Hess, K. L., Hu, X., Lansky, A., Mermin, J., & Hall, H. I. (2017). Lifetime risk of a diagnosis of HIV infection in the United States. *Annals of Epidemiology, 27*(4), 238–243. https://doi.org/10.1016/j.annepidem.2017.02.003

Joint United Nations Programme on HIV/AIDS. (2017, January). *90–90–90—an ambitious treatment target to help end the AIDS epidemic.* Retrieved from https://www.unaids.org/en/resources/documents/2017/90-90-90

Kaiser Family Foundation. (2020, March 9). *Women and HIV in the United States.* Retrieved from https://www.kff.org/hivaids/fact-sheet/women-and-hivaids-in-the-united-states/

Kapadia, F., & Landers, S. (2019). Ending the HIV epidemic: Getting to zero and staying at zero. *American Journal of Public Health, 110*(1), 15–16. https://doi.org/10.2105/AJPH.2019.305462

Kedia, S. K., Dillon, P. J., & Basu, A. (2019). A qualitative exploration of "mother first" identity and antiretroviral adherence among African American women living with HIV in the Mid-South region of the United States. *Health Communication,* 1–10. https://doi.org/10.1080/10410236.2019.1623641

Kennedy, V. L., Serghides, L., Raboud, J. M., Su, D., Blitz, S., Hart, T. A., … Loutfy, M. R. (2014). The importance of motherhood in HIV-positive women of reproductive age in Ontario, Canada. *AIDS Care, 26*(6), 777–784. https://doi.org/10.1080/09540121.2013.855295

Knowlton, A. R., Arnsten, J. H., Gourevitch, M. N., Eldred, L., Wilkinson, J. D., Rose, C. D., & INSPIRE Study Team. (2007). Microsocial environmental influences on highly active antiretroviral therapy outcomes among active injection drug users: The role of informal caregiving and household factors. *Journal of Acquired Immune Deficiency Syndromes, 46*, S110. https://doi.org/10.1097/QAI.0b013e31815767f8

Lazarus, J. V., Safreed-Harmon, K., Barton, S. E., Costagliola, D., Dedes, N., del Amo Valero, J., & Rockstroh, J. K. (2016). Beyond viral suppression of HIV – the new quality of life frontier. *BMC Medicine, 14*(1), 94. https://doi.org/10.1186/s12916-016-0640-4

Lillie-Blanton, M., Stone, V. E., Snow Jones, A., Levi, J., Golub, E. T., Cohen, M. H., ... Wilson, T. E. (2010). Association of race, substance abuse, and health insurance coverage with use of highly active antiretroviral therapy among HIV-infected women, 2005. *American Journal of Public Health, 100*(8), 1493–1499.

Lipira, L., Rao, D., Nevin, P. E., Kemp, C. G., Cohn, S. E., Turan, J. M., ... Williams, E. C. (2020). Patterns of alcohol use and associated characteristics and HIV-related outcomes among a sample of African-American women living with HIV. *Drug and Alcohol Dependence, 206*, 1–9. https://doi.org/10.1016/j.drugalcdep.2019.107753

Lipira, L., Williams, E. C., Huh, D., Kemp, C. G., Nevin, P. E., Greene, P., ... Rao, D. (2019). HIV- related stigma and viral suppression among African-American women: Exploring the mediating roles of depression and ART nonadherence. *AIDS and Behavior, 23*(8), 2025–2036. https://doi.org/10.1007/s10461-018-2301-4

Losina, E., Schackman, B. R., Sadownik, S. N., Gebo, K. A., Walensky, R. P., Chiosi, J. J. Freedberg, K. A. (2009). Racial and sex disparities in life expectancy losses among HIV-infected persons in the United States: Impact of risk behavior, late initiation, and early discontinuation of antiretroviral therapy. *Clinical Infectious Diseases, 49*(10), 1570–1578. https://doi.org/10.1086/644772

Matthews, T., Baken, D., Ross, K., Ogilvie, E., & Kent, L. (2019). The experiences of patients and their family members when receiving bad news about cancer: A qualitative meta-synthesis. *Psycho-Oncology, 28*(12), 2286–2294. https://doi.org/10.1002/pon.5241

Mazanderani, F., & Paparini, S. (2015). The stories we tell: Qualitative research interviews, talking technologies and the 'normalization' of life with HIV. *Social Science & Medicine, 131*, 66–73. https://doi.org/10.1016/j.socscimed.2015.02.041

Murphy, D. A., Roberts, K. J., & Herbeck, D. M. (2011). HIV disease impact on mothers: What they miss during their children's developmental years. *Journal of Child and Family Studies, 20(*3), 361–369. https://doi.org/10.1007/s10826-010-9400-9

Muze, R., & Onsomu, E. O. (2017). Our children, our hope: Voices of African American mothers living with HIV and rearing uninfected children. *Journal of Community Health Nursing, 34*(3), 160–168. https://doi.org/10.1080/07370016.2017.1340770

National Prevention Information Network. (2019, March 21). National HIV Prevention Conference: Closing plenary session. Retrieved from https://www.facebook.com/watch/live/?v=426124004860555&ref=watch_permalink

Nesheim, S. R., FitzHarris, L. F., Lampe, M. A., & Gray, K. M. (2018). Reconsidering the number of women with HIV infection who give birth annually in the United States. *Public Health Reports, 133*(6), 637–643. https://doi.org/10.1177/0033354918800466

Noblit, G. W., & Hare, R. D. (1988). *Meta-ethnography: Synthesizing qualitative studies.* Thousand Oaks, CA: SAGE.

Okoro, O., & Odedina, F. (2017). HIV treatment in African American women—care that makes a difference. *Journal of Racial and Ethnic Health Disparities, 4*(3), 376–384. https://doi.org/10.1007/s40615-016-0238-8

Peltzer, J. N., Ogawa, L., Tusher, S., Farnan, R., & Gerkovich, M. M. (2017). A qualitative description of HIV-infected African American women's experiences of psychological distress and their coping strategies. *Journal of the Association of Nurses in AIDS Care, 28*(2), 226–237. https://doi.org/10.1016/j.jana.2016.09.010

Persson, A. (2013). Non/infectious corporealities: Tensions in the biomedical era of 'HIV normalization.' *Sociology of Health & Illness, 35*(7), 1065–1079. https://doi.org/10.1111/1467-9566.12023

Popay, J., Rogers, A., & Williams, G. (1998). Rationale and standards for the systematic review of qualitative literature in health services research. *Qualitative Health Research, 8*(3), 341–351. https://doi.org/10.1177/104973239800800305

Rao, D., Desmond, M., Andrasik, M., Rasberry, T., Lambert, N., Cohn, S. E., & Simoni, J. (2012). Feasibility, acceptability, and preliminary efficacy of the Unity Workshop: An internalized stigma reduction intervention for African American women living with HIV. *AIDS Patient Care and STDs, 26*(10), 614–620. https://doi.org/10.1089/apc.2012.0106

Reif, S., Wilson, E., McAllaster, C., & Pence, B. (2019). The relationship of HIV-related stigma and health care outcomes in the US Deep South. *AIDS and Behavior, 23*(S3), 242–250. https://doi.org/10.1007/s10461-019-02595-5

Robinson, K., Fial, A., & Hanson, L. (2019). Racism, bias, and discrimination as modifiable barriers to breastfeeding for African American women: A scoping review of the literature. *Journal of Midwifery & Women's Health, 64*(6), 734–742. https://doi.org/10.1111/jmwh.13058

Schutz, A. (1962). *Collected papers, Vol. 1: The problem of social reality*, edited by M. Natanson. Hingham, MA: Kluwer Academic.

Sleijpen, M., Boeije, H. R., Kleber, R. J., & Mooren, T. (2016). Between power and powerlessness: A meta-ethnography of sources of resilience in young refugees. *Ethnicity & Health, 21*(2), 158–180. https://doi.org/10.1080/13557858.2015.1044946

Sontag, S. (1989). *AIDS and its metaphors.* New York: Penguin Books.

Thomas, J., & Harden, A. (2008). Methods for the thematic synthesis of qualitative research in systematic reviews. *BMC Medical Research Methodology, 8*(1), 45. https://doi.org/10.1186/1471-2288-8-45

Tufts, K. A., Wessell, J., & Kearney, T. (2010). Self-care behaviors of African American women living with HIV: A qualitative perspective. *Journal of the Association of Nurses in AIDS Care, 21*(1), 36–52. https://doi.org/10.1016/j.jana.2009.07.006

Turan, B., Smith, W., Cohen, M. H., Wilson, T. E., Adimora, A. A., Merenstein, D., … Turan, J. M. (2016). Mechanisms for the negative effects of internalized HIV-related stigma on antiretroviral therapy adherence in women: The mediating roles of social isolation and depression. *Journal of Acquired Immune Deficiency Syndromes, 72*(2), 198–205. https://doi.org/10.1097/QAI.0000000000000948

United Nations Children's Fund. (2019, July). *Elimination of mother-to-child transmission.* Retrieved from https://data.unicef.org/topic/hivaids/emtct/

United Nations. (2015). *Transforming our world: The 2030 agenda for sustainable development.* Retrieved from https://doi.org/10.1891/9780826190123.ap02

Vyavaharkar, M., Moneyham, L., Corwin, S., Tavakoli, A., Saunders, R., & Annang, L. (2011). HIV-disclosure, social support, and depression among HIV-infected African American women living in the rural southeastern United States. *AIDS Education and Prevention, 23*(1), 78–90. https://doi.org/10.1521/aeap.2011.23.1.78

Walker, L. (2020). Problematizing the discourse of 'Post-AIDS.' *Journal of Medical Humanities, 41*(2), 95–105. https://doi.org/10.1007/s10912-017-9433-9

Webel, A. R., Cuca, Y., Okonsky, J. G., Asher, A. K., Kaihura, A., & Salata, R. A. (2013). The impact of social context on self-management in women living with HIV. *Social Science & Medicine, 87*, 147–154.

Webel, A. R., & Higgins, P. A. (2012). The relationship between social roles and self-management behavior in women living with HIV/AIDS. *Women's Health Issues, 22*, e27–e33. https://doi.org/10.1016/j.whi.2011.05.010

9 "YOU FUCKING DESERVE HIV"

Seeking PrEP Information, Disciplinary Power, and Queer Technologies of the Self on /r/AskGayBros

Roberta Chevrette

"I am a bottom, and while I do not demand condoms, I do not take cum in the ass whatsoever … I am not a slut," announces one individual. Another responds, "That doesn't make much sense. Just because you don't let guys breed you doesn't stop you being a slut." So begins an unfolding online dialogue in a post about Pre-Exposure Prophylaxis (PrEP) on the subreddit /r/AskGayBros. Given its ability to reduce the risk of HIV transmission from sex by about 99% when taken daily (Centers for Disease Control and Prevention, 2019), PrEP, primarily marketed to gay and bisexual men, has been heralded as a way to bring about the "end of AIDS" (Kane, 2019). Unfortunately, those utilizing Truvada, the drug most commonly associated with PrEP, have indicated that their experiences with the medication have included stigmatization (Calabrese & Underhill, 2015; Grimm & Schwartz, 2019) and uncertainty (Schwartz & Grimm, 2016). Dominant narratives regarding HIV prevention and PrEP are constructed by the government, health, and service agencies and focus primarily on biomedical discourses (Spieldenner, 2017; Treichler, 1987). However, biomedical discourses do not fully encompass the experiences of PrEP users, nor do they completely reflect common narratives about PrEP within LGBTQ (lesbian-gay-bisexual-transgender-queer) communities. For this reason, there is a need for expanding forms of research that can integrate "biomedical, personal and social contexts" to understand LGBTQ experiences related to sexual health and decision-making (Spieldenner, 2014, p. 13).

While extant research has included interviews and surveys of gay men taking PrEP (Grimm & Schwartz, 2019; Halkitis et al., 2018; Koester, Erguera, & Myers, 2017), there is an under-researched population of individuals seeking and sharing information about experiences with this drug on social media and other digital platforms. Following the federal approval of PrEP in 2012, blogs such as "My PrEP Experience" (2015) and "I'm Still Josh" (2019), as well as various LGBTQ-oriented subreddits, have provided forums where "at-risk" individuals narrate their experiences of medical professional interactions and social pressures from both heterosexual and LGBTQ communities. Examining discourses

DOI: 10.4324/9781003000945-12

produced by, and in, online spaces offers insight into integrating the biomedical, personal, and social in the everyday experiences of those taking, or considering taking, this medication. Interactive online spaces also reflect discursive trends in gay communities, including the daily communication of those concerned about HIV exposure. This chapter engages in a critical qualitative analysis of conversations about PrEP in one such space, the subreddit /r/AskGayBros. Using the framework of Foucault's (1988c) technologies, I identify how disciplinary structures are reproduced in these conversations through technologies of production, power, and signs, as well as how PrEP can be utilized as a queer technology of the self through which individuals navigate and resist dominant discourses of health, sexuality, and heteronormativity. This investigation is an important step in illuminating the role of PrEP/Truvada as it relates to sexual health, sexual practices, and queer lives in a "post-AIDS" world.

Disciplinary Power, LGBTQ Sexual Health, and Queer Interventions

Foucault's theorizations of governmentality and biopolitics are useful for understanding how LGBTQ individuals negotiate sexual behavior and health decisions within larger regimes of power. Governmentality emphasizes that the regulation of individuals' conduct is not merely produced by governing authorities such as formal representative bodies of the state. Instead, individuals consent and participate in their own governance through processes including normalization and judgement, which serve to regulate behaviors, disciplining their own and others' bodies (Foucault, 1977). As a disciplinary discourse, the historical pathologization and labeling of same-sex attraction as a disease encouraged gay men to regulate their behavior in various ways, including seeking a "cure" for their same-sex attraction (Wahlert, 2013), living closeted lives (Sedgwick, 1990), and moving to "gay ghettos" (Levine, 1979). The theorization of biopolitics further illuminates how state power extends to control populations by regulating physical and political bodies (Foucault, 2004). The workings of biopower are evident in the U.S. nation-state's failure to effectively respond to the HIV/AIDS crisis at the time of its emergence in the 1980s (e.g., France, 2016). Together, U.S. citizens' own judgments and the lack of federal resources and attention marked LGBTQ and other "at-risk" populations as less worthy of life.

Foucault's (1988c) theorization of technologies offers a way to examine how regulatory systems related to the discursive legacy of the HIV/AIDS epidemic continue to impact LGBTQ populations. Foucault suggested that subjectification occurs through four main technologies: technologies of production, technologies of power, technologies of signs, and technologies of the self. I employ this framework to examine how contemporary gay subjects navigate contradictions inherent in "post-AIDS" discourses. Among these contradictions is that, through successful treatments, it has become possible to live a healthy life as a person who is HIV positive, yet HIV stigma remains pervasive. This impacts individuals' access to and attitudes regarding prevention and treatment options.

Foucault's theorization of technologies emphasizes the discursive production of subjects rather than viewing the self as "the site of an interiority" (Halperin, 2007, p. 6) – that is, the site of an *a priori* existence of the subject. Attending to sexuality as not only an interior identity, but as also externally produced through technologies of discourse is important for inquiring into the subjective lives of LGBTQ individuals as they navigate stigmatized sexual landscapes. Dominant discourses of sexuality "place contemporary gay subjects under many kinds of personal, political, epistemological, analytical, and ethical pressure" (Halperin, 2007, p. 108). As such, confusion, stress, and uncertainty about one's sexual identity and practices, along with – and in relation to – material structures of oppression and homophobia, have frequently characterized LGBTQ experiences, impacting individuals' understandings of sex, self, and agency.

Encounters with health systems and biomedical discourses in the U.S. have further contributed to both the lived uncertainties and discursive production of subjectivities experienced by gay and bisexual men and other men who have sex with men. As Halperin (2007) notes:

> The medical establishment in the United States never told [gay men] it was safe to have sex, let alone that sex was good for us. They still have not given us a green light to practice unprotected oral sex (even without ejaculation). Nor did they say we could have as many sexual partners as we wanted so long as what we did with them was safe. They have never endorsed condomless sex among HIV-positive men or agreements among HIV-negative partners in a stable relationship to have unprotected sex with each other [....] The [U.S.] American medical establishment never even told us it was safe to kiss.
> (p. 19)

Given that normalizing discourses about HIV, risk and gay men's sexualities have historically been laden with cisheteropatriarchal assumptions, and have failed to engage with the realities of people's lived experiences, "it is gay men themselves who have continued to define, and to redefine, the limits of safety through an ongoing history of sexual experimentation and mutual consultation" (Halperin, 2007, p. 20). My inquiry into men's online discussions of PrEP in the /r/AskGayBros forum thus seeks to understand how PrEP use is being defined by and creating new definitions of self for individuals taking this medication. This analysis also offers insight into normalizing discourses of sex and safety within gay communities and the various technologies through which PrEP users navigate these discourses.

I come to this study shaped by my experiences as a bisexual, white, cisgender woman who lost her father to AIDS (see Chevrette, 2020), and whose research focuses on the rhetorical production of identities, belongings, and subjectivities through difference. From this subject position, I am strongly invested in the production of "livable lives" for LGBTQ persons (Butler, 2007, p. 88) and believe a queer standpoint is instrumental to this endeavor (see Layne, 2017). Among the many perspectives offered by the queer theory are: recognizing a "diversity of sexual and intimate relations as worthy of respect and protection," resisting "the notion that the state should be allowed to accord legitimacy to some kinds of consensual sex but not others," insisting that "much of what [is] taken to be morality, respectability, and decorum [is], in practice, a way of regulating sexual pleasures and relations," refusing heteropatriarchal cultural norms as "the standards by which queer life should be measured," and demanding "that any vision of sexual justice begin by considering the unrecognized dignity of [queer] outcasts, the ways of living they represent, and the hierarchies of abjection that make them secondary, invisible, or deviant" (Warner, 1999, pp. 88–89). I recognize that focusing on gay men's online discussions of PrEP does not reflect experiences of women taking the medicine, or queer and trans persons who may not be able to access this treatment due to their subject positions and social and geographic locations. However, I am interested in the material and discursive possibilities PrEP enables for men who are able to, and choose to , utilize it, along with challenges they face as they negotiate relationships with providers, relational and/or sexual partners, and LGBTQ communities. To address how marginalized individuals navigate and resist power structures and at times reproduce them, the following questions guided my research: How do online communities create spaces of agency for gay men to produce and access knowledge related to PrEP? What disciplinary discourses of sex, health, and sexuality are evidenced in communication about PrEP on /r/AskGayBros? And how does PrEP use enable gay men to engage in technologies of the self related to sex, sexuality, and sexual health?

Analyzing Discursive Technologies in PrEP Discussions on /r/AskGayBros

Reddit, launched in 2005, is a popular online platform and discussion hub for a wide variety of topics. The platform works by establishing communities called "subreddits," denoted by "/r/[name of subreddit]." Reddit users can subscribe to and receive news feeds from subreddits of interest, each acting as its own online community forum. All posts are anonymous, showing only the poster's username, and, following certain guidelines, any user can create a subreddit community. /r/AskGayBros was established in 2012 and has 180,000 members at the time of this writing. The "Community Details" description reads, "This is where you can ask the manly men for their opinions on various topics," followed by the advice: "AskReddit style questions. AMA. ELI5. Everything in between" (*AskGayBros*, 2019). In online contexts, "AMA" means "Ask me anything," while "ELI5" is shorthand for "Explain like I'm 5." This description suggests that all questions are welcome, and simple explanatory responses are encouraged.

In the Wiki tab on /r/AskGayBros, an additional description appears that provides one "correction" to the description cited above. This one reads, "[W] elcome to /r/askgaybros, where a bunch of manly (actually most of us are pretty fem) men answer your questions!" (*AskGayBros*, 2019). Quick links direct users to frequently asked questions including sections on coming out, relationship advice, and sexual health advice, a "best of section" containing posts on a variety of topics, a glossary of terms commonly utilized in gay and queer communities, and a "guide to safe sex" that opens to a thread titled: "If you have to be a slut, be a safe(r) slut: The guide you didn't learn in sex ed for reducing (not eliminating) your odds of acquiring/transmitting STDs" (*AskGayBros*, 2019). In their resistance to gendered and sexual normativities, these informative pages establish a queer tone for the forum. However, the participatory elements of the platform mean that conversations that unfold within the forum do not always follow this same tone, at times reinscribing heteronormative and homonormative discourses. For example, despite the sex-positive approach evidenced in the "safe(r)" sex guide foregrounded on the /r/AskGayBros homepage, numerous user comments within discussion threads nonetheless depict sex as unsafe and/or morally questionable unless it occurs within normative parameters such as a long-term, mutually exclusive relationship.

To establish the dataset, a search was performed for all threads containing conversations about PrEP; this was subsequently narrowed to the most recent year of posts at the time of data collection in 2019. This yielded 65 threads, ranging from four individual posts on the shortest thread to 191 posts on the longest. I open-coded approximately ten percent of the data to establish initial codes (Charmaz, 2014), which were organized in relation to the four technologies defined by Foucault (1988c): technologies of production, technologies of power, technologies of sign systems, and technologies of the self. I then used focused coding to code the rest of the data in NVivo, writing memos and adding a few additional codes to capture new themes discovered during analysis (Charmaz, 2014). In total, there were approximately 30 codes and 50 sub-codes, which aided in developing an integrated understanding of the operations of these four technologies. Data collection did not require informed consent from participants in this Reddit community because this data is publicly available. However, because of the sensitive nature of the information discussed, I have chosen not to identify data excerpts with usernames to further preserve anonymity. Online language conventions vary from formal writing; rather than "correct" users' language, I have elected to retain the format of the original posts, including (mis)spellings, punctuation, and capitalization.

My discussion turns first to technologies of production. Here, I establish how the platform of Reddit, and the /r/AskGayBros subreddit specifically, enables certain modes of interaction and allows community members to engage in knowledge production. Next, I address technologies of power, examining how dominant discourses regarding sex and sexuality impact individuals' encounters with healthcare systems and LGBTQ communities. Turning to technologies of signs, I focus on how "HIV/AIDS," "PrEP," and "condoms" operate as interconnected signs that frequently align with heteronormative and homonormative discourses. I also examine how queer signifiers are used to resist dominant discourses. The final section of the analysis focuses on technologies of the self, addressing how individuals utilize /r/AskGayBros to seek sexual health guidance from a broader LGBTQ community. I further address how PrEP can enable feelings of agency and bodily ownership for its users and assist in challenging sexual normativities. In conclusionIn the conclusion, I highlight the necessity of queer critique as it relates to LGBTQ sexual health in the "post-AIDS" era.

Technologies of Production: "Can Someone Explain Prep to Me Like I'm an Idiot?"

According to Foucault, (1988c), technologies of production "permit us to produce, transform, or manipulate things" (p. 18). Technologies of production include explicit or implicit rules that regulate organizational processes and systems. In the case of /r/AskGayBros, there are technologies of production specific to Reddit as a social media platform, including the rules of Reddit themselves, such as the use of up- and down-voting on posts. These rules establish guidelines for interaction and regulate the manner in which posts circulate and appear. Subreddits, including /r/AskGayBros, are also an element of Reddit's technologies of production in that they allow users to converge around a common interest. As a platform, Reddit thus enables the production of communities of users, or publics (see Warner, 2002), formed by their attention to, and participation in ensuing conversations.

Turning to technologies of production within the /r/AskGayBros community, one significant aspect of conversations generated on /r/AskGayBros is how they enable users to engage in technologies of knowledge production, including asking and answering questions. Overall, the kinds of questions about PrEP on /r/AskGayBros included questions about how and where to get it, its cost, its effectiveness, possible side effects, the history of the drug's development, and others' personal experiences with it. For example, one user posted, "I've heard about getting PrEP free but I'm not sure how to actually go about it." Another asked, "I was wondering if any of you had advice on dealing with the initial side effects, how long they lasted for, and also if you have any other experiences whilst on PrEP I'd love to hear!" Often emphasis was placed on gaining insight from those who had experiential knowledge, as seen in the example above. In response to such queries, other users offered information about PrEP along with other sexual health information. While many short responses drew only from personal experience (for example, "one thing that helped me with the nausea was eating applesauce"), other responses provided detailed information and links to additional research, generating a substantive archive of health information. In several lengthy threads, participants extensively discussed PrEP's cost and accessibility (which varied depending on global location); its development, patenting, and approval; studies on effectiveness, side effects; and more. Other sexual health information shared by /r/AskGayBros participants ranged from questions to ask your doctor, to questions to ask your sexual partners, to rates and risks of HIV transmission and other STIs.

Further technologies of production can be evidenced in established norms for interaction on this subreddit, which serve to govern talk in particular ways.

Findings demonstrated that /r/AskGayBros users utilized several strategies to correct or challenge others' claims, and that these produced specific forms of interaction that at times contributed to the overall production of knowledge. The most prevalent strategy of governing talk, which I identified as "chiding," was a form of online scolding to criticize other posts or participants. Examples included telling others to "stop complaining," "do some research," or to not "get triggered by facts." A different strategy, which I coded as "calling out," was evidenced when participants challenged other posters' "bad" behavior,; for example, telling someone that their comment to another person was "super unnecessary," or "a jerk comment." Another form of calling out took was when individuals directly pointed out elements of homophobia or other oppressive attitudes implicit in others' comments. For example, one person responded to a comment placing blame on HIV-positive persons by saying, "your blaming the patient bullshit ... is either fueled by ignorant bigotry, cold indifference or both." These norms of interaction, while different from the straightforward sharing of information evidenced in certain other posts, still provided a means of producing knowledge by attempting to correct inaccurate information or harmful attitudes.

By providing a platform for seeking and sharing information, experiences, and attitudes, /r/AskGayBros and its technologies of production enable users to expand their capacity to make choices regarding PrEP and other aspects of sexual health. As gay, bisexual, and other men who have sex with men ask and answer one another's questions on /r/AskGayBros, they share specialized information in a manner that other LGBTQ individuals can access. The individuals on this subreddit thus engage in agentic acts that enable access to knowledge outside of dominant power structures and, in so doing, produce alternate systems of discourse.[1] In this regard, sharing health information in this online community is a means of countering the anti-LGBTQ bias and/or lack of knowledge about LGBTQ sexual health within healthcare institutions that prevent knowledge about PrEP from being more widespread among medical and other communities. As discussed in the following section, healthcare systems and regulatory discourses about sex are among the technologies of power that /r/AskGayBros community members navigated, resisted, and at times reproduced.

Technologies of Power: "Should I Trust My Doctor's Advice?"

Technologies of power "determine the conduct of individuals and submit them to certain ends of domination" (Foucault, 1988c, p. 18). Healthcare organizations and insurance providers are among the structures gay men seeking to use PrEP must navigate; these institutions formalize hierarchical relationships between patients, providers, and the state. Moreover, these organizations institutionalize barriers to access, including, but not limited to, cost. Concerns about costs expressed by /r/AskGayBros users ranged from expensive copays, to finding "programs to help pay for prep," to comparisons of prices in different countries, as seen, for example, in one poster's query, "why does PrEP cost 2000 in the US and 8 in Australia?" Responses also reflected geographic and cultural impediments to access; for example, in a thread where several persons living in countries with universal healthcare discussed receiving PrEP for free, one user asked participants to consider that "as a latino living in Latinoamerica ... not everyone has access to HIV medicines and can be open about his status to family." A similar sentiment was expressed by a different poster who stated, "I'm a college student currently in a country that doesn't have access to PrEP, [and] there's a very real possibility my family would disown me if they found out I was gay *and* HIV positive." Such comments offer important indicators regarding how PrEP use can be limited by intersecting barriers to access that reproduce normative systems.

Technologies of power further include the establishment of hierarchies of relationships and knowledges. Power imbalances define provider-patient relationships, and because individuals seeking to use PrEP must have an Rx from a provider, many conversations focused on how individuals navigated various hurdles they faced in this relationship. First, it was evidenced in some threads that providers were hesitant, or even refused, to write prescriptions unless they deemed the patient's level of "risk" to be sufficiently high, a concern evidenced in a thread titled, "Help! Doc won't give me prep." Another person recounted, "Today I went to the doctor and described my situation. She told me that I was low risk and that I wasn't eligible for PrEP." Such comments indicated that it could be difficult for individuals deemed "low-risk" by certain medical professionals to access PrEP unless there were mitigating factors. For example, one /r/AskGayBros user noted that although they did use condoms, the fact that the condom could break or be taken off (what is referred to as "stealthing") created a significant amount of stress for them. Their, and their doctor "was compassionate of me being prone to anxiety so prescribed me PREP."

A second issue /r/AskGayBros users highlighted was providers' lack of knowledge about PrEP. For gay and bisexual men, interactions with medical providers are regulated by uneven relationships in knowledge and power, despite providers' frequently not being trained in LGBTQ health information (Morris & Roberto, 2016). For patients interested in using PrEP, their provider holds the "expert" position, yet often lacks knowledge about PrEP (Grimm & Schwartz, 2019), which can leave potential users with unanswered questions. Several threads contained original posts where individuals expressed a lack of knowledge or confusion about PrEP tied to information they had received, or not received, from their providers. Some noted their doctors did not know the protocols. As one commenter described, "PrEP isn't big in my area and a lot of doctors and people don't really know about it so it was a process of getting it." Another explained that their doctor "didn't give me very much information about what to expect." Moreover, due to the role of healthcare professionals in the historical oppression of LGBTQ people and the biases gay men frequently face when seeking treatment (Dean, Victor, & Guidry-Grimes, 2016; Ussher, 2009), some /r/AskGayBros community members explicitly indicated their distrust of the information being provided to them by their doctors. For those whose doctors were, in their own words, "lousy," "not that informed," "bad," "dismissive," or "not appropriate," asking other members of the /r/AskGayBros online community offered a means of checking whether the information they had received was accurate, and provided an agentic means of navigating unequal power structures embedded within health systems.

Technologies of power also include processes of normalization and judgment that produce subjects, regulate sex, and police desire and (hetero)sexualities (Foucault, 1977, 1988a). A few /r/AskGayBros community members explicitly noted their concerns regarding doctors' stigmatizing perceptions based on their sexual identities or practices. One individual explained their choice to use Planned Parenthood, instead of their primary care provider, for PrEP because they are "non-judgmental." At the same time, a different person shared that their new primary care doctor "asked me if I have HIV three times across 2 appointments." Judgments regarding gay sexual practices and identities impact individuals' interactions with other medical professionals as well; in one /r/AskGayBros comment, the user described having had "poor support" related to sexually transmitted infections "from both my psychologist and my psychiatrist, who instead preferred to assume I had done bareback and proceed to lecture me about the importance of safe sex." In these cases, assumptions from medical providers regarding patients' sexual practices seem to limit the ability to provide care responsive to individual needs.

Discourses regulating sex, and types of sex, come not only from heteropatriarchal and biomedical discourses, however; they also come from within LGBTQ communities. I found such discourses recurring within the data set, and organized this data around four separate but frequently intersecting codes. The first, regulating condomless sex, appeared in a plethora of posts advocating condom use as the only legitimate means of protection. Examples included directives such as "wrap it up," and "use a condom it's just smart," as well as assertions like "condomless sex is not safe sex, period," and "if someone refuses to use condoms, that's your cue to not have sex with them." The second, regulating monogamy, captured how some /r/AskGayBros participants advocated monogamy as the preferred, desired, or only "safe" form of relationship. This was expressed in sentiments such as, "why not just like, not hook up all over the place and get into a monogamous relationship instead?" Another post capturing the regulation of both condomless sex and monogamy stated: "All sex without a condom is unsafe outside of an exclusive relationship." The third regulatory discourse, regulating types of sex, came up in discussions of preferences for and risks of different types of sex, including anal sex, oral sex, and masturbation. While individuals may, of course, choose their own preferred sex practices, it is a regulatory discourse when claims are made that a certain type of sex is uniformly unsafe (i.e., "I don't do anal," or "not ANAL"). The final means of regulating sex evidenced in conversations on /r/AskGayBros was what I called "stranger danger." Several people expressed concern over hook-up culture and casual partners, arguing that sex "is dangerous on 'one night stands,'" and offering advice to others to "not fuck dozens of total strangers." Many of these regulatory discourses echo those found in "straight" culture, and place constraints on individuals' behavior through processes of normalization and judgment. Therefore, individuals seeking to use

PrEP must navigate assumptions regarding using condoms, seeking monogamy, avoiding certain types of sex, and not hooking up that come from their providers, heterosexual communities, and from within LGBTQ communities.

Foucault (1972) conceived of power as not just regulatory in a top-down fashion, but also as productive in that "it traverses and produces things, it induces pleasure, forms knowledge, [and] produces discourse" (p. 119). Although the term "power" is most frequently associated with critiques of domination, the productive elements of power mean that it can also be deployed in a positive sense, that is, as a means of resistance. One means of resistance to the technologies of power permeating healthcare systems and organizations was /r/AskGayBros users' assertions of their rights to health and treatment. Critiquing the U.S. healthcare system, one user noted, "almost every industrialized nation treats healthcare as a right, and they focus on preventing disease." Such critiques frequently aligned with critiques of capitalism, with one common theme being that "healthcare shouldn't be earned." One of the longest threads I encountered examined the "profoundly broken" U.S. health system, reflecting the salience of this topic for individuals seeking information about PrEP, and LGBTQ communities more broadly. AskGayBros subreddit users also explicitly engaged in discursive resistance to regulatory discourses of sex and sexualities. In the next section, I expand on these forms of resistance in the next section after first addressing continuities and shifts in the signifying power of HIV/AIDS in "post-AIDS" times.

Technologies of Signs: "Does Anyone Else Think that PrEP Is a Curse in Disguise?"

Technologies of sign systems refer to the systems governing the use of "signs, meanings, symbols, or significations" (Foucault, 1988c, p. 18). Technologies of signs frequently intertwine with technologies of power, given that power is reproduced through discourse. In conversations on /r/AskGayBros, among the signs holding prominent discursive positions were "AIDS," "PrEP," and "condoms." These terms were the most frequently repeated ones throughout the threads (in addition to "sex" and "people"), and all are entangled with the regulatory discourses about sex and sexuality mentioned above. The first of these, "AIDS," is particularly charged, having a long history of entangling discourses of disease, danger, fear, and punishment, specifically in relation to the gay male body and its being marked as deviant (Herek & Capitanio, 1999; Treichler, 1987). As Spieldenner (2014) notes, "[I]n the history of the HIV epidemic, gay men have been closely affiliated with the public view of the disease—including being stigmatized along with people living with HIV/AIDS" (p. 12, see also Gere, 2004; Herek & Glunt, 1988). For this reason,

> the medical and biological reality of HIV as a disease exists alongside a multitude of social, cultural and symbolic meanings [that] transform our understanding of the disease, its pathology, its infectiousness, the transmission routes and associated risks, and even the people who catch the disease. (p. 13)

In a number of instances, HIV was rhetorically associated with infection, (irrational) fears, and judgmentsjudgements. Some individuals expressed that fears of contracting HIV prevented them from engaging in sex at all; as noted by one /r/AskGayBros participant: "I am scared to attempt to even have sex period." A different user similarly stated, "I am very worried about getting something. I've only had intercourse (with condom) once in my life." There are numerous ways to engage in sex that limit risks of HIV transmission; however, as Treichler (1987) pointed out,

> our social constructions of AIDS … are based not upon objective, scientifically determined "reality" but upon what we are told about this reality: that is, upon prior social constructions routinely produced within the discourses of biomedical science (AIDS as infectious disease is one such construction). (p. 35)

Dominant discourses surrounding HIV/AIDS can lead to, as one /r/AskGayBros post put it, "emotional fear tak[ing] over facts," which can significantly impact the sex lives of gay, bisexual, and other men who have sex with men.

Anxiety was a prevalent theme in many of the original posts from gay men seeking information about PrEP despite the fact that, in several threads, the men asking questions regarding whether they should get PrEP were in very low-risk situations. For example, in one post, the original poster expressed concern about a recent hookup in which they had used a condom with a partner who "claimed to be negative, on PrEP, and that he got tested three weeks prior." After hearing from several others in the thread that there was nothing to worry about, the original poster agreed,

> yeah, if I think about it, the HIV would have to beat PrEP (assuming he takes it regularly), beat the condom, and then beat the lower odds of infecting a top, so rationally speaking the risk is probably very low.

Although expressions of anxiety regarding safer sexual practices intersected with the aforementioned technologies of power, they can also be seen as tied to discourses of homophobia that depict LGBTQ sex and, specifically, HIV/AIDS as deviant.

Further sedimenting links between HIV/AIDS and fear with the discursive construction of HIV-positivity as deviance is usingthe use of the terms "clean" and "dirty" to describe partners or potential partners, sometimes in tandem with racialized or classed assumptions. For example, one individual described a recent sexual partner as likely to have been HIV-negative because they were "a nice guy and seemed legit and clean cut." On the other side of this value-laden dichotomy was the use of the word "contaminated" to describe persons with HIV-positive statuses. The use of these binaristic terms clearly reflects stigmas associated with HIV positive status, as seen, for example, in a post stating: "People with HIV obviously don't have the best decision-making ability, it is unwise to rely on such a person to truthfully disclose their affliction." Another individual argued that "anyone who is infected" has "certain character traits," including "poor judgment, poor decision making, intentionally reckless or self-destructive behavior or a propensity to disregard their own health and wellbeing." Illuminating the extent of negativity towards HIV-positive persons within LGBTQ communities (see O'Brien, 2020), one /r/AskGayBros user stated, "My concern is solely for neg people, and the world will be a better place when all the poz scum finally die off." Such language frames HIV/AIDS as the responsibility and "fault" of those who have contracted it.

As an HIV-prevention medicine, PrEP is situated within these already existing technologies of signs. Spieldenner (2016) has written about how Truvada and PrEP are constructed as signs of deviance, identifying how discourses including slut-shaming and grieving the loss of condoms function to discipline PrEP users. These discourses were evidenced in some /r/AskGayBros users' stances against PrEP, and their responses to individuals seeking information. One person, for example, criticized another poster by saying,

> you are talking about bareback in a sort of romanticized way like guys on PrEP are all having some kind of beautiful intimate sex with each other, when in reality it's just a bunch of grimey guys on Grinder propositioning men they barely know.

A different individual suggested that PrEP had "made people sluttier." Another, in response to an individual's query about getting on PrEP to expand their range of sexual partners to include those choosing not to use condoms, stated, "I'm sorry you don't know how to say 'no' and mean it." In an especially hostile response to others' advocacy of PrEP, one individual noted, "smh [shaking my head] I'm ready for a super-AIDS to take all you hoes out." These kinds of comments evaluate PrEP users as "bad" and improper subjects engaged in deviant sexual behavior. From a biomedical perspective, the symbolic construction of PrEP in this manner is a significant issue given that "gay men exposed to stigmatized messages about PrEP—such as the myth that people on PrEP are promiscuous—[are] significantly less likely to be interested in learning more about PrEP" (Grimm & Schwartz, 2019, p. 1181). As Grimm and Schwartz (2019) note, "[S]tigma can negatively impact access to health resources, undermine social relationships that are important for keeping individuals healthy, contribute to psychological and physical stress, and adversely affect a multitude of psychological and behavioral processes" (p. 1181).

The stigma of PrEP stems from its rhetorical associations with HIV and condomless sex (as well as from its association with queer sexual practices in general). At times, this association was made quickly in passing; at other times, it was explicitly spelled out, as seen in a post stating:

> HIV incubated quietly for a decade before the bodies started to pile up. When the next lethal megavirus emerges (and it will), PrEP won't save us.

> The condom-free crew will have already infected millions of our neighbors and partners. We can only hope that it won't be as deadly as the AIDS complex.

As seen in this comment, as a sign, "HIV" could thus be mobilized to counter the value of PrEP while simultaneously stigmatizing its users, illustrating how HIV stigma easily extends into "queer-shaming and the pathologization of queer sex and sexualities" (O'Brien, 2020, p. 33). Also shown in this comment is how critiques of PrEP users frequently collapsed PrEP use into a debate over condom-use and barebacking, as evidenced in another of the longest threads analyzed, titled: "Does anyone else in here think that PrEP is a curse in disguise for our community?" In this thread, the original poster expressed concerns that PrEP would lead to a decline in condom use that could threaten LGBTQ communities. In such conversations, those arguing the pro-condom position tended to employ a rhetoric of responsibility, as seen, for example, in the comment: "Having condomless sex with random partners would be considered irresponsible for a straight man or woman. What makes you or any gay man so special that you should be immune to judgment?"

The pathologization of gay identities and sexual practices was evidenced in posts on /r/AskGayBros in which "deviant" sexual behaviors – including the desire to engage in condomless sex – were described as resulting from psychological factors. One individual argued that "many rejected, wounded, outcast gays lose all ability to delay gratification. It is the textbook response to protracted emotional abuse." Another noted, "There is also something to be said with promiscuous men there is sometimes an element of narcissist and obsession with vanity." Yet another stated, "it's like the desire to have unsafe sex is completely endemic." Other posts reflected value-laden judgments regarding sexual behaviors and identities through the use of terms including "psycho," "debased," "creepy," and "sinister." The discursive construction of persons with HIV-positive statuses, PrEP users, and others engaging in behaviors outside of the regulatory discourses of sex in this manner aligns with the rhetorics of "deservingness" that suggest HIV/AIDS was a punishment for improper sexual behavior, which fueled mainstream responses to the crisis, and against which queer activists had to fight. Unfortunately, this discursive construction of HIV as punishment was even, at times, repeated by individuals who seemed to be attempting to dismantle "anti-poz" attitudes. For example, one /r/AskGayBros user expressed their frustration with the original poster's concern about contracting HIV by saying: "OH FUCKING CHRIST YOU'RE ALREAY ON GODDAMN PREP AND YOU USED A FUCKING CONDOM THAT WAS SLIGHTLY TORN!!!!! YOURE CHANCES ARE SLIM TO FUCKING NONE. YOU FUCKING DESERVE HIV JUST FOR YOUR GODDAMN IRRATIONAL PARANOIA FUCK."

Technologies of signs are not only a means of replicating dominant systems, however; they are also a means of resisting them. Some /r/AskGayBros users explicitly challenged the discourses denigrating PrEP use. One person, for example, using the calling-out strategy discussed earlier, commented, "the opposition to PrEP is rooted in plain old sex negativity and slut shaming. At some unconscious level, a lot of these anti-PrEP fear mongers believe that gay men who have condomless sex *deserve* to be punished with STIs." Other individuals called attention to positive aspects of PrEP, including its high rate of effectiveness for preventing HIV transmission, and the fact that PrEP users are regularly screened for STIs. A number of forum users also resisted the connection of HIV/AIDS with deviance. One man, for example, shared a link to a study regarding the "0% likelihood of HIV transmission" from undetectable partners (see Rodger et al., 2019), stating, "guess what – here I am three years later, happily committed and living with an HIV+, undetectable man, enjoying amazing, unprotected sex every day."

A final technology of signs reflected on /r/AskGayBros was the use of queer signifiers, which can also be viewed as a form of resistance in their disruption of gendered norms. Although the name of the sub-reddit, "AskGayBros," itself suggests a particular relationship to a normalized form of masculine relating, and there were moments where heteromasculinist assumptions and language were reinscribed in individual users comments, more often, these were disrupted through the use of queer signifiers and the embrace of queer masculinities. Identifying oneself by sexual positions as a "top" or "bottom," and using other terms widely recognized within LGBTQ communities was common on /r/AskGayBros. In some posts, men referred to other men in the thread as "babes," "queens," or "ladies," all of which are terms employed in queer communities in ways that frequently (though not always) counter cisheteronormative gendering practices. Also observed was the use of phrases common in queer communities such as "Yaas Kween" to express excitement, "U ok Hun?" as a means of mitigating a particularly negative post, "thx fam" to indicate gratitude for others' responses, or "bitch bye" as a means of ending a conversation. Public expressions of same-sex attraction are also a form of queer signification insofar as this disrupts regulatory norms in which sex is presumed to be both heterosexual and private. This was seen in several comments such as, "I m a cocksucker, what can I say?" and "Guy had a huge, beautiful, hung dick, Looked so delicious couldn't stop daydreaming about it." One /r/AskGayBros user ended their post with, "Hoe long and get fucked. ~an ethical slut." In the face of technologies of power-producingpower producing the regulatory discourses about sex described above, embracing "sluttiness" as a positive virtue of/for the self signifies resistance to these norms.

Technologies of the Self: "How Has PREP Changed Your Life?"

In Foucault's (1988c) conceptualization, technologies of the self

> permit individuals to effect by their own means or with the help of others a certain number of operations on their own bodies and souls, thoughts,

> conduct, and ways of being, so as to transform themselves in order to attain a certain state of happiness, purity, wisdom, perfection, or immortality.
> (p. 18; see also Foucault, 1988b, 2005)

In the previous sections, I have addressed how technologies of production, power, and signs subject individuals to disciplinary structures and the ways individuals resist this subjectification. Foucault (1982) proposed two meanings of the word "subject": subject to or dependent on another's control; and consciously producing one's own identity through self-knowledge. In keeping with the second meaning, technologies of the self address individuals' abilities to shape their own behaviors, subjectivities, and futures. Each of the agentic behaviors identified in previous sections, such as the use of /r/AskGayBros as a community for producing knowledge, and the challenging of dominant systems of power and signs, can also constitute a technology of the self. Here, I turn to two themes not yet addressed above, addressing how gay guidance constitutes an act of agentic subject formation and how PrEP itself offers its users a technology through which they can transform their relationship to self and others.

I have identified how information seeking and sharing constitutes a technology of production on /r/AskGayBros. Findings further indicated that sexual health queries on /r/AskGayBros were distinct in that users were not simply seeking biomedical information. Instead, in posting questions about PrEP use on /r/AskGayBros, individuals specifically sought experiential knowledgeinformation from others, a finding termed *gay guidance*. As one person stated, "I have asked [a doctor] who said I should be fine, but they aren't the ones who know all the ins and outs of PrEP." Instead, individuals were interested in acquiring firsthand accounts from others in similar situations. While this is similar to other online health communities where individuals come together to discuss illness experiences (Yan et al., 2016), it is also different given that LGBTQ individuals face challenges from the healthcare system, and from their communities, that are specific to the marginalized status of their sexual identities and practices (Dean, et al., 2016; Ghabrial, 2016; Ussher, 2009). As a technology of the self, seeking and receiving gay guidance is, thus, a means of navigating societal discourses "surrounding the practice and management of the gay self" (Halperin, 2007, p. 108).

Political and personal pressures placed on LGBTQ individuals from oppressive and homophobic societal structures as they intersect with signifying systems regarding sex, safety, and HIV/AIDS risk also place individuals under what Halperin (2007) refers to as "epistemological" pressure. On /r/AskGayBros, individuals were able to find relief from, and transform, feelings of confusion, stress, and uncertainty by seeking and receiving community guidance and reassurance. The desire for reassurance was sometimes directly stated in comments such as "I could use some reassurance or some advice on what to do." It was also indicated by questions like "can anyone relate?" or statements such as "I have a serious question that I would love answered to ease my mind." In response, /r/AskGayBros members offered assurances to original posters including "I can relate," "I understand," "you're being perfectly reasonable," "You're doing great!" and "You're not only a good man, you're a good human. (Even better: into nails!)." Gay guidance did not only come in the form of simply offering reassurances, however; I also found that one form of guidance was correcting misinformation, including challenging mistaken assumptions about PrEP.

Turning to PrEP itself as a technology, my findings further indicate that PrEP can enable feelings of agency and bodily ownership in its users, and assist in challenging sexual normativities. For some, PrEP provides an additional measure of protection that can help them feel confident engaging in sex, as reflected in several conversations on /r/AskGayBros where individuals spoke of getting on PrEP primarily to "ease the discomfort and anxiety" associated with fear of HIV transmission. Some men further described how being able to engage in sex with or without condoms due to being on PrEP enabled a sense of agency and ownership over their own bodies, frequently utilizing the phrase "peace of mind" to describe PrEP's impacts on their sexual behavior. One individual noted, "I can tell you that the peace of mind that came from fucking on PrEP (with and without condom) was incredibly liberating and lead to the best sex I ever had." A different poster commented, "Now I take responsibility of my own health, and it feels good. I do fuck raw sometimes, but not always." Another stated, "It feels amazing, I get to enjoy my body and be as responsible as I want with it." These comments challenge and reframe discourses suggesting PrEP users are not being responsible, while also simultaneously emphasizing gay pleasure.

Emphasizing pleasure in discussions about LGBTQ sexual health is important to integrate personal and social experiences and practices with biomedical discourses. In the medical field, "questions of sexuality and pleasure tend to be largely absent from current debates on PrEP" (Brisson & Nguyen, 2017, p. 1074). As it connects to pleasure, I found a range of experiences for PrEP users on /r/AskGayBros: some used it to provide an additional layer of protection or "failsafe" in casual hook-ups with condoms, others used it in committed relationships with HIV-negative or HIV-positive partners, others used it because they preferred sex without a condom. Understanding the use of PrEP as a technology requires engaging with the full range of these subject positions in a non-pathological manner. As Race (2009) indicates,

> HIV education has in fact been most effective when it has foregrounded and incorporated the embodied pleasures of endangered groups. The history of HIV prevention may be understood as a series of struggles on the part of affected groups to elaborate bodily practices capable of mediating between pleasure and safety. Here, health does not stand in opposition to pleasure. (pp. 1–2)

Conversations about safer sex that do not include a range of embodied pleasures – including the simple fact that, yes, some people prefer sex without condoms – are not reflective of lived experiences of LGBTQ sexualities, sexual practices, and sexual health.

As a technology of the self, PrEP also encompasses queer potentialities. As Brisson and Nguyen (2017) note, PrEP use may, for some, constitute "an act of resistance to the critics advocating for condom-centered sexual practices" (p. 1074). Being able to more safely practice sexual practices long deemed to be "high risk" may, thus, constitute a form of queer resistance and an engagement in "non-shaming sexual practice" that allows individuals to "explore new paradigms of queer pleasure but also to explore the self and sexual empowerment" (O'Brien, 2020, p. 133). This includes, as one /r/AskGayBros participant put it, the ability of LGBTQ persons to make "conscious decision[s] about the level of disease risk they are willing to tolerate in the pursuit of pleasure." HIV prevention practices produce "subjects and technologies together" (Brisson & Nguyen, 2017, p. 1069). As a technology that materially enables risk-reduction, PrEP may also present a means of challenging the discursive construction of HIV/AIDS as an always lingering, unspoken, terrifying presence, and the "shame-inducing power" of these discourses (Halperin, 2007, p. 93). Removing the shame associated with queer sex, queer desires, and the still-powerful signification of "HIV = death," in an era when that is no longer the case with access to appropriate treatment, has the potential to transform not only the self, but also society.

Conclusion

Online health discussions enable individuals to acquire knowledge, seek support, and make sense of their own experiences; they also contain "culturally embedded symbols that reveal personal and social beliefs" (Spieldenner, 2014, p. 14). This examination of discussions of PrEP on /r/AskGayBros offers insight into knowledge acquisition, sensemaking, and support as they relate to the social construction of health, risk, and sexuality in contemporary gay communities. This is significant given that biomedical advances including PrEP and antiretroviral therapy have enabled imaginaries of "a future with no substantial increase in HIV incidence: hence, the notion of the end of AIDS" (Koester et al., 2017, p. 23), and yet, this future has failed to materialize. In other words, despite certain medical breakthroughs, "we have not witnessed equivalent breakthroughs at the societal level" (Koester et al., 2017, p. 23). This failure can be directly tied to the discursive technologies analyzed here, as well as material impediments to access mentioned in a number of /r/AskGayBros conversations. Although technologies of production, power, signs, and the self were separated in the discussion to parse out specific discursive strategies, the technologies intertwine and reinforce one another. As PrEP users and individuals seeking information about PrEP navigate regulatory discourses about sex that influence their encounters with providers and their communities, online spaces of gay guidance, such as /r/AskGayBros, fulfill an important role in allowing community members to engage in knowledge production. Conversations in these spaces can reflect but also challenge heteronormative and homonormative assumptions about sexuality and, in doing so, generate spaces of queer possibility.

One function of queer critique, according to Butler (2007), is to interrogate "the terms by which life is constrained in order to open up the possibility of different modes of living; [...] to establish more inclusive conditions for sheltering and maintaining life" (p. 4). Butler further argues that queer critique

> must be situated within the context of lives as they are lived and must be guided by the question of what maximizes the possibilities for a livable life, what minimizes the possibility of unbearable life or, indeed, social or literal death.
>
> (p. 8)

The insights this analysis offers regarding the challenges faced by gay men seeking information about PrEP are significant given the "ideological links between 'post-AIDS' culture, homonormativity, and the disavowal of HIV-positive masculinities" (O'Brien, 2020, p. 131) that, indeed, can contribute to social or literal death. The continued biopolitical stigmatization of certain LGBTQ identities and practices as deviant from both within and outside gay communities, and the still-powerful rhetorical alignment of HIV/AIDS with discourses of fear, irresponsibility, and punishment means that there are gaps between material and discursive realities that can influence practices of disclosure and prevention, leaving many young gay men confused about, and afraid of, sex. As indicated in the analysis, lacking information regarding LGBTQ sexual health, experiencing difficulties navigating healthcare systems, navigating regulatory discourses about sex, and feeling emotions such as anxiety and shame – all of these things can limit an individual's ability to have a healthy and satisfying sex life.

In the case of PrEP, although technologies of signs align PrEP with condomless sex – and, therefore, irresponsibility and heightened HIV risk – equating the drug only with condomless sex does not capture the full range of experiences of those taking the medicine. In the findings, a number of individuals said they were on PrEP and also used condoms. Moreover, in their dismissal of other viable safer sex practices, pro-condom rhetorics are not reflective of the various preventative strategies utilized within LGBTQ communities. Although condoms offered the only HIV prevention technology recommended by public health agencies at the beginning of the HIV/AIDS epidemic, prevention strategies have evolved, with developments in biomedical technologies and practices originating within LGBTQ communities, including serosorting, positioning strategies, external ejaculation, and more. The expansion of options from wearing "a condom every time" to a "wider range of possibilities not only affects sexual choices but also generates debate, conflict and even confrontation as choices must be negotiated between sexual partners and in the broader communities that have concerns about HIV transmission" (Brisson & Nguyen, 2017, pp. 1068–1069). Challenging homonormative and assimilatory discourses and countering "the figuring of HIV/AIDS as punishment for non-assimilation" (O'Brien, 2020, p. 126) is, thus, essential to expanding queer possibilities.

Queer standpoints "served as the basis for much of the AIDS activism movement" (Warner, 1999, p. 90). In today's "post-AIDS" culture, there remains a need for continuing to queer our discussions of LGBTQ health. Constructing understandings of "safe" sex through biomedical discourses and limiting "expert" knowledges to those produced by health authorities who frequently lack lived experience is one means by which the medical community avoids the "unpleasant realities of gay men and HIV prevention" (Spieldenner, 2017, p. 126). These include safer sex strategies developed within LGBTQ communities that do not always rely on monogamy, abstention, or condom use. Given the intersecting technologies of production, power, and signs that shape the encounters of gay and bisexual men with the medical establishment, furthering LGBTQ technologies of the self remains "a central problem, a collective project, even an urgent political necessity" (p. 108). Seeking and receiving gay guidance in anonymous online communities should be seen as part of this collective project to increase individual sexual agency, foreground marginalized knowledges, and enhance queer lives.

Although some members of LGBTQ communities currently define prEP in ways that reflect normalizing assumptions, it is also creating new definitions of self for some individuals who choose to use it. For those who choose to take the medicine, PrEP thus constitutes a health decision and a political act. By this, I do not mean to glamorize the taking of PrEP by framing it as a liberatory impulse rather than an HIV prevention option, medical necessity, or means of survival. I do, however, believe that given the intersections of the biomedical, personal, and social contexts that continue to produce dominant understandings of gay sexualities and sexual behaviors as deviant – particularly in the context of HIV-risk – that to live a queer life is "to live a life politically, in relation to power, in relation to others, in the act of assuming responsibility for a collective future" (Butler, 2007, p. 39). By providing a means of navigating heteronormative and homonormative discourses that produce queer sex as deviant and dangerous, PrEP can enable gay men to feel empowered in their sexual relationships and behaviors.

Acknowledgments

This chapter has greatly benefitted from the support of Robert B. Layne II, whose insights helped shape the conceptualizations found here. I also thank the editors for their generous feedback and commitment to this project.

Note

1 In the context of this essay, "agency" refers to the "human capacity to enact choices in negotiating structures" (Dutta, 2011, p. 9) This does not, however, suggest that agency is solely determined by individual choice; as Hanchey (2016) argues, recognizing agency "as a collective attribute rather than individual [...] is integral to transformative efforts for social change" (p. 13). In this case, individual /r/AskGayBros users may increase their capacities to act in relation to dominant structures, while the forum itself may increase collective agencies by providing a place to access marginalized knowledges.

References

Brisson, J., & Nguyen, V.-K. (2017). Science, technology, power and sex: PrEP and HIV-positive gay men in Paris. *Culture, Health & Sexuality, 19*(10), 1066–1077. doi: 10.1080/13691058.2017.1291994

Butler, J. (2007). *Undoing gender.* New York: Routledge.

Calabrese, S. K., & Underhill, K. (2015). How stigma surrounding the use of HIV preexposure prophylaxis undermines prevention and pleasure: A call to destigmatize "Truvada whores." *American Journal of Public Health, 105*(10), 1960–1964.

Centers for Disease Control and Prevention. (2019). PrEP. Retrieved from https://www.cdc.gov/hiv/basics/prep.html

Charmaz, K. (2014). *Constructing grounded theory.* Thousand Oaks, CA: Sage.

Chevrette, R. (2020). Blinded by acceptance: Straight fragility, shame, and the dangers of postqueer politics. *QED: A Journal in GLBTQ Worldmaking, 7*(1), 100–107.

Dean, M. A., Victor, E., & Guidry-Grimes, L. (2016). Inhospitable healthcare spaces: Why diversity training on LGBTQIA issues is not enough. *Journal of Bioethical Inquiry, 13*, 557–570.

Dutta, M. J. (2011). *Communicating social change: Structure, culture, and agency.* New York: Routledge.

Foucault, M. (1972). *The archaeology of knowledge,* trans. A. Sheridan. New York: Routledge.

Foucault, M. (1977). *Discipline and punish: The birth of the prison,* trans. A. Sheridan. New York: Random House.

Foucault, M. (1982). The subject and power. *Critical Inquiry, 8*(4), 777–795.

Foucault, M. (1988a). *The history of sexuality, volume 1: An introduction,* trans. R. Hurley. New York: Random House.

Foucault, M. (1988b). *The history of sexuality, volume 3: The care of the self,* trans. R. Hurley. New York: Random House.

Foucault, M. (1988c). Technologies of the self. In L. H. Martin, H. Gutman, & P. H. Hutton (Eds.), *Technologies of the self: A seminar with Michel Foucault* (pp. 16–49). Amherst, MA: University of Massachusetts Press.

Foucault, M. (2004). *The birth of biopolitics: Lectures at the College de France, 1978–1979.* M. Sellenart (Ed.), trans. by G. Burchell. New York: Picador.

Foucault, M. (2005). *The hermeneutics of the subject: Lectures at the College de France, 1981–1982.* F. Gros (Ed.), trans. by G. Burchell. New York: Picador.

France, D. (2016). *How to survive a plague: The inside story of how citizens and science tamed AIDS.* New York: Knopf.

Gere, D. (2004). *How to make dances in an epidemic: Tracking choreography in the age of AIDS.* Madison: University of Wisconsin Press.

Ghabrial, M. A. (2016). "Trying to figure out where we belong:" Narratives of racialized sexual minorities on community, identity, discrimination, and health. *Sexuality Research and Social Policy 14*(1), 42–55. doi: 10.1007/s13178-016-0229-x

Grimm, J., & Schwartz, J. (2019). "It's like birth control for HIV": Communication and stigma for gay men on PrEP. *Journal of Homosexuality, 66*(9), 1179–1197. doi:10.1080/00918369.2018.1495978

Halkitis, P. N., Jaiswal, J., Griffin-Tomas, M., Krause, K. D., D'Avanzo, P., & Kapadia, F. (2018). Beliefs about the end of AIDS, concerns about PrEP functionality, and perceptions of HIV risk as drivers of PrEP use in urban sexual minority men: The P18 cohort study. *AIDS Behavior, 22*(11), 3705–3717. doi:10.1007/s10461-018-2218-y.

Halperin, D. M. (2007). *What do gay men want? An essay on sex, risk, and subjectivity.* Ann Arbor: The University of Michigan Press.

Hanchey, J. (2016). Agency beyond agents: Aid campaigns in sub-Saharan Africa and collective representations of agency. *Communication, Culture, & Critique, 9*, 11–29.

Herek, G. M., & Capitanio, J. P. (1999). AIDS stigma and sexual prejudice. *American Behavioral Scientist, 42*, 1130–1147. doi:10.1177/0002764299042007006

Herek, G. M., & Glunt, E. K. (1988). An epidemic of stigma: Public reactions to AIDS. *American Psychologist, 43*, 886–891.

I'm Still Josh. (2019). Retrieved from https://imstilljosh.com/

Kane, J. (2019, May 14). What Trump's PrEP deal means for the spread of HIV. *Public Broadcasting Service.* Retrieved from https://www.pbs.org/newshour/health/what-trumps-prep-deal-means-for-the-spread-of-hiv

Koester, K. A., Erguera, S. A., & Myers, J. J. (2017). "PrEP makes my relationship even more normal:" The discursive production of hope in the context of HIV pre-exposure prophylaxis among young adults with partners living with HIV infection. In A. Persson,& S. D. Hughes (Eds.), *Cross-cultural perspectives on couples with mixed HIV status: Beyond positive/negative* (pp. 23–36). Switzerland: Springer.

Layne II, R. (2017). *The communicative constitution of reproduction and reproductive genetic testing for sex and gender minorities: A queer standpoint approach.* (Unpublished doctoral dissertation). University of Utah. Salt Lake, UT.

Levine, M. P. (1979). Gay ghetto. *Journal of Homosexuality, 4*(4), 363–377. doi:10.1300/J082v04n4_04

Morris, M., & Roberto, K. R. (2016). Information-seeking behavior and information needs of LGBTQ health professionals: A follow-up study. *Health Information and Libraries Journal, 33*, 204–221. doi:10.1111/hir.12139

My Prep Experience. (2015). Retrieved from http://myprepexperience.blogspot.com/

O'Brien, C. (2020). HIV and AIDS in Irish theatre: Queer masculinities, punishment, and 'Post-AIDS' culture. *Journal of Medical Humanities, 41*(2), 123–136. doi:10.1007/s10912-017-9439-3

/r/AskGayBros. (2019). Retrieved from https://www.reddit.com/r/askgaybros/

Race, K. (2009). *Pleasure consuming medicine: The queer politics of drugs.* Durham, NC: Duke University Press.

Rodger, A. J., Cambiano, V., Bruun, T., Vernazza, P., Collins, S., Degen, O., … Lundgren, J. (2019). Risks of HIV transmission through condomless sex in serodifferent gay couples with the HIV-positive partner taking suppressive antiretroviral therapy (PARTNER): Final results of a multicentre, prospective, observational study. *The Lancet, 393*(10189), 2428–2438. doi:10.1016/S0140-6736(19)30418-0

Schwartz, J., & Grimm, J. (2016). Uncertainty in online US news coverage of Truvada. *Health Communication, 31*(10), 1250–1257.

Sedgwick, E. K. (1990). *Epistemology of the closet.* Berkeley: University of California Press.

Spieldenner, A. (2014). Statement of ownership: An autoethnography of living with HIV. *The Journal of Men's Studies, 22*(1), 12–27. doi: 10.3149/jms.2201.12

Spieldenner, A. (2016). PrEP whores and HIV prevention: The queer communication of HIV Pre-Exposure Prophylaxis (PrEP). *Journal of Homosexuality, 63*(12), 1685–1697. doi:10.1080/00918369.2016.1158012

Spieldenner, A. (2017). Infectious sex? An autoethnographic exploration of HIV prevention. *QED: A Journal in GLBTQ Worldmaking, 4*(1), 121–129.

Treichler, P. (1987). AIDS, homophobia and biomedical discourse: An epidemic of signification. *Cultural Studies 1*(3), 263–305.

Ussher, J. M. (2009). Heterocentric practices in health research and health care: Implications for mental health and subjectivity of LGBTQ individuals. *Feminism & Psychology, 19*(4), 561–567. doi:10.1177/0959353509342933

Wahlert, L. (2013). Anti-love or anti-"lifestyle": Historical reflections on reparative therapies for homosexuality. *American Journal of Bioethics, 13*(11), 36–38. doi:10.1080/15265161.2013.840869

Warner, M. (1999). *The trouble with normal: Sex, politics, and the ethics of queer life.* Cambridge, MA: Harvard University Press.

Warner, M. (2002). *Publics and counterpublics.* Brooklyn, NY: Zone Books.

Yan, Z., Wang, T., Chen, Y., & Zhang, H. (2016). Knowledge sharing in online health communities: A social exchange theory perspective. *Information & Management, 53*, 643–653. doi:10.1016/j.im.2016.02.0010378-7206/2016

10 Intimacy Uncertainty and Post-AIDS Discourse

HIV and the Role it Plays as an Uninvited Third Party in Serodiscordant Relationships

Scott A. Eldredge

HIV has, today, morphed from a near-certain death sentence to a chronic, almost invisible condition (U.S. Department of Health and Human Services [HHS], 2020). Since protease inhibitors were first introduced in 1996, people living with HIV can now expect to live long, largely healthy lives. With this shift in medical outcomes associated with HIV, the term "post-AIDS" began to creep into the medical lexicon, and with it, the notion that HIV was no longer a threat. With the 1998 publication of his oft-cited book, *Dry Bones Breathe*, Rofes discusses the meanings and distinction of "end of AIDS" rhetoric as it relates to the very real health crisis AIDS presented during the 1980s and the early 1990s. In this context, the "end of AIDS" means the end of AIDS-as-crisis conceptualization of the disease, and Rofes (1998) presents the ongoing frustration of activists and those who work in advocacy that argue AIDS is not over, and the crisis is ongoing. As Rofes (1998) relates, the AIDS-as-crisis construct served as the catalyst mobilizing a host of social services primarily targeting white, urban, middle-class gay men, but the rhetoric of crisis and death has done little to highlight the ongoing threat HIV presents, particularly for women and people of color.

Today, over 20 years beyond the inflection point brought on by the protease inhibitor moment, popular culture continues to characterize HIV as a crisis, dying, and death, and, simultaneously, that we are now living in a post-AIDS era, particularly in countries with access to robust public health services (O'Brien, 2013, 2020). Popular culture effectively tells us we have arrived in a post-AIDS world because we no longer acutely witness HIV ravage white, urban, gay men. The loss of urgency carried by post-AIDS discourse could be interpreted as encouraging us to believe that society's immediate and pressing concerns, even those for the LGBTQ community, are not about HIV (Román, 2000). As a public, post-AIDS discourse continues to take an end-of-AIDS perspective, the implication becomes that public policy de-emphasizes support for HIV treatment, prevention, and research. For example, the United Nations launched its 17 Sustainable Development Goals (SDGs) to Transform Our World in 2015 (United Nations, Department of Economic and Social Affairs, 2020). These SDGs serve as policy benchmarks for all members of the United Nations; critics argue that they represent a shift away from advocating for an HIV exceptionalism

DOI: 10.4324/9781003000945-13

public policy response that requires HIV to be addressed through health interventions that are "beyond normal" versus interventions for other types of diseases and health concerns (O'Connell, 2020).

As post-AIDS discourse affects public policy decisions regarding HIV treatment and prevention, writers continue to highlight the contradictions presented by the end-of-AIDS themes found within that discourse. HIV prevention efforts still focus on individuals managing their own behaviors, such as practicing sexual behaviors commonly identified as safe-sex techniques (i.e., condom use), and perhaps taking one of the two anti-HIV drugs approved for use as a pre-exposure prophylactic (PrEP). According to Walker (2020), the 1996 introduction of antiretroviral drugs represents a biotechnical solution to AIDS. Still, this approach to public health efforts ignores the social and symbolic realities and the complex effects of the stigma, associated with HIV. Some argue this approach amounts to a singular focus on a common gay identity, with the LGBTQ community often being lumped into one, central identity (Dowsett, 2009). However, the LGBTQ community encompasses a wide diversity of people with different serostatuses, ethnicities, ages, generations, and relationship practices. Despite this diversity, prevention efforts lack the nuance needed to better address the psychosocial realities faced by this multifaceted community (Dowsett, 2009). Because anti-HIV drugs are dispensed as both a treatment for people living with HIV (PLHIV) as well as a prophylactic that prevents HIV transmission, it could be argued that public health efforts today are primarily focused on directing a simple, singular message to a mass audience, centered on the notion that taking this drug means HIV is no longer an issue, effectively continuing the "end of AIDS" themes found within this post-AIDS discourse.

We are left, then, with a gap in how we conceptualize this disease, leaving treatment and prevention efforts without the context and insight into the lived experiences of PLHIV and HIV-negative persons. Because illness is an interdependent phenomenon and HIV is a chronic, communicable disease, effective communication surrounding treatment and prevention efforts must consider the relational experiences of both PLHIV and those who are HIV-negative. For PLHIV, they must navigate their identity and sense of self, which will, in turn, affect how they manage their disease. For those that are HIV-negative, the virus becomes a significant issue as they attempt to initiate and maintain intimate relationships with a partner who is living with HIV. In particular, the HIV-negative partners of gay men living with HIV are almost completely absent from any type of public discourse on HIV. Faced with ongoing stressors and stigmatization of their relationships and sexual identities, gay men engaged in romantic partnerships with men living with HIV must, on a daily basis, deal with the effects of a disease they do not actually have. However, as these HIV-negative men continue to struggle with realities they must face, the rhetoric surrounding HIV in a post-AIDS world leaves no place for discussing the psychosocial aspects of the disease and what it means for relationship functioning. We have effectively told them you can just take a pill (i.e., Walker's, 2020 biotechnical solution) or use a condom, and HIV will no longer be a problem for anyone, whether you are living with HIV or are HIV-negative. To better manage and ultimately overcome HIV, we must first understand the full range of people impacted by HIV and include discussions of those impacts in our public discourse. For the HIV-negative partners of men living with HIV, we need to explore and understand their lived realities and move beyond the post-AIDS discourse focused on how HIV is easily removed from their lives. While we are socialized to follow particular relational scripts, HIV-related uncertainties disrupt those storylines. The participants in the study presented herein are left without the tools, skills, concepts, and imagery that may help them manage and regulate intimacy with their relational partners. Given that the following narratives occur within a societal structure bounded by end-of-AIDS and post-AIDS discourse, the purpose of the study reported in this chapter is to explore the intimacy-related uncertainties felt by HIV-negative gay men who are the partners of PLHIV and to understand the role HIV plays in their uncertainty management efforts.

Literature Review

HIV as an Interdependent Phenomenon

A patient's relationship and communication with a spouse or partner impacts how they conceptualize illness and health care. In close relationships, one partner's stress can be shared or can affect the other partner directly or indirectly (Goldsmith, 2009; Westman & Vinokur, 1998). However, most research looking at how people cope with illness-related stress focuses on an individual's response to stress, even though stress is a shared experience in interdependent relationships. Further, responding to and coping with stress is done through interactions with others (Afifi, Hutchinson, & Krouse, 2006); stress is managed through communication.

Chronic illness and its uncertainties introduce stress into close relationships and influence the day-to-day lives of relational partners in many ways. Stressors from illnesses affecting the relationship are not solely felt by the patient. When someone suffers a spinal cord injury, is diagnosed with cancer, or tests positive for HIV, the primary story told is often that of the patient; however, even though not diagnosed with an illness, the patient's partner must figure out how to navigate the effects of illness in their own unique manner (Goldsmith, 2009). Essentially, the patient has a healthcare provider available to treat the symptoms and side effects that come with being sick; the partner, while not actually being sick, still has to deal with the challenges brought on by their partner's illness, often without asking for help and receiving little attention from healthcare providers (Kuyper & Wester, 1998).

While advanced treatment protocols have made living with HIV more akin to a chronic condition, HIV – being an infectious disease carrying with it high levels of social stigma – brings with it a unique set of circumstances that couples experiencing other serious illnesses may not face. Committed, romantic partners where one partner is living with HIV and the other is HIV-negative must address issues of intimacy, including sex and risk of HIV infection; they must decide about HIV disclosure to family and friends; they must investigate issues surrounding reproductive decisions; they must anticipate disability or death; and they must negotiate caregiving concerns (Derlega, Winstead, Oldfield III, & Barbee, 2003; Kalichman, 2000; Wrubel & Folkman, 1997).

Each of these circumstances introduces additional illness-related stress into the relationship, thereby having the potential to exacerbate the effects of illness and create additional relational stress. For example, disclosing one's HIV status has been shown to be an acute and recurrent stressor for both the person living with HIV and their partner (Holt et al., 1998). For the HIV-negative partner, the partner living with HIV also carries with it meaning that has implications for the negative partner. Essentially, disclosure of the partner's HIV status also says something about the HIV-negative partner. In this way, the negative partner must deal with the effects of a disease without actually having the disease. In this situation, stress arises from the fallout of managing disclosure.

Gay, male, mixed-status couples must deal with the illness effects, stigma, and social isolation often associated with the disease to successfully maintain their relationship and prevent relational decline (Haas, 2002). For these mixed-status couples, social support provided by the HIV-negative partner is important to relationship maintenance as the couple handles the illness stressors (Haas, 2002). Relational partners, as opposed to close friends and family, are the primary and irreplaceable source of social support for both partners (Haas, 2002). However, providing social support is also complicated because the stressors associated with illness are interpreted, made sense of, and responded to by both partners. In this way, the illness impacts partners directly, making the partner more than just a source of social support, but rather a co-participant in the illness experience (Goldsmith, 2009).

HIV, Uncertainty, and Intimacy

The way illness is felt within a close, romantic relationship is a complex, shared experience that gives rise to varying levels of uncertainty felt by the relational partners. Uncertainty Reduction Theory discusses uncertainty in terms of an individual's ability to predict the future behavior of another (Berger & Calabrese, 1975). Uncertainty, in this context, is a negatively oriented state of not knowing information about another person. When considering uncertainty within the context of illness and health, uncertainty is defined as the inability to determine the meaning of illness-related events (Mishel, 1988). The communicative behaviors associated with navigating illness-related uncertainties and providing social support become an important buffer for the relational partners against the negative effects associated with the disease. This communication helps individuals living with HIV manage uncertainty (Brashers, Neidig, & Goldsmith 2004). When HIV-related prevention recommendations are limited to discourse on PrEP and condom usage, it neglects the uncertainties that may play a role in influencing the adoption or rejection of these recommended methods for HIV prevention.

While relational uncertainty is defined in terms of the uncertainties partners engaged within a relationship, have about themselves, their partner, and the status of the relationship (Knobloch & Solomon, 1999), the intrusion and disruption that an HIV diagnosis brings to a relationship gives rise to uncertainties related to intimacy (Beckerman, 2002). Intimacy has been defined and conceptualized exhaustively in the literature (Reis, 1990). For the purposes of this study, intimacy is comprised of the following five components: Closeness, a feeling of union between two people who spend time with one another and influence each other's behaviors and beliefs; Openness, the willingness of partners to reveal private information about themselves to each other; Trust, the feeling that a relational partner will keep us safe; Affection, the positive feelings we have for another person that are communicated to that person with various actions; and Mutuality, when relational partners acknowledge and value the bond that exists between them (Solomon & Theiss, 2013).

With HIV being a constant consideration, the very presence of HIV introduces uncertainties felt by the relational partners that are related to the components of intimacy. To understand the progression of intimacy within relationships, it is also helpful to consider how relationships begin and develop over time. Knap (1984) proposes a model of relational development that includes stages involving initiation, experimenting, intensifying, integrating, and bonding. Each stage of the model represents increasing intimacy between the individuals involved in the relationship by communicating and performing behaviors that reduce uncertainty, increase closeness and mutuality, and develop an identity as a social unit.

Relational Scripts and Post-AIDS Discourse

"Once upon a time." "Happily ever after." These are the familiar openings and closings to the common fairy tale archetype, and, with some slight modification to the pronouns involved, these stories follow a pattern where a boy dreams of growing up and, while pursuing a grand, life-changing adventure, meets the man of his dreams, falls in love, and lives happily ever after. What actually happens in the "happily ever after?" The desire and pursuit of a long-lasting, intimate relationship certainly are not confined to heterosexual couplings, and gay men can relate to stories of catching a potential partner's eye at a dinner party, pursuing flirtatious opportunities, long late-night talks on the phone, dreaming of marriage, planning for the future, and growing old together. In following these types of relational scripts, gay men are no different from their heterosexual counterparts (Peplau & Fingerhut, 2006). We know that relationships grow, intensify, develop, change, and even dissolve over time. Considered against the backdrop offered by post-AIDS discourse where pharmaceuticals have removed the threat HIV presents, it would seem pursuing relationships modeled after these scripts certainly does not – and need not – include thoughts regarding the risks of contracting or transmitting HIV. However, even as post-AIDS narratives dismiss the notion of HIV as a threat to health and well-being, HIV-negative individuals, as well as PLHIV, continue to confront myriad social, emotional, and biological uncertainties brought on by the disease.

Gay culture has also allowed for the freedom to choose non-traditional relationship styles, including consensual nonmonogamy and polyamory. Research in queer theory identifies egalitarian and non-gendered cultural values driving the development of queer dating and relational scripts that reject traditional, heterosexual relational norms (Lamont, 2017). In structuring their relationships, gay men often find themselves vacillating between heteronormative conceptualizations of relationships and the more open, culturally-based relational scripts found within the LGBTQ community (Butler, 2004). In many cases, gay men choose to change and modify their relationship style with their partner over time. For example, younger gay men may start with a monogamous relationship, moving to an open relationship where the partners negotiate rules and boundaries around sex outside the partnership (Pawlicki & Larson, 2011; Philpot et al., 2018; Wheldon & Pathak, 2010). While gay men have the freedom to choose from various relationship styles, they also don't have clear social norms to follow about how relationships are "supposed" to form (Butler, 2004). In addition, they may also feel pressure to conform to the scripts found within the LGBTQ community (Lamont, 2017). For example, many gay men desire a heteronormative, monogamous relationship yet often perceive open relationships to be the expected norm among gay men and potential partners.

Many factors affect relationships, and on top of these relational scripts, gay men entering into committed, romantic partnerships with another man also encounter an additional unique set of conditions. Romantically paired men must navigate a world where their relationship will often be stigmatized, misunderstood, discriminated against, and, the advent of same-sex marriages notwithstanding, limited in the formal recognition society offers heterosexual marriages (Peplau & Fingerhut, 2006). Any of these factors alone is certain to add additional stressors to the relationship. Still, in addition to these situations, gay men also must navigate a world where being gay is often associated with HIV.

Gay men remain one of the groups at greatest risk for contracting HIV (HHS, 2020), and the simple act of giving blood is restricted if one identifies as gay.[1] In addition, gay men are encouraged to get tested for HIV infection regularly, often several times a year, depending on their sexual habits. Set against post-AIDS discourse, critics argue that end-of-AIDS rhetoric represents a conscious rejection of the connection between gay identity and HIV, which, in turn, allows for the decline in research and activism related to HIV prevention and treatment (Butler, 2004). For the HIV-negative man, every potential romantic partner represents both the possibility of a fulfilling relationship as well as a potential threat to their health and well-being. After all, who wants to think about disease when trying to find your Prince Charming? Catching a disease that, at best, will mark you as sick and require constant treatment or, at worst, kill you is not exactly something that helps set a romantic mood. And yet, as society declares this the post-AIDS era, gay men must still consider that Prince Charming just may be a PLHIV.

Against this backdrop of stigmatization, an ever-present disease threat, myriad relationship choices, and a post-AIDS discourse dismissing the disease as any real threat that HIV-negative men attempt to form close, romantic partnerships. In seeking insight into the relationships of HIV-negative, gay men form with PLHIV, this study posed the following questions:

RQ1: What are the HIV-related intimacy uncertainties felt by the HIV-negative, gay partners of PLHIV?
RQ2: What role does HIV play in the relationships of gay men in serodiscordant, romantic partnerships?

Methods

Drawing on data collected through in-depth, semi-structured interviews, this study explores the experience of nine HIV-negative partners of gay men living with HIV. For inclusion in this effort, the men identified as being in a romantic partnership were ones where the couple had to: (1) both be at least 18 years of age, (2) both identify as gay, (3) both have a male gender identity, (4) both identify as being in a committed, romantic partnership and (5) have one partner identify as a PLHIV and the other as HIV-negative. As part of data collection, both partners agreed to be interviewed, with data collected on the partner who was a PLHIV reported on separately.

The following demographics characterize the nine individuals included in this chapter. Eight of the participants identified as white. One participant identified as Latino. The average age of the participants was 45 years (range 26–66 years). One participant reported he had finished high school. One participant had an associate's degree. Two participants had bachelor's degrees. Four participants had master's degrees, and one participant had a doctoral degree. The average length of time these men identified being in a committed, romantic relationship with their partner was 7.5 years (range 2–17 years).

To develop a deeper understanding of participants' experiences, the researcher followed additional grounded theory techniques for data analysis as outlined by Charmaz (2006), generating a written account of the results of this analysis and a discussion of those results. All nine participants reviewed the composite findings to establish the credibility of the report. Pseudonyms have been used in reporting the findings to protect the participants' identities.

Results

For the men participating in this study, the relational uncertainties brought on by HIV becoming a seemingly chronic, manageable condition are most associated with intimacy between the partners. As David discusses the sexual difficulties he and his partner experienced, he reveals the threat to overall intimacy he felt between himself and his partner. David and his partner had been in an on again-off again-on again relationship, and his partner contracted HIV in the few months when they were not together. When they got back together, his partner had not yet been diagnosed, and the shock of the diagnosis took a toll on the connection they had established.

> Well I think with ... I think that had an impact on non-sexual intimacy. I think there was a shift. It's really hard to put into words, but there was a palpable shift for me in terms, um, [pause] ... I don't know it seemed to have some kind of significance in how we would then be with each other. So, with intimacy, it was about sex, but that also filtered into just connection.

As David discussed how the uncertainties associated with the mechanics of sexual intimacy turn to broader concerns of emotional intimacy within the overall relationship, he described a very definite shift in how the partners related to one another after his partner's HIV diagnosis. In addition, David's quote also demonstrates the difficulty in making sense of this shift in intimacy. It is this kind of psychosocial concern that is absent from the post-AIDS discourse. David's quote goes beyond the idea that you can take a pill or use a condom to deal with issues of sexual intimacy. You can't take a pill to fix emotional connections.

HIV Slows the Progression of Intimacy

For these HIV-negative men, meeting a man living with HIV requires them to stop and think about whether they want to truly get close to this individual. These men need to consider potential consequences – physical, social, and emotional – that come with being in an intimate relationship with someone who has a chronic illness, particularly one that is stigmatized, contagious, and potentially life-threatening. This is a unique consideration when positioned against the heteronormative scripts describing relationship growth and progression. With some of the men in the present study, entering into a relationship with a PLHIV was a conscious choice. These men met their partners when their partners already identified as a PLHIV; HIV already had a starring role in the relationship when it began. Intellectually, they know that today HIV is treatable and survivable. PLHIV can and do live long, healthy lives. However, HIV became the central, most salient point of consideration when these men assessed their relationship options.

Tim and his partner met through mutual friends 11 years prior to his interview. His partner was diagnosed with HIV nearly 30 years ago, but he has never really experienced severe sickness from the disease and is today on antiviral medication. Tim described an extended, flirtatious courtship with his future partner that preceded them actually dating. Their first date, dinner, and a movie came later. Deciding to date this man was, for Tim, a very considered decision. Two of his previous partners died of AIDS, so he felt there was quite a bit to consider before entering into a relationship with another man living with HIV.

> I wasn't sure at the moment, at that point in time. He was very open about being HIV-positive, and I had to think a lot about whether I wanted to get

> involved because I'd been involved in [City, State] with somebody in the 80s who, when the test first came out, found out he was positive, contracted AIDS fairly early on, um, and passed away. And I drove him to the hospice, and went through the wringer. And then had a few friends here in [current location] in the early 90s who passed away. A guy that I was dating ... there was a lot of ... I just questioned myself, do I, you know, want to get involved with someone who is HIV-positive, and, because I don't want to lead anybody on. I just had to weigh everything, the costs and benefits of this, and am I prepared to deal with possible events in the future? Illness, just like I had to deal with in the past. I did a lot of soul searching about that stuff.

Throughout the description of how they met and the questioning of whether he could enter into a relationship with yet another man living with HIV, Tim struggled with whether he should make himself emotionally vulnerable to such a relationship. Tim's uncertainty centers on the question of whether entering into a relationship with this man would protect him from the emotional harm he had experienced in the past. As Tim demonstrates, past experiences and conceptualizations about HIV directly affect his decision to pursue a relationship with a PLHIV. In Tim's case, it is not just stories about people's experiences with HIV or even his past understanding of the potential course of the disease in the other person. For Tim, he felt no recognition that he had arrived in a post-AIDS world. Tim's considerations about a potential relationship were based on his own past relational experiences where AIDS was a factor and the very real presence of HIV with his current partner.

Similar to Tim's experience of an extended courtship prior to a first date, Carlos and his partner spent the six months prior to their first date interacting only online. On that first date, Carlos describes kissing his partner for the first time, and it is apparent that even at those most romantic moments, HIV lurked in Carlos' thoughts.

> It was just the perfect day for him to tell me, in other words. And, um, he caught me on a day that I wasn't with my walls up and protecting myself all the time. And when he told me [that he was HIV-positive], and then I thought about all the stuff we talked about and everything. I basically became more comfortable, and he was looking toward the view of the city and the sun just hit him perfectly. I remember that, and I was like, 'Damn! He looks nice even though he has that bug in him!' But, um, and I just leaned over and gave him a kiss.

For Carlos, the mood was right, the setting was perfect, and he felt that connection with his partner. The moment of the first kiss in a new relationship may commonly be thought of as a signal pointing to a progression of intimacy as the couple's feelings of closeness intensify. However, for Carlos, even as the desire to connect with his partner won out, HIV intruded on his thoughts. Providing insight into his personal attitudes about the virus, Carlos refers to HIV as a "bug" in his partner, even though his partner still "looks nice." Even though the medical community has signaled the end of AIDS, Carlos still had to overcome the negative conceptions he carried regarding HIV. Carlos eventually was able to further develop his relationship with his partner; however, his story demonstrates how uncertainties and negative preconceptions associated with HIV may slow relationship progression, taking more time and effort for intimacy to develop than would be expected without the presence of HIV.

For both Tim and Carlos, HIV was there with that initial sense of attraction, forcing a more considered approach to the idea of dating someone who was living with HIV. It seemed to take longer for their attractions to ignite, and they moved much slower when initiating a relationship because their partner was living with HIV when they first met. In these cases, HIV served as a mechanism for slowing down the progression of intimacy between the couple; its potential illness effects and issues associated with HIV were central features in the decision-making process to even consider starting a relationship with a PLHIV.

While HIV presents an issue to be considered when deciding to begin a relationship, it also affects the pace at which the relationship intensifies. For Tim and his partner, several months went by before there was any kind of sexual contact.

> We waited a couple of months actually before we had sex which is weird in the gay community, too. A lot of people kind of have sex, and then introduce themselves afterwards. [laughs] For us it was the other way around. We got to know each other.

Because of HIV, Tim and his partner made the conscious decision to wait to have sex, and as he mentions, he feels he and his partner went against the common relationship patterns followed by most other gay men.

All relationships move through periods of intensification that may involve relational turbulence. Still, for Carlos, HIV was consistently at the center of his thoughts and decisions to get more intimate with his partner, as he consternated over how it might look to family and friends that he was dating a PLHIV.

> I was always thinking, 'What would the family say? What would my friends say?" And, "How would I fit into my social circle?" I was basically a semi-popular kid here in downtown [City] and, um, and then my family had me as the Golden Boy. They had me on a pedestal, and every move I made was the perfect one. I was thinking about all this stuff ... literally got me thinking. For a while there, we didn't have sex, because I was just, like, too much ... too much pressure, and so little time for me to learn all this stuff, and for me to feel comfortable.

Carlos struggled with what dating a PLHIV would say about him. He worried about the stigma associated with the disease, and his mind went to a place where he imagines or questions what his friends and family would think if he became a PLHIV. He mentioned that he is seen as perfect, so that contracting HIV would damage that image of perfection. This seemed overwhelming for him, so sex was out of the question until he could figure out how to deal with these uncertainties. Abstinence is obviously an effective HIV prevention method, and only then could Carlos assure himself that he remained HIV-negative. He is denied the potential for sex as a method to bring him and his partner closer and intensify the bond between them. By delaying the progression of intimacy, he only had to deal with the effects of the disease on his partner without any personal repercussions associated with being sick.

Sex, in relation to intimacy, is a behavior used to express affection for the relational partner. It works to form the bond that results in and reinforces feelings of closeness (Leigh, 1989). Another participant, Peter, discussed the importance of sex and how it plays a significant role in establishing the connection between himself and his partner.

> I think there's no more intimate thing than letting someone inside you, and I got to a point where I was just very much in love with this man. I wanted to experience that. I wanted him inside of me. I wanted a piece of him. It might sound odd, but that's kind of how I feel.

Peter identified the significant role sex performs in intensifying the relationship. However, both Tim and Carlos chose to delay having sex with their partners and, thus, delay the progression of intimacy as they sought to manage the relational uncertainties brought on by the presence of HIV.

Once the decision was made to have sex, the study participants still proceeded slowly. For all the men in this study, the use of condoms was emblematic of how HIV presents a barrier to getting closer. Peter's quote is part of a larger discussion regarding not using condoms with his partner. For Peter, the decision to use condoms has always been an easy decision when having sex outside of a committed relationship. However, in his comments regarding sex with his partner, he discusses the downsides of using them. Condoms, then, represent both a physical and psychological barrier to intimacy. Like Peter, another participant, John, also describes the barriers to intimacy that result from condom use.

> But your question was, why unprotected sex? Why is that important? It's an intimacy thing. I would say [partner] and I are pretty kinky individuals, so, like, randomly having sex somewhere that isn't our home could happen, and if you've got to kind of like whip out condoms it can kill the mood. It really can. It's nice to just not have to worry about it. Well … it's, it would be nice. The best thing would be if no one had to worry about it. I still have to worry about it.

For another example, Carlos described the disruptive nature associated with condom use.

> Even though you don't think about it, but you can see the reaction, the way they move, when they're reaching over for the condom. You can see they're like, "Oh, we have to go through all this process just to get something."

In relating these difficulties with condoms, Peter, John, and Carlos identified how intimacy is controlled by HIV. The presence of HIV necessitates using a condom, requiring the partners to move more slowly, and, in Carlos' words, "go through all this process." It directly affects the partners' efforts at affection and closeness and causes the partners to interrupt an intimate moment to make accommodations for the unwelcome third party that is HIV.

While Carlos is now on PrEP, it is important to note that his decision to have unprotected sex as the receptive partner was made prior to him going on antiviral medication for prophylactic purposes. Even though his partner was taking antiviral medication and his viral load was undetectable, Carlos described the tension he and his partner experienced while having sex for the first time after deciding to forgo a condom.

> My whole body was shaking, because I was like, and he was like, "You don't feel comfortable, [Carlos]." And I was like, "I do, to certain degree, it's just that my body is like, ehh." But my mind was feeling comfortable. We did it the first time, and he, of course, ejaculated outside. He was like, "How do you feel? How do you feel?" And, for that one day, I thought that I should go and get tested for some reason, because I was petrified. I thought I was like, "What was I thinking?" Of course, I had to wait more time, so I was like, "Okay. Fine. I'm going to wait," and I was like, "[Partner], let's use condoms now to see if everything is still okay." Everything came out fine, and I was negative, and he was like, "Are you comfortable? Are you okay? We can use condoms if you still want to." I was like, "I feel more comfortable. I feel more safe. I feel like you will respect the one thing that we agreed on, that you will ejaculate outside when we bareback, and if you want to ejaculate inside, you will always use a condom. And so he's respective of that, and for that, I am truly grateful to him.

For Carlos, he and his partner's first experimentation with forgoing a condom resulted in significant anxiety related to sex and intimacy for both partners. Carlos' partner already carried with him concerns about the possibility of transmitting the virus to Carlos. For his part, Carlos had to deal with the fear and uncertainty that came with potentially exposing himself to the virus. Even though a post-AIDS worldview would suggest that pharmaceuticals have removed the threat posed by HIV, it still sits at the center of issues salient to conceptualizations of intimacy within these relationships, causing these men to both reflect on their past experiences and understandings of the illness, as well as contemplate both their personal future and the future of their relationships. While these men work to resolve the uncertainties they have about intimacy with a PLHIV, post-AIDs rhetoric actually serves to discourage the development of any models of relational functioning that may help them manage their uncertainties. If we have reached the "end of AIDS," it would seem there is no need to talk about how to deal with these feelings.

HIV Diagnoses Disrupt Established Relational Patterns

While some participants highlighted ways that the presence of HIV at the start of the relationship slows the initiation and progression of intimacy, other men in this study began their relationships with both partners being HIV-negative, and it was later that their partner became infected with the virus. In some cases, the couple had discussed and set up rules for an open relationship, while other couples engaged in sex outside the relationship without explicitly designating the relationship as open until after one partner was diagnosed. After the HIV diagnosis, these men found it difficult to manage new intimacy-related uncertainties and establish new relational norms. At the time of his interview, Andrew and his partner had been together for a total of 11 years, and his partner was diagnosed seven years into their relationship. For both Andrew and his partner, being monogamous was an understood aspect of the relationship, even though they had never explicitly discussed it, and they both recognized that each occasionally engaged in sex outside of the relationship. Once HIV came along, they felt the need to formally recognize the relationship as open, but specific rules around being non-monogamous remain unspoken between the couple. Here, Andrew discusses uncertainties and changes to sexual practices brought on by HIV, but it is apparent that the disruption to the couple's existing intimacy patterns has been difficult to address.

> Well, I mean, you know, just sort of fooling around not, not going, not going the full distance, just for, just for safety's sake, slam on the brakes, or something like that … especially when he wasn't on meds. Um, but, I mean, we weren't completely abstinent just … just limited our activities to some of the less risky things. But, yeah, it was definitely work still, uh … maybe a year ago … still sort of thinking maybe we don't know … we don't want to do that … I don't just want to do that to you.

Andrew noted that even after three years following his partner's diagnosis, they would not engage in certain sexual practices. It took three years to get comfortable with certain aspects of sex and physical intimacy. This speaks to the difficulties in re-establishing or maintaining intimacy because HIV was introduced after patterns and norms were set. Andrew also acknowledged that HIV prevents some sexual activities between himself and his partner because those activities raise the risk of transmitting the virus. Andrew does not "begrudge him wanting to do some things that we can't at the moment." Within their relationship, Andrew and his partner found that HIV dictated how they expressed and maintained connection and intimacy, leaving them to try and discover new ways to maintain their closeness.

Caleb and his partner had been together for 17 years, and his partner was diagnosed with HIV nearly 15 years into their relationship. Like Andrew and his partner, Caleb and his partner didn't explicitly talk about the opening up of the relationship, even though Caleb knew his partner did engage in extra-relational sex. As of this interview, Caleb and his partner were still working through some of the intimacy-related difficulties brought on by his partner's HIV diagnosis, even though they now do discuss their extradyadic sexual encounters.

> So, it did cause, I think some problems between us as far as that goes. And it's taking some time for us to try to figure out where we're going to go with it, and we're still kind of figuring that out, two plus years later. We're still trying to figure out where we're going to go with, with, with how we're going to have sex, how we're going to do it.

According to Caleb, the couple has very different personalities that drive very different needs, desires, and approaches to sex and intimacy. Because of this, the couple spent quite a bit of time working to develop agreed-upon norms around initiating sex. When HIV intruded on the relationship, those agreed-upon rules suddenly changed.

> So, the first couple years of our relationship, he got to the point where he was like, "I'm always initiating. Why are you never initiating?" So, then we got to the point where he's like, "I'm not going to initiate. So, if you want to have sex, you have to initiate. So, if we go a week not having sex, it's your fault because you didn't initiate." So, we still have those kinds of things sometimes, but uh, it's hard for me I guess, being more the reserved person, to be the initiative person, so, so, we still have that area to go. And I think the HIV may have, let me go back to old behaviors a little bit because, okay, how are we going to have sex now? What are we going to do? If we're only going to do this little quick thing then it's easier to kind of do that kind of thing and so, um, so we have to kind of come back to where we were before which has taken a little bit of time to do that.

As Caleb described, HIV allowed him to fall into previous relationship patterns that the couple had already discussed and worked to change. Specifically, the responsibility for initiating sex became a point of contention in their relationship. With Caleb having difficulty taking responsibility for intimacy and the partners struggling with issues of mutuality regarding sexual practices, Caleb and his partner worked to change that. Caleb became more comfortable initiating sex, but when HIV came along, it brought uncertainty about sex and intimacy with it. The previously agreed-upon rules had not taken into account HIV. With HIV now a factor, reverting to old relationship patterns where a different kind of uncertainty was present was easy to do.

As previously noted, David's partner contracted HIV during a short break in their relationship. Prior to the HIV diagnosis, David always insisted on a monogamous relationship even though his partner had expressed an interest in an open relationship. However, with HIV being introduced, David described a change to their agreed-upon relationship rules.

> Prior [to the HIV diagnosis], he had always been interested in that [an open relationship]. I insisted on it not. So, then I said I want that [after the HIV

> diagnosis]. I need that in order to keep this relationship going. I think, at the time, I felt, um … [pause] I needed to go out and meet other people, and I needed to experience sex. I don't know why exactly. I don't think there's a rational reason I can give you other than maybe it was simply I needed or wanted a, [pause] venue to express my stress or frustration, [pause] whatever emotions I was feeling at the time.

David also described the struggle he and his partner had with determining what this virus meant for the sexual aspects of their relationship.

> I just didn't know what it meant for us. I remember thinking well it shouldn't mean anything for us, but it did. And, um, [pause] it primarily concerned me from a sexual standpoint. It concerned me, what that meant for our sex life. I don't think I had concerns, at least conscious concerns, at that point. I wasn't concerned with him dying or anything like that. I knew enough about it to not be scared of that. Um, but it was around intimacy and how could we now be intimate, and now that we would always have to use a condom if I didn't want to become infected. And those are huge concerns.

David earlier described the shift in intimacy within his relationship. Once HIV became a part of his relational reality, David's shift away from monogamy was his way of dealing with the changing dynamics around the closeness and mutuality he had shared with his partner. Sex before HIV was associated with intimacy. After HIV disrupted the relationship, sex became an emotional release. The presence of HIV changed the intimacy-related norms the couple had patterned for the relationship.

David, Caleb, and Andrew all hint at a larger concern growing out of the uncertainties regarding sex. Sex is one aspect of intimacy, and, as these men discuss concerns with the mechanics of sex, they also reveal broader concerns regarding overall intimacy, not just sexual intimacy, within the relationship. HIV had the effect of forcing them to leave behind or change the path they had already established toward fostering and reaffirming intimacy between themselves and their partner. For all of these couples, the HIV diagnosis occurred 12 years or more after the first antiretroviral drugs were introduced and ten years after the declaration of the end-of-AIDS and the term "post-AIDS" appeared in medical discourse. PrEP (pre-exposure prophylaxis) and PeP (post-exposure prophylaxis) were readily available at the time of these interviews. Even years after their partners' diagnoses, the men still had difficulty managing the intimacy-related uncertainties wrought by HIV.

HIV Creates Doubts Regarding Commitment

The men participating in this study also recognize the doubts their partners, as PLHIV, may have regarding the negative partners' commitment to the relationship. There was a reluctance to delete his profiles on websites and smartphone apps designed for meeting and dating other men for Carlos' partner. Carlos described how he interpreted this behavior.

> At first, I think he just thought that I was going to, like leave him. He had the websites still open because he thought eventually I was going to go, and he would have to have a rebound or something. But once I assured him that I was with him, that I was getting comfortable, that I was comfortable ... now he doesn't worry about that.

Carlos described his partner's previous struggles with feelings of being tainted and not worthy of a relationship. Because of HIV, Carlos' partner had difficulty believing that Carlos could commit to a lasting relationship with a PLHIV. Carlos went on to describe how he had to work continuously at reassuring his partner of his commitment to the relationship to combat his partner's feelings of unworthiness.

> What I mean by responsibility is that you have to always maintain the relationship. You have to make sure that he, that individual, feels loved. That he feels that you appreciate him, and I, like, on that, on that area, I have to admit, but I do let him know that I care about him.

For Carlos, demonstrating to your partner that feeling of mutuality, that you both are committed and involved in the relationship, is a duty that is essential to the health of the relationship, particularly when HIV creates uncertainties in the partner living with HIV about how committed the HIV-negative partner is to the relationship.

Peter and his partner met via a dating app specifically for gay men, with his partner's positive HIV status indicated on his profile. Their relationship progressed from casual hookups to "friends with benefits" to a committed partnership. As Peter previously discussed, sex is an important part of bonding and maintaining closeness for the couple. However, as he continued to discuss sex, it is apparent that the risk of transmission is a concern of his partner's, and it represents an overall threat to the connection the men share.

> I don't think I was ever concerned that I'd get HIV from him. One of my concerns was from a perspective of being in a relationship ... was how he felt about being in a serodiscordant relationship and whether he would feel ... some of what I hear as I read is that some folks don't want to be in a relationship with someone who is negative because they fear they would give them HIV, and that would be devastating.

All the men participating in this study discussed their partners' fears regarding transmitting the virus to their negative partner. This fear is in tension with the negative partners' desires to be close to the PLHIV. This tension becomes a source of uncertainty threatening intimacy within the relationship, and, as

Peter's quote above demonstrates, this fear of passing along the virus also involves an additional thought. It is one thing to fear transmitting the virus; it is another to fear being in a relationship because of being afraid of transmitting the virus. In this way, HIV creates doubt in the HIV-negative partners' minds about the stability or the mutuality of commitment each partner has to the relationship. It is interesting to consider a post-AIDS worldview in light of this finding. Regardless of the effectiveness of available prevention methods, HIV is still a communicable disease. PLHIV still carry uncertainties and fears related to infecting others. As Peter notes, his partner would be "devastated" if Peter was diagnosed with HIV, yet Peter is more concerned about his partner's commitment. Post-AIDS rhetoric seems to reinforce this tension as the medical community and popular culture portray HIV as no longer a threat. As the men in this study illustrate, these fears and uncertainties directly affect core relationship functions, and they attempt to manage these uncertainties without alternate cultural scripts to guide them.

Tim discussed how he learned over the years that comments his partner makes that involve a particular side effect of his medication represent fears his partner has regarding Tim's commitment to the relationship. Tim describes how he must work at reassuring his partner that he is committed for the long term:

> The main problem is the side effect of the meds he takes is lipodystrophy [i.e., abnormal distribution of fat]. He's very conscious about body image, and he had to basically kind of have liposuction done. I supported him, helped pay for that, uh, so that's more of an issue is his … his self-image because of that. One of the things that I try to reassure him is that I'm okay with that. That doesn't affect my attraction to him at all. Um, I know it is something that bothers him, so I try to, um, make that not a concern if I can.

While this side effect is related to his partner's body image issues, it also speaks to his partner's fear of feeling unattractive and the uncertainty of what that could mean for intimacy within the relationship. Tim explained how he allays his partner's fears.

> I think I've done it a number of times. I've heard him say, "I hate the way my body looks," and that's a cue. When we were in … and I think when we were in Florence [Italy] we were having a dinner … and I brought it up again and said, "I know that you're concerned about this, but I'm telling you I love you and it makes no difference to me. You're no less attractive to me. I still think you're hot, and I still love you and don't worry about it for my sake or in terms of our relationship."

With Tim addressing the mutuality the two men share regarding their commitment to one another, he works to address his partner's uncertainties, foster their emotional connection, and reinforce their bond.

Steve's partner identified as a PLHIV when they met. At the time of this interview, Steve's partner was suffering from extensive side effects from HIV and other serious autoimmune conditions, and kidney failure. With his partner dealing with multiple, severe, acute health conditions, Steve explains how his partner questioned Steve's commitment: "I think his concerns are then with me. I think he probably is concerned if I'm going to leave him." Because Steve's partner has experienced so many overwhelming and debilitating effects of illness, he knows that Steve also experiences the overwhelming nature of the disease. Steve recognizes that this instills a fear in his partner that he may decide one day that dealing with constant, demanding, acute disease just involves too much emotional effort to stay in the relationship. This is not an unfounded fear. As Steve related in the following, relationships can just be too difficult to deal with.

> It's draining. Yeah. Because you know what happens? After all the lovey-dovey stuff like that, it's, ah, truly it becomes, are you going to be there for that person? You know. Are you going to truly be there? And I don't know if the reward is worth, if there's, the reward is worth the work to get to that. What I'm trying to say is, where I am right now, do I have enough of that fulfillment from the relationship I have with my own kids, or with my friends that I ***need*** [emphasis added by participant] a relationship? Probably not. It may change. And that's another thing I've learned. Your opinions change very quickly in life. What I thought five years ago is vastly different than what I think so now. But um, but where I am is, I would never be in another relationship. It's draining. It's totally draining.

Steve and his partner have battled through years of debilitating side effects from his partner's illnesses, including some beyond HIV. As those illnesses grew more serious and debilitating, Steve described the catastrophic effects his partner's health issues have had on intimacy and their relationship.

> In essence, it is like, grieving your relationship every day. You don't have a relationship anymore. You can't. You know? You're not two healthy, independent people growing together. You're with somebody who is fighting to survive.

The overwhelming nature of the disease at this very acute stage completely destroys intimacy, and with it, the sense that there is much of a relationship at all.

Intimacy Promoting Communication and Behavior

While all the participants in this study discussed uncertainties and challenges related to sex and intimacy, Tim was the only participant to discuss ways he and his partner successfully manage their uncertainties related to HIV while still finding ways to establish, maintain, and strengthen their feelings of closeness, mutuality, and intimacy. As he discussed how he and his partner have developed and opened up their sex lives to other kinds of activities, Tim's experience stood out as a negative case in relation to the other participants. In a way, the constraints to sexual activity imposed by HIV required them to be more creative, but ultimately, it led to greater satisfaction with their sex life.

> How has it changed? It's gotten a little more adventurous in some aspects. We're both interested in leather, sort of, in general, which we didn't do at first. That's almost another coming out, when you're interested in BDSM [Bondage & Discipline; Domination & Submission; Sadism & Masochism]. Um, so it took us a while to open up about that and those interests to each other. Yeah, and, and, you know, doing and experimenting more stuff with what we wanted to do together.

Tim also described how he helps his partner by helping him set up his medications each week.

> The one thing that I do every week is that he has, uh, a set of meds that he takes. And a little box for every day of the week, morning and evening and so every week, every Sunday, I do his meds. He asked me to do that very early in the relationship. Um, I thought okay I'll do this. It kind of, in a way, I don't forget that he's HIV-positive, and it's one of the ways, drudgery sort of things that he doesn't like to do. I think he wanted me to, [pause] and we didn't talk about it. I think he wanted me to have some type of part in his healthcare. We're sharing a life together, and part of that is taking care of each other, and being there for each other. I see doing that as, uh, sort of symbolic of that.

While they still had to consider HIV, Tim and his partner opened up to each other about their sexual interests. They found new ways to incorporate the necessary aspects of managing HIV into their relationship in meaningful ways. While opening up their sex lives to new experiences helps address uncertainties related to physical intimacy, the simple act of Tim organizing his partner's medication addresses needs associated with emotional intimacy. Because of this, HIV, rather than continuing to be a source of intimacy uncertainty that must be removed from the relationship, serves as a mechanism to actually reinforce their commitment to one another, promote intimacy within their relational lives, and help cement the feelings of closeness and mutuality they desire.

Discussion

More than 20 years after the medical establishment declared the "end of AIDS," HIV continues to play a role in our intimate lives, particularly in those of gay men. The purpose of this study was to explore the uncertainties felt by HIV-negative gay men who are in a romantic partnership with a PLHIV. Sex is an important arbiter of intimacy, and there exists an extensive body of literature identifying the role sex plays in helping romantic partners express and maintain emotional closeness (Leigh, 1989). Because of this, understanding the role HIV plays in the intimate lives of serodiscordant gay couples helps provide insight as to why, despite the availability of effective treatment and prevention methods, HIV infects over 37,000 people in the United States each year, with men who have sex with men accounting for 69% of all new diagnoses (Centers for Disease Control and Prevention, 2020). As the narratives of the participants in this study demonstrate, HIV exerts a social influence on the relational dynamics of these couples, not only complicating the physical aspects of sex but also disrupting the emotional pathways the couples use to foster connection. The effects of these social influences are significant, as the above statistics demonstrate. The biotechnical solutions offered by condoms and pharmaceuticals haven't stopped the spread of HIV, despite their demonstrated effectiveness.

HIV as Intimacy Regulator

In the field of clinical psychology, clinicians often treat clients, both couples and individuals, facing intimacy issues by helping find ways to regulate intimacy (Prager, 2000). According to Prager (2000), "Effective intimacy regulation seems to involve a rhythm of intimate contact alternating with more separateness in which partners' needs are fulfilled and in which conflict and recrimination are minimized" (p. 241). Each couple possesses an optimum mode where they determine the timing, pace, and depth of intimacy-promoting behaviors. The key to effective intimacy regulation is the control partners exert over behaviors designed to promote intimacy.

For this study's participants, HIV intrudes on the couple's sense of intimacy and causes uncertainties in ways that make it more difficult for the couple to share aspects of their lives that contribute to a close, intimate relationship. For couples experiencing the intrusion of HIV, they perceive HIV as taking the control of intimacy regulation away from the partners, limiting their options for intimacy-promoting behaviors. HIV demands specific behavior changes related to their intimacy, affecting the pace at which intimacy is developed over the course of the relationship, the timing and type of intimate behaviors they engage in, and the depth of intimacy between the partners. HIV, in this sense, becomes the intimacy regulator between mixed-status couples, and the uncertainties associated with this intimacy disruption propel the men to choose behaviors that hopefully minimize the disruption and HIV's power over the relationship.

Intimacy and Uncertainty Management

As the participants attempt to make sense of the intimacy-related uncertainties they feel, tensions arise between their strategies to prevent the transmission of HIV and the desire for closeness and affection. For David, he repeatedly insisted on a monogamous relationship prior to his partner's HIV diagnosis. However, after his partner became infected, he then needed the emotional release provided by sex outside the relationship. His need for the closeness and commitment sex helps to foster with his partner sits in tension with his need for physical intimacy to occur without the threat of HIV. Research into how HIV status can influence sexual decision-making has found that many gay men seek out sexual partners that have a concordant serostatus because they feel more relaxed and have less anxiety about sex, whether they are HIV-negative or a PLHIV (Bird et al., 2017).

All the men participating in this study discussed the fear their partners experienced about potentially transmitting the virus to them. Many discussed how condoms acted as a barrier to both physical and emotional intimacy. Much research has investigated the "barebacking" phenomenon. While there are a variety of reasons gay men forgo using a condom, the condom is seen as a barrier to not just physical intimacy, but emotional intimacy as well is common (Starks, Pawson, Stephenson, Sullivan, & Parsons, 2018). This need to remove the physical barrier that is a condom so that it will remove any emotional barriers to intimacy between the couple is held in tension with the desire the PLHIV has to protect the HIV-negative partner from contracting HIV.

Forgoing condoms was important to intimacy and connection for the men in this study, which is consistent with other studies indicating gay men, regardless of HIV status, see condoms as a barrier to intimacy in committed partnerships, but absolutely necessary when engaging in casual sex (Starks et al., 2018). It would seem HIV forces a situation with no good choices: use a condom and lessen the intimacy, or forgo a condom, increase sexual anxiety, and risk transmission, thereby impacting intimacy. Either choice limits the intimacy regulation options available to the couple and puts HIV in control.

Despite living in a "post-AIDS" society, the continued negative conceptions (i.e., stigma) and fears associated with contracting HIV continue to impact relationships at a macro and micro level. For all of the participants interviewed, the struggles with intimacy stem from the unsatisfactory solutions they have for managing their uncertainties. They can use condoms to protect against the transmission of the virus, but they detract from intimacy. They can delay sex or have sex with other people, but this removes an important behavior to establishing and maintaining closeness. Their relationships are often stigmatized by society at large, but if they choose to have open relationships, follow heteronormative relationship patterns, take PrEP, or forgo condoms, they risk further stigmatizing their relationships and adding additional stressors to their lives. As Mishel (1990) points out, theories of uncertainty make no effort at explaining how uncertainties evolve over time; yet, studies have shown that chronically ill patients tend to appraise uncertainty more positively the longer they live with uncertainty. Rather than something to be removed, chronically ill patients view uncertainty as part of the rhythm of life, and this process of forming a new perspective regarding uncertainty is normal for chronically ill patients unless it is blocked or prolonged in some way (Mishel, 1990).

The participants in this study demonstrated the difficulty associated with the process of forming a new perspective regarding uncertainty. In some cases, the process of incorporating successful uncertainty management practices into their relationship was still a work in progress even after several years. However, the experience of Tim and his partner highlight the important role communication plays in helping the couple reframe HIV-related uncertainties and incorporate HIV into their daily lives. In particular, self-disclosure and the perceptions of a partner's self-disclosure have been shown to be intimacy-promoting communication, increasing feelings of relationship satisfaction, love, and commitment (Rubinsky & Hosek, 2020; Sprecher & Hendrick, 2004). For Tim and his partner, sharing confidences related to interests in leather and BDSM became an act of vulnerability, demonstrating trust in each other and thereby promoting a stronger, more intimate bond. Rather than limiting their options for sex and intimacy, BDSM has offered sexual activity that the couple could perform without adjusting or compromising for HIV. Other participants' struggles stemmed from HIV's disruption to their preferred sexual practices and patterns. HIV made it difficult to do what they had always done. In contrast, Tim and his partner sought alternative sexual practices that did not require catering to HIV or disrupting their current sexual desires.

During their interview, several participants noted the importance of demonstrating support and care for their partner. In particular, Tim described how sharing a life with his partner involved Tim taking responsibility for organizing his partner's medications each week. The gesture may seem small, but it serves as a significant point of communication for the two, signaling commitment and mutuality to each other. For Tim's partner, asking Tim to take part in this small activity serves as a request that Tim be interested in and understanding of what it is like to be a PLHIV. For Tim, it allows him to demonstrate support for his partner and take part in his illness experience that is, at the same time, unthreatening to both Tim's sense of self and his personal identity as a healthy person. Future research should focus on the ways in which couples have incorporated new sexual practices and relationship rituals to reframe their outlooks and perspectives on uncertainty related to HIV.

Intimacy, Uncertainty, and Post-AIDS Discourse

One goal of the present study involved exploring uncertainties held by the HIV-negative partners in mixed-HIV status couples. These data contribute to Mishel's Uncertainty in Illness theory and Brashers' Uncertainty Management theory by extending the notion of illness-related uncertainty from primarily a patient-oriented perspective to one that looks at the illness-related uncertainties of the partners of patients, specifically within the context of HIV in the current study. Previous studies investigating HIV and uncertainty have found that PLHIV hold uncertainties regarding unclear relational implications and unknown impacts on long-term relationships as a result of their HIV infection (Brashers et al., 2003). The present study helps to shed light on uncertainty sources within mixed-status relationships by identifying intimacy as a primary source of uncertainty for the HIV-negative partner.

Approximately 20 years after Rofes' work, we find that we still don't have ways to help these men and their partners effectively deal with these situations. As Walker (2020) points out, the rhetoric around antiretroviral drugs has supported and driven notions of the end-of-AIDS found in post-AIDS discourse. In reality, the post-AIDS discourse has actually had a role in allowing us to not think about the difficult issues presented by the social realities associated with living with HIV. The term "post-AIDS" means HIV is gone, or, at a minimum, is elsewhere (e.g., the Global South or other marginalized populations), and mainstream culture has forgotten about it (Petrus, 2019). The reality is the issues associated with intimacy, and relational functioning are harder to address. These are potentially more individualized, and the feelings associated with them are not always easily made sense of. As Walker (2020) suggests, simple, straightforward biotechnical solutions aren't available for these situations. Where post-AIDs discourse is about sex without fear of disease, it neglects to discuss emotional connection without fear of disease.

The advent of anti-HIV drugs succeeded in expanding the nature of uncertainties faced by those confronted with the disease. At that time, Rofes (1998) reflected on the changes in his own relationship with a partner living with HIV. He had already been dealing with the sexual implications of partnering with a PLHIV; however, as the imminent threat of his partner's death from HIV abated, the couple recognized shifts in how they related to one another, the roles they had adopted within the relationship, and how they navigated their intimate lives with one another (Rofes, 1998). Much like the men participating in this study, Rofes discussed how these changes were unexpected and difficult to rationalize, leaving both partners with uncertainties that required outside help to understand and learn to manage. As post-AIDS discourse began declaring the "end of AIDS," Rofes, more than ever before, found the disease impacting his relationship in significant ways and, now more than 20 years after that "end-of-AIDS" moment Rofes (1998) writes about, gay men are still struggling to manage uncertainties related to HIV and intimacy, both physical and emotional, as they attempt to form and maintain committed, romantic partnerships.

Note

1 The FDA has announced a relaxing of its restrictions on gay men being allowed to donate blood, in light of the coronavirus disease 2019 (COVID-19) pandemic. Now, instead of one year, if a male has had sex with another male, he need only wait three months to donate blood. See https://www.fda.gov/news-events/press-announcements/coronavirus-covid-19-update-fda-provides-updated-guidance-address-urgent-need-blood-during-pandemic

References

Afifi, T. D., Hutchinson, S., & Krouse, S. (2006). Toward a theoretical model of communal coping in post-divorce families and other naturally occurring groups. *Communication Theory*, *16*, 378–409.

Beckerman, N. L. (2002). Couples coping with discordant HIV status. *AIDS Patient Care and STDs, 16*(2), 55–59.

Berger, C. R., & Calabrese, R. J. (1975). Some explorations in initial interaction and beyond: Toward a developmental theory of interpersonal communication. *Human Communication Research, 1*, 99–112.

Bird, J. D., Morris, J. A., Koester, K. A., Pollack, L. M., Binson, D., & Woods, W. J. (2017). "Knowing your status and knowing your partner's status is really where it starts:" A qualitative exploration of the process by which a sexual partner's HIV status can influence sexual decision making. *The Journal of Sex Research, 54*(6), 784–794.

Brashers, D. E., Neidig, J. L., & Goldsmith, D. J. (2004). Social support and the management of uncertainty for people living with HIV or AIDS. *Health Communication, 16*, 305–331.

Brashers, D. E., Neidig, J., Russell, J., Cardillo, L., Haas, S., Dobbs, L., Garland, M., McCartney, B., & Nemeth, S. (2003). The medical, personal, and social causes of uncertainty in HIV illness. *Issues in Mental Health Nursing, 24*(5), 497–522.

Butler, P. (2004). Embracing AIDS: History, identity, and post-AIDS discourse. *JAC, 24*, 93–111.

Centers for Disease Control and Prevention. (2020). *HIV Basics.* Retrieved from https://www.cdc.gov/hiv/basics/statistics.html

Charmaz, K. (2006). *Constructing Grounded Theory.* Thousand Oaks, CA: Sage.

Derlega, V. J., Winstead, B. A., Oldfield III, E. C., & Barbee, A. P. (2003). Close relationships and social support in coping with HIV: A test of sensitive interaction systems theory. *AIDS and Behavior, 7*(2), 119–129.

Dowsett, G. W. (2009). Dangerous desires and post-queer HIV prevention: Rethinking community, incitement and intervention. *Social Theory & Health, 7*(3), 218–240.

Goldsmith, D. J. (2009). Uncertainty and communication in couples coping with serious illness. In T. D Afifi, & W. A Afifi (Eds.), *Uncertainty, information management, and disclosure decisions: Theories and applications.* New York: Routledge.

Haas, S. M. (2002). Social support as relationship maintenance in gay male couples coping with HIV or AIDS. *Journal of Social and Personal Relationships, 19*, 87–111.

Holt, R., Court, P., Vedhara, K., Nott, K. H., Holmes, J., & Snow, M. H. (1998). The role of disclosure in coping with HIV infection. *AIDS Care, 10*, 49–60.

Kalichman, Seth C. (2000). HIV transmission risk behaviors of men and women living with HIV-AIDS: Prevalence, predictors, and emerging clinical interventions. *Clinical Psychology: Science and Practice, 7*(1), 32–47.

Knap, M. L. (1984). *Interpersonal communication and human relationships.* Boston, MA: Allyn & Bacon.

Knobloch, L. K., & Solomon, D. H. (1999). Measuring the sources and content of relational uncertainty. *Communication Studies, 50*(4), 261–278.

Kuyper, M. B., & Wester, F. (1998). In the shadow: The impact of chronic illness on the patient's partner. *Qualitative Health Research, 8*(2), 237–253.

Lamont, E. (2017). "We can write the scripts ourselves:" Queer challenges to heteronormative courtship practices. *Gender & Society, 31*(5), 624–646.

Leigh, B. C. (1989). Reasons for having and avoiding sex: Gender, sexual orientation, and relationship to sexual behavior. *Journal of Sex Research, 26*(2), 199–209.

Mishel, M. H. (1988). Uncertainty in illness. *Journal of Nursing Scholarship, 20*, 225–232.

Mishel, M. H. (1990). Reconceptualization of the uncertainty in illness theory. *Journal of Nursing Scholarship, 22*, 256–262.

O'Brien, C. (2013). Performing POZ: Irish theatre, HIV stigma, and "post-AIDS" identities. *Irish University Review, 43*(1), 74–85.

O'Brien, C. (2020). HIV and AIDS in Irish Theatre: Queer Masculinities, Punishment, and 'Post-AIDS' Culture. *Journal of Medical Humanities, 41*(2), 123–136.

O'Connell, G. (2020). Introduction: Framing 'Post-AIDS' and Global Health Discourses in 2015 and Beyond. *Journal of Medical Humanities, 41*(2), 89–94.

Pawlicki, P., & Larson, P. (2011). The dynamics and conceptualizations of non-exclusive relationships in gay male couples. *Sexual and Relationship Therapy, 26*(1), 48–60.

Peplau, L. A., & Fingerhut, A. W. (2006). The close relationships of lesbians and gay men. *Annual Review of Psychology, 58*(1), 405–424. doi: 10.1146/annurev.psych.58.110405.085701

Petrus, J. (2019). Discussing the undiscussable: Reflecting on the "end" of AIDS. *GLQ: A Journal of Lesbian and Gay Studies, 25*(1), 67–72.

Philpot, S. P., Duncan, D., Ellard, J., Bavinton, B. R., Grierson, J., & Prestage, G. (2018). Negotiating gay men's relationships: How are monogamy and non-monogamy experienced and practiced over time?. *Culture, Health & Sexuality, 20*(8), 915–928.

Prager, K. J. (2000). Intimacy in personal relationships. In C. Hendrik, & S. S. Hendrick (Eds.), *Close relationships: A sourcebook* (pp. 229–242). Thousand Oaks, CA: Sage.

Reis, H. T. (1990). The role of intimacy in interpersonal relations. *Journal of Social and Clinical Psychology, 9*(1), 15–30.

Rofes, E. (1998). *Dry bones breathe: Gay men creating post-AIDS identities and cultures.* New York: Routledge.

Román, D. (2000). Not-about-AIDS. *GLQ: A Journal of Lesbian and Gay Studies, 6*(1), 1–28.

Rubinsky, V., & Hosek, A. (2020). "We have to get over it": Navigating sex talk through the lens of sexual communication comfort and sexual self-disclosure in LGBTQ intimate partnerships. *Sexuality & Culture, 24*, 613–629.

Solomon, D. H., & Theiss, J. (2013). Intimacy and interpersonal communication. In D. H. Solomon & J. Theiss. *Interpersonal communication: Putting theory into practice* (pp. 264–291). New York: Routledge.

Sprecher, S., & Hendrick, S. S. (2004). Self-disclosure in intimate relationships: Associations with individual and relationship characteristics over time. *Journal of Social and Clinical Psychology, 23*(6), 857–877.

Starks, T. J., Pawson, M., Stephenson, R., Sullivan, P., & Parsons, J. T. (2018). Dyadic qualitative analysis of condom use scripts among emerging adult gay male couples. *Journal of Sex & Marital Therapy, 44*(3), 269–280.

United Nations Department of Economic and Social Affairs. (2020). Retrieved from https://www.un.org/development/desa/disabilities/envision2030.html

U.S. Department of Health and Human Services (2020). Retrieved from https://www.hiv.gov/hiv-basics/overview/about-hiv-and-aids/what-are-hiv-and-aids

Walker, L. (2020). Problematizing the discourse of "post-AIDS." *Journal of Medical Humanities, 41*(2), 95–105.

Westman, M., & Vinokur, A. D. (1998). Unraveling the relationship of distress levels within couples: Common stressors, empathic reactions, or crossover via social interaction? *Human Relations, 51*, 137–156.

Wheldon, C. W., & Pathak, E. B. (2010). Masculinity and relationship agreements among male same-sex couples. *Journal of Sex Research, 47*(5), 460–470.

Wrubel, J., & Folkman, S. (1997). What informal caregivers actually do: The caregiving skills of partners of men with AIDS. *AIDS Care, 9*(6), 691–706.

11 The Experience of Building and Testing a Visual Health Literacy Resource for HIV Prophylaxis

Sachiko Terui and Joy V. Goldsmith

It was career day, 1986. I chose to attend the *author* session. My girlfriends were also going, which made it the obvious selection for the afternoon slot. Those two hours changed me. I was in central Kansas, a small town. Everyone white and straight (i.e., white and performing the part of straight). And this woman, Beverly Barbo, wasn't talking about writing. She really was talking about the horror of seeing her son change and suffer and die from something called AIDS. It was the first time I had heard of this illness. Coming of age in the 80s, death from HIV and then AIDS was an inevitability. Ms. Barbo's talk and book (*The Walking Wounded*) taught me about a thing I didn't know existed. I could never have guessed in 1986 that now, in 2020, I would be a health communication researcher, have the gift of a colleague like Sachiko, or have the opportunity to be part of a research project about HIV – an illness that is now fully treatable if the resources for care are available.

***

We sat in Sachiko's office listening spellbound to Donna, a Community Health Worker. A student in Sachiko's class facilitated the connection for us as part of a health promotion assignment. Donna was uniquely invested in stopping HIV transmission in Memphis. She was telling us it was a public health crisis and that our city was unfortunate in holding the position of 7th highest transmission rate in the country. For both of us, we felt far away from the HIV community, advancements in treatment, and tools to limit new transmissions. This was a wheelhouse that wasn't either of ours. And honestly, we knew very little about HIV when this journey with Donna began. We still feel like this is a health crisis that we know too little about. Donna was describing this medicine called PrEP, and explained that it would protect people from acquiring the HIV virus. PrEP, in her descriptions, seemed to be integrated into HIV services in other parts of the country, but not in the southeastern states. It sounded like she was describing something akin to magic. PrEP sounded not real. And not believable.

DOI: 10.4324/9781003000945-14

Donna continued. From a biomedical perspective, HIV had become a chronic rather than deadly disease, and people living with HIV can have a full life if they can continue to take treatments/remain "in care." Pharmaceuticals make it possible to prevent people from acquiring HIV. Despite the medical technology, the number of new HIV diagnoses are not decreasing drastically in our region of the country. "We need more energy focused on the social and psychological work. The people here see HIV as highly stigmatized, and many times they don't know how to get resources. People living with HIV don't want others to know that they have HIV. That has been a huge barrier in treatment and prophylaxis. We have to have more conversations about HIV. We have to start talking. It can't be about judgement of behaviors." Donna repeated this multiple times and guided us in joining the post-AIDS discourse.

HIV Transmission in the South

Poverty and limited access to education are two variables that are strongly correlated with human immunodeficiency virus (HIV) occurrence and reduced utilization of pre-exposure prophylaxis (PrEP) (Denning & DiNenno, 2017; Siegler et al., 2018). PrEP (brand name Truvada) contains two medicines (tenofovir and emtricitabine) and was approved as an HIV medication by the U.S. Food and Drug Administration in 2012. Taking PrEP daily protects individuals from acquiring HIV, and its recognized effectiveness in reducing HIV acquisition has led the federal government to increase efforts to promote its use (HIV.gov, 2016). Despite these efforts, PrEP is not very well known among people in the general public and healthcare providers and healthcare workers (Collier et al., 2017). PrEP use throughout the southern states has been low, particularly in impoverished communities and among African American populations (Siegler et al., 2018). High HIV acquisition and the relatively limited use of PrEP in this region set the stage for the current public health crisis.

According to the federal Centers for Disease Control and Prevention (CDC), approximately 1,122,900 people in the United States are currently living with HIV, and 37,600 new HIV diagnoses are reported each year (CDC, 2017a). Efforts to reduce new HIV cases have been made over the past decade, but positive progress has been unequally experienced in the South. HIV disparities are more prevalent among individuals in underserved populations (CDC, 2017b). The number of individuals receiving an HIV diagnosis is highest in the southern states, compared with other regions in the U.S. (HIV.gov, 2017). In an effort to mitigate this public health crisis, scholars (e.g., Osborn et al., 2007; Tique et al., 2017) have identified *health literacy* as one of the key factors contributing to HIV prevalence.

Health Literacy

The CDC (2017c) and the Patient Protection and Affordable Care Act of 2010, Title V, define health literacy as "the degree to which an individual has the capacity to obtain, communicate, process, and understand basic health information and services to make appropriate health decisions" (para. 1). The study of health literacy has been expanded and continues to have different meanings depending on who is involved in the matter and in what context (Parnell, 2015). Despite the different foci and contexts, scholars commonly agree that (a) health literacy is positively correlated with the use of preventive services and the quality of healthcare individuals receive (Berkman et al., 2011); (b) low health literacy is closely associated with misperceptions about disease/illness and its treatments (e.g., HIV/AIDS), even among individuals living with such health challenges (Kalichman et al., 2000); and (c) those with low health literacy tend to experience adverse mental and physical health outcomes and have a shorter life expectancy (Baker et al., 2007; Wolf et al., 2005). These ties between health literacy and health outcomes have attracted scholars and practitioners to establish hundreds of measurement tools to assess health literacy levels, hoping to accommodate and assist individuals in need.

Baker's health literacy model describes the relationship among individual capacities, health-related spoken and written communication, and health outcomes (Baker, 2006). In accord with the Institute of Medicine and nursing and health literacy researchers (Yuen et al., 2015), the synergy among those receiving care, providing care, and the resources provided by health systems converge to either establish or remove health literacy barriers. Baker identifies not only (1) individual capacity as a primary factor in gaining needed health information, but also the (2) complexity and difficulty of written and spoken messages, (3) cultural factors, and (4) system barriers. The first construct, individual capacity to gain resources, is predicated on conceptual knowledge of health issues impacting the patient and caregiver. The second construct, written and spoken communication, consists of the quality of materials and conversations about caregiver concerns, which heavily influence caregiver understanding and preparedness. The third construct addressing cultural barriers is one that the caregiver, provider, and healthcare system bring to any interaction. The fourth and final construct addresses health outcomes, which are influenced by access to and understanding health-related information (Berkman et al., 2011). Addressing all four constructs is an important but challenging task to achieve among stakeholders and frontline workers in the field.

> Donna sat with us in our offices and we talked through a possible intervention effort that would engage our students with their community peers. Knowing as much or less than our students knew about HIV in that moment, we asked Donna to integrate herself into our courses for the next two semesters and support a project that would ultimately reach hundreds of people in the city to engage in conversations, which emphasize the nature of HIV disease and the available resources for care and prevention, while acknowledging and making attempts to reduce stigma. She agreed. She was the best kind of partner to a researcher. She had all the hook-ups to health information, practical knowledge, HIV testing, a world of STD resources, and very skilled engagement as a human communicator. We were nervous

> about the course being heavily wrapped around the HIV intervention but decided to move ahead with this clear purpose, hoping that framing the course as an engaged learning experience would make the research design possible and create positive influence on health in our surrounding communities. On the first day of class, the very first words we uttered were about the HIV intervention at the center of the course. We invited students to consider this carefully and urged them determine if this was a focus they could support for the entirety of the term.

Education-based health interventions have been reported as an effective tool to address concerns pertaining to low health literacy in the context of the HIV crisis (Osborn et al., 2007; Sani et al., 2016). Despite promising, positive evidence of equipping a community with accurate information about prevention methods, resources, treatment, and skills to manage health (Hicks et al., 2006), it is also known that three factors – (1) HIV stigma and misconceptions, (2) distrust toward healthcare professionals, and (3) dissatisfaction in patient-provider interactions – contribute to diminished care (Schulz & Nakamoto, 2013). These barriers are especially present among underserved populations (Dixon et al., 2016). The culture of silence pertaining to sexual health and abstinence-based sex education deprive opportunities for individuals to effectively seek, communicate, and utilize quality information to protect themselves (Hood & Friedman, 2011). Promoting communication on sexual health has been identified as a powerful intervention to improve sexual health behaviors, modify misconceptions, reduce stigma, and increase knowledge (Friedman et al., 2016). Accordingly, we developed a communication-centered HIV and PrEP intervention by adopting a peer-delivered intervention called the Social Network Strategy (SNS) (CDC, 2005). This chapter describes the process of developing this intervention and examines the effectiveness of a customized visual aid in the intervention efforts.

Social Network Strategy and HIV Prophylaxis

According to a CDC HIV Surveillance report (CDC, 2017b), 61.8% of the individuals who received new HIV diagnoses are between 20 and 29 years old. Given the racial characteristics of these individuals (45.24% African American, 26.55% Caucasian, and 22.13% Hispanic), our students and their peers and families in Memphis, Tennessee, are a demographic match for vulnerable populations. To reach a wide range of Memphians with our health communication intervention, we adapted the SNS (CDC, 2005) as a community engagement course project.

The SNS is an evidence-based approach to promote HIV testing among hard-to-reach populations (CDC, 2005). The goals of SNS include identifying persons with undiagnosed HIV and linking them to HIV testing, counseling, and referral. SNS health practitioners enlist HIV-positive individuals and HIV-negative persons at high risk (*Recruiters*) to recruit individuals in their social, sexual, and drug-use network (*Network Associates*) based on two ideas: (a) people in the same network tend to share similar risks and risk behaviors; and (b) individuals in the same social network have existing, trusting relationships that can influence one another.

Researchers have reported the effectiveness of SNS: results indicated significantly increased reach to individuals who were unaware of their HIV status and who were not under care, compared with other methods (Girault et al., 2015; Kimbrough et al., 2009; Lightfoot et al., 2018). Following SNS principles, the individuals identified as *recruiters* in these studies are predominantly ones within specific identity categorizations, such as men who have sex with men (MSM), drug users, and sex workers. Despite the strengths of SNS, it still has limitations. First, using such categorizations (i.e., MSM) in recruiting efforts contributes to the stigma attached to HIV (Smith, 2007) and creates barriers for HIV interventions (Mahajan et al., 2008). Because sexual intercourses among individuals without such categorizations is the second most common channel of HIV transmission (CDC, 2016), and these individuals are less likely to be tested compared to MSM (Linley et al., 2016; Woodring et al., 2014), individuals without such categorized identities are also at risk. Implementing the SNS intervention without applying categorizations also creates promising recruiting results for individuals both with and without such categorized identities (Gwadz et al., 2017).

Second, SNS's principle to connect people living with HIV and individuals at risk with healthcare systems is a reactive approach and does exert significant influences on prevention. Therefore, we executed an SNS intervention in which recruiters reached out to individuals in their social networks for possible testing, counseling, and referral while educating those peers about HIV infection and resources for prevention and treatment. Our intervention aims to break the culture of silence and promote conversations about sexual health. Communicating HIV risk without such categorization and promoting conversations about sexual health can create opportunities, regardless of identities and health statuses, to obtain accurate information about HIV and available resources for prevention and treatment. Thereby, the conversation itself can deconstruct stigmas and misconceptions attached to HIV/AIDS.

In addition to connecting network associates with testing, counseling, and referral, the recruiters in the study communicated the risk of HIV and preventive resources, including the information about PrEP through peer training. Involving peers in HIV preventive intervention is identified as a promising practice (Ergene et al., 2005). We sought to provide insights into the effectiveness of SNS and to examine the opportunities to create theory-based behavioral interventions.

Peer Health Communication Intervention

We adopted the SNS (CDC, 2005) and decided to join our students in Health Communication courses across two semesters to conduct a communication-centered intervention to increase health literacy and knowledge about HIV and resources to create positive impacts on behavior. During the first semester of the project, we engaged two classes, totaling 64 students. In the following semester,

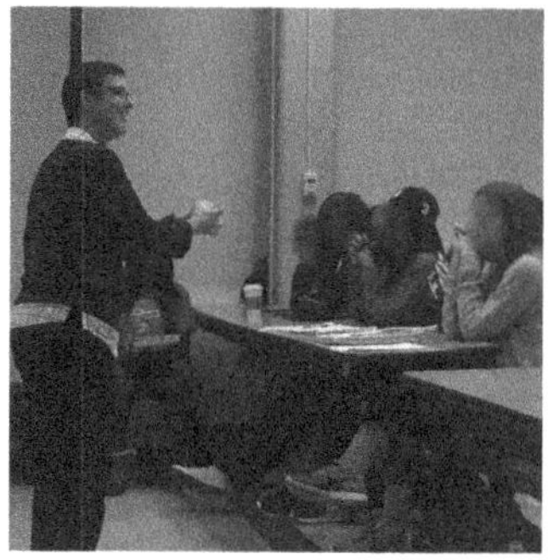

Picture 11.1 Donna providing training sessions.

we enlisted 44 students in one class as student-interventionists. In both semesters, the engagement project was integrated immediately into the first moments of the course. The schedule was built around HIV content, health literacy, visits from Donna, regular discussions about questions related to recruiting and maintaining participants, and the best approach to administer the conversation about HIV and PrEP (see Picture 11.1). We reminded students that *they* were the intervention and that their relationship with the peer was central to delivering the health information and resources.

Students completed the CITI training program for human subjects research at the beginning of each semester. Donna visited each HC class to provide training sessions (90 minutes × 2), in which students learned about HIV, its history, preventive and treatment resources (free testing and counselling) and medication (PrEP), and relevant science, as well as strategies for communicating HIV information to their network associates. Donna and her colleagues provided free HIV testing, mental health counselling, and a range of medications (including PrEP) for this project. We instructed students to frame the training content in culturally appropriate ways for their network associates so as to minimize possible resistance. Each student recruited between five and eight network associates. Students utilized health communication concepts and delivered the training content to their network associates in face-to-face meetings.

Assessing the Intervention

Network associates' knowledge about HIV was examined with ten items on a Likert scale, constructed with help from Community Health Workers, ranging from strongly disagree (1) to strongly agree (5). A higher score indicates better knowledge about HIV and PrEP. Moreover, we assessed network associates' reactions toward our HIV intervention with seven items on a Likert scale, constructed based on iterative discussions with Community Health Workers and a small group of undergraduate students, anchored by strongly disagree (1) to strongly agree (5). Higher scores indicate positive reactions toward the HIV intervention participants received from their peers.

We also adopted Miller and Adame's (2016) scales to examine participants' perceived Vested Interest (VI) or personal stake in a matter. *Severity* indicates perceived potential of negative consequences of HIV; *salience* is associated with the level to which HIV is an evident, relevant, and/or a pronounced issue; *certainty* involves the level of confidence attached to the probability of exposure (Petrocelli et al., 2007); *immediacy* is the temporal dimension associated with the perceived time before consequences of HIV arise; *self-efficacy* involves perceptions of one's ability to protect oneself from HIV; and *response-efficacy* indicates one's perceived effectiveness of coping behaviors related to recommended actions (Witte et al., 2001). Higher scores indicate higher vestedness and probabilities for these network associates to take the recommended actions. Participants were asked to respond to six VI variables using a Likert scale anchored by strongly disagree–strongly agree. Because many people, including health professionals, do not know about PrEP (Collier et al., 2017), we included the response-efficacy variable in T1 and 2 only to avoid unnecessary confusion among participants. Each VI variable achieved acceptable to good reliabilities: severity (six items; α = 0.832); salience (four items; 0.913); certainty (three items; α = 0.732), immediacy (four items; α = 0.711), self-efficacy (seven items; α = 0.840), and response-efficacy (five items; α = 0.885). The reliability number is based on the data obtained in the second semester.

We also asked about five outcome variables in the last of the three surveys, addressing whether or not (1) they had an HIV test after hearing about HIV and PrEP from their peer; (2) they contacted a PrEP coordinator after hearing about HIV and PrEP from their peer; (3) they are currently taking PrEP; (4) they talked about HIV prevention with at least one person who is important to them after hearing about HIV and PrEP from their peer; and (5) they know their HIV status. Participants provided dichotomous answers to these questions. All survey items were modified to a 6th grade reading level to meet plain language needs (Doak et al., 1996).

In the first semester, we used paper surveys, and our students shuttled the data back to us on three different occasions. Ultimately the students themselves contributed their ideas about the SNS in this project (Terui et al., 2019). The first round of the study is reported elsewhere (Terui et al., 2020). During the next semester, our collection strategies were refined to lighten the load on student recruiters, so we digitized surveys. Across two semesters, our students ultimately recruited a total of 695 community members to receive a face-to-face communication intervention about HIV education, prevention, and treatment that emphasized PrEP.

> Our students trusted Donna. On her second visit to our classes, she asked if they themselves wanted a testing event. They could come alone, bring a friend for testing, or send a friend. They wanted to do it. We knew we needed two private spaces, which we had a ton of in our academic building.

But our administrator at the time said, "No." There was "too much risk of HIPAA violations" to perform these tests and counseling sessions in our building. A colleague of ours expressed concern that our classes were now involving testing, and pressed us on showing her our IRB for the project, though the testing had nothing to do with the research project. Furthermore, a coordinated testing event (for HIV and other STIs) at our branch campus, which was well-attended by students, was forcefully moved by an administrator there because it was too uncomfortable for them. We were really stunned. And saddened. And then something pretty great happened. We asked the university library if we could have a testing event there. They welcomed us immediately. We were given two large study rooms on the third floor. Because the walls were glass, we covered them with opaque paper and masking tape. Students came alone, with friends, and sent acquaintances for this free opportunity. Other testing days followed. Donna was incredible. She and her colleagues even went to our students' and recruits' homes to complete tests. Many students brought friends, were tested themselves, or had conversations about testing and where to get it done for free as a result of this unexpected set of opportunities that grew from the engaged research project in class. We hadn't planned to test. But students requested it, and Donna was thrilled to do it.

Visual Health Literacy Aid

Because health literacy barriers have been identified as a significant cause of HIV transmission (Dawson-Rose et al., 2016), we thought about advancing the project in the second semester. Health information, a pillar of health literacy, can support health knowledge, decision-making, and behavior. Despite abundant health information materials pertaining to HIV prevention and PrEP, less is known about developing ***health-communication***-driven materials featuring plain language and visual health literacy practices appropriate to specific audiences.

We determined to create a visual health literacy (VHL) resource for a group of students to implement in the peer intervention. A control group would use the former strategy of a range of resources and conversation only. But the VHL group would additionally utilize the VHL resource, share one with the participant, and give an additional one for the participant to pass on to someone else. To explore the reduction of health literacy barriers surrounding HIV and PrEP, we created and developed a visual aid that would include content about (1) HIV infection and transmission, (2) PrEP, (3) HIV misconceptions, (4) local resources for obtaining support (map, phone numbers, free-testing sites, Community Health Worker contacts), and a (5) feedback/worksheet area for users. We wanted to see if this resource impacted the larger intervention compared with the former strategy.

Through collaboration with Community Health Workers (Donna and her colleagues) who promote HIV testing and coordinate PrEP for clients and researchers with expertise in visual communication, message design, and strategic communication, the authors developed a visual aid to assist student-interventionists. To strive to meet health literacy demands of this health information, we designed our visual aid using the Health Literacy INDEX (Kaphingst et al., 2012) and describe those elements below.

Kaphingst Guidelines and Resource Creation

Kaphingst and colleagues produced ten criteria with related topics to aid in the construction of health information. They describe the lack of consensus on the best way to assess the health literacy demands of health information material and created an INDEX of indicators that serves as a comprehensive tool to evaluate and guide health information creation (Kaphingst et al., 2012). As we created the health literacy visual resource for the HIV PrEP project, we used the INDEX to guide our construction of the piece. Those criteria and our attempt to fulfill them are described here.

Plain language. Though only one aspect of material and communication that minimizes health literacy barriers, plain language is essential in creating health information. Health organizations, including the National Institutes of Health and the American Medical Association, have recommended that the level of educational preparation of sixth grade serve as the cut-off for language complexity (Hersh et al., 2015). The Plain Language Act was included as part of the Affordable Care Act and was signed into legislation in 2010 by President Obama. This law requires that government agencies employ understandable language to communicate with the public. Though the Act did not include regulation, it did emphasize the imperative for plain language and gave rise to an expansion of resources to be used throughout a host of industries and in all government agencies. This underscored the already occurring shift in the healthcare industry to make the language more culturally and linguistically accessible for users.

We sought to include text in short sentences, with few syllables per word, without jargon, incorporating an active voice. Across iterations, we would test the text for grade and readability level using an automated readability calculator until we achieved a sixth-grade or lower level.

Clear purpose. We aimed to build a resource that would ultimately support this particular peer intervention, which meant the piece needed to resonate with student recruiters and those recruited by them. We wanted people to see themselves in this health information. But more specifically, and to inform the content, we identified the purpose of the piece to include information about HIV and transmission facts; PrEP as a medication to protect people from the acquisition of HIV; and immediate local resources for obtaining support (i.e., map, phone numbers, free-testing sites, Community Health Workers' phone numbers). We limited and emphasized key points, stated the purpose of the piece on the outer cover, and supported the purposive content within using visual elements such as boxes and bullets to organize space, white areas to guide the human eye, unified fonts throughout, and a simplified color scheme.

After meeting with a colleague in digital media design, we decided to seek out a noted influencer from the campus community to appear on the cover of the visual aid resource. We filled out the required media requests to gain access to this influencer's visage. After three weeks of follow-up phone calls and inquiries, it was clear that media machine and this well-known figure were distancing themselves from the invitation. There was zero response from those related offices, and we were on to Plan B. At the time, Joy was teaching a capstone course full of seniors. They all agreed to be photographed, signed media releases, and posed together in group arrangements, and our Film and Video colleague captured the photos and edited them. We also realized that if the university media offices were involved in the creation of the resource, it could take a very long time to complete its production. The vetting process and the branding would not only slow down the work, but also alter its content and our intent. So we determined to produce it ourselves. And really, Sachiko made the execution of the resource happen. We struggled to free the funds to produce the resource, even though these funds had been deposited to our school as a grant award. Nothing came with ease. Except the work with and through our students.

Supporting graphics. The overall design of the visual aid establishes a sequence of six clearly numbered elements. Large blue circles with the number of elements offer structure and a sight pathway through the two-sided resource. Element one incorporated icons that communicated (1) the only transmission routes for the virus, as well as those (2) behaviors that cannot serve as transmission routes but have been erroneously thought to be pathways for the virus. See Figure 11.1 for the first element. Element four presents a color map of the Memphis area that incorporates red numbered dots correlating with free testing sites, their hours, and addresses/phone numbers (Figure 11.2).

Throughout the resource, there are three different images of our students; they represent the faces of our community members. In the end, we felt these people – our own students – were the most effective influencers. Our students were impacted by the teaching content and research project and greatly impacted the community members they recruited. As Donna had been essential to the project, we included her photo to personalize her role in facilitating testing and PrEP acquisition (Figures 11.3 & 11.4).

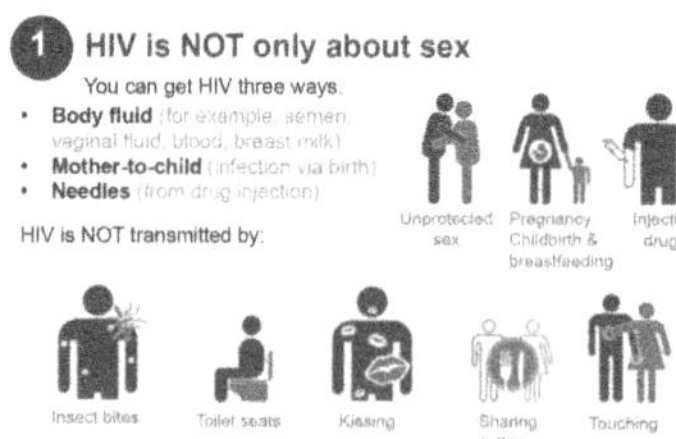

Figure 11.1 First element showing the ways HIV is transmitted.

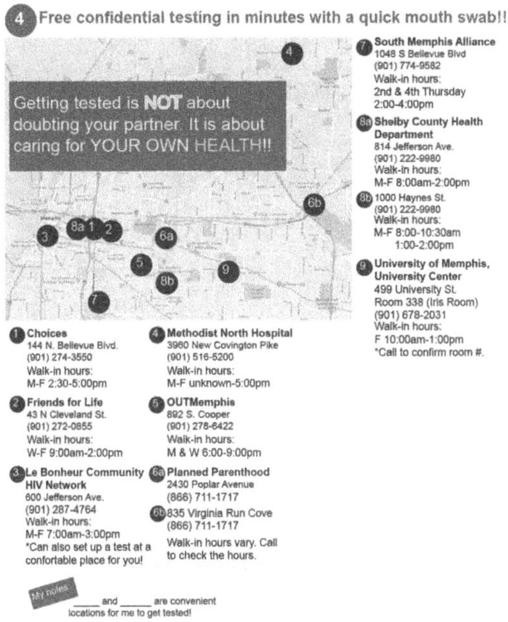
4 Free confidential testing in minutes with a quick mouth swab!!
Getting tested is NOT about doubting your partner. It is about caring for YOUR OWN HEALTH!!
4
6b
3
8a
1
2
6a
5
9
8b
7
1 Choices
144 N. Bellevue Blvd.
(901) 274-3550
Walk-in hours:
M-F 2:30-5:00pm
2 Friends for Life
43 N Cleveland St.
(901) 272-0855
Walk-in hours:
W-F 9:00am-2:00pm
3 Le Bonheur Community HIV Network
600 Jefferson Ave.
(901) 287-4764
Walk-in hours:
M-F 7:00am-3:00pm
*Can also set up a test at a confortable place for you!
4 Methodist North Hospital
3960 New Covington Pike
(901) 516-5200
Walk-in hours:
M-F unknown-5:00pm
5 OUTMemphis
892 S. Cooper
(901) 278-6422
Walk-in hours:
M & W 6:00-9:00pm
6a Planned Parenthood
2430 Poplar Avenue
(866) 711-1717
6b 835 Virginia Run Cove
(866) 711-1717
Walk-in hours vary. Call to check the hours.
7 South Memphis Alliance
1048 S Bellevue Blvd
(901) 774-9582
Walk-in hours:
2nd & 4th Thursday
2:00-4:00pm
8a Shelby County Health Department
814 Jefferson Ave.
(901) 222-9980
Walk-in hours:
M-F 8:00am-2:00pm
8b 1000 Haynes St.
(901) 222-9980
Walk-in hours:
M-F 8:00-10:30am
1:00-2:00pm
9 University of Memphis, University Center
499 University St.
Room 338 (Iris Room)
(901) 678-2031
Walk-in hours:
F 10:00am-1:00pm
*Call to confirm room #.
My notes
____ and ____ are convenient locations for me to get tested!

Figure 11.2 Free resources for testing and consultations along with a map.

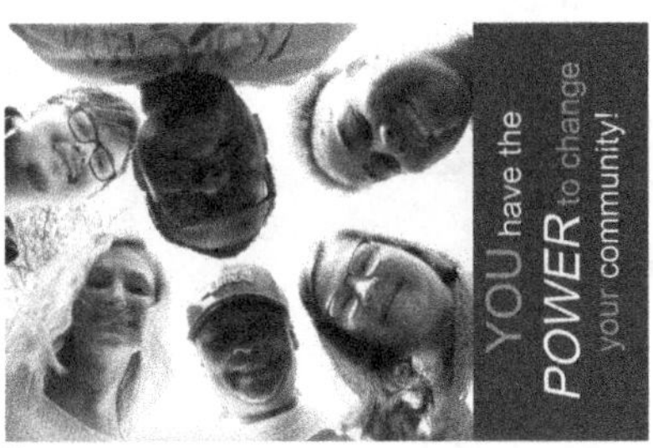
YOU have the POWER to change your community!

Front cover

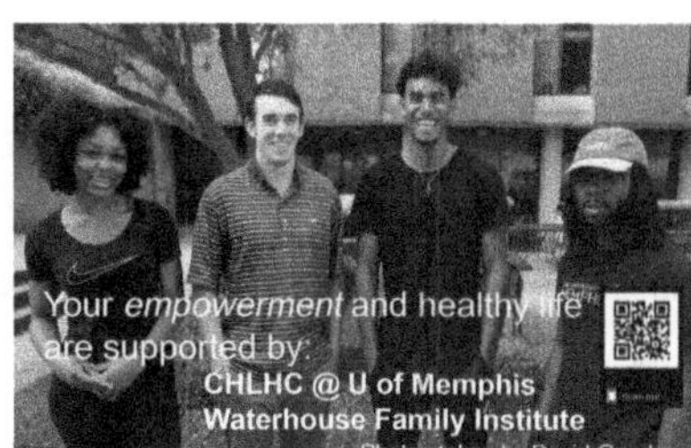
Your empowerment and healthy life are supported by:
CHLHC @ U of Memphis
Waterhouse Family Institute
Photos taken by David Goodman

Back cover

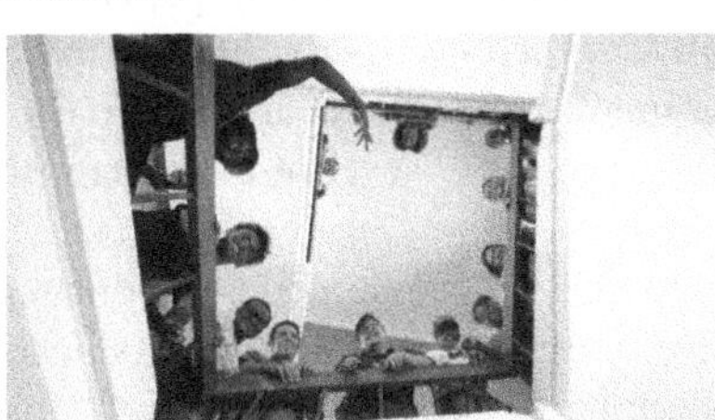

Within the visual aid

Figure 11.3 Pictures featuring our students.

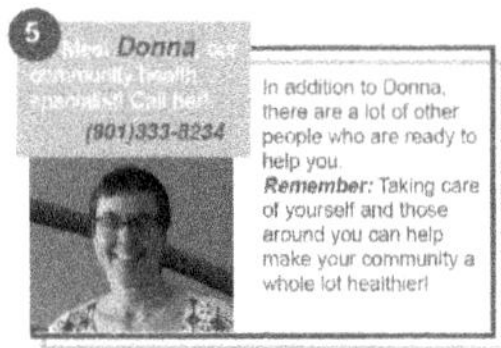

Figure 11.4 Donna's picture with her contact information.

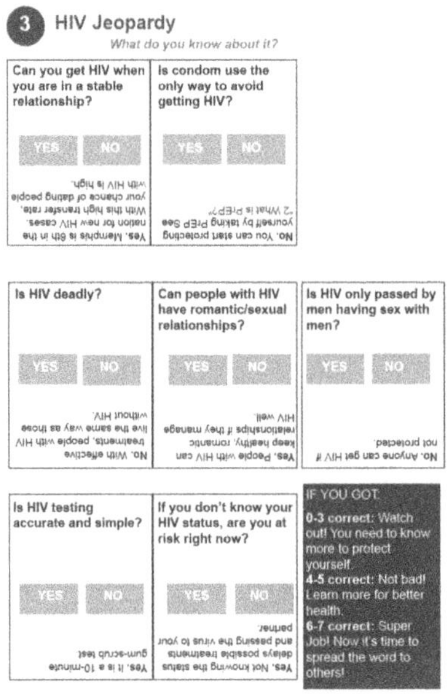

Figure 11.5 HIV Jeopardy as an interactive strategy.

User involvement. Interactive strategies and user responses were an aspect of the INDEX we wanted to employ, even though this was a fold-up paper visual aid. Element three presented "HIV Jeopardy," which invites the user to answer questions about HIV transmission and treatment, and includes answers to those questions, as well as a scoring chart to gauge the user's level of understanding (Figure 11.5).

Skill-based learning. Engaging behavioral skills is a powerful component of any intervention resource. We included a five-point prompt that presents behavioral directives that begin with the words "know," "get," "talk," "contact," and "consider." With each directive, the steps to take to accomplish this list of actions are provided. Across these five actions, getting tested for HIV, sharing knowledge with others, and reaching out to Donna are emphasized (Figure 11.6).

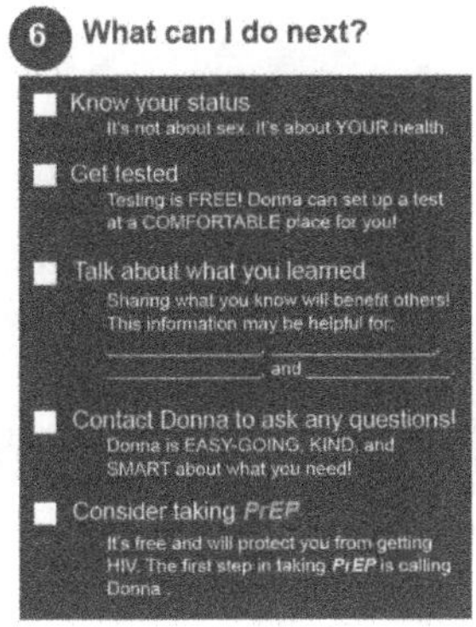

Figure 11.6 Behavioral directives prompts.

Audience appropriateness. We wanted the resource to be both discrete and appealing. We examined many different media pieces that employed varying sizes, shapes, colors, and techniques in opening and closing portions of the piece. Knowing we were attempting to impact the cycle of silence about HIV and its transmission, it was a trifurcated line to walk – discretion, normalization, and information in the form and content of the visual aid. In the end, we elected to produce a two-sided 8" × 11" piece that folded down to a 2" × 3" small, rectangular, business-card size, with cardstock covers (Figure 11.7).

We incorporated the colors of our school heavily on the piece to visually identify with our own students and the surrounding community but opted to sponsor the production through a foundation to avoid significant delays of vetting via marketing and branding departments for the university. In essence, we identified through colors with the students and their peers but did not align ourselves with the school.

> Sachiko spent hours wrangling with three different printing agencies, seeking the best price and timeline for the project so we could meet our research/teaching deadline. Finally, and due to cost, we chose to have the inside of the piece printed by one company, and the outer cardstock covers created by another. Sachiko assembled the resource covers, folded the paper, and managed all 250 copies of the visual aid by hand at her kitchen table.

Instructions. We emphasized testing to address the criteria of instruction. Correlated with the map were 11 different testing sites; their locations, hours, and phone numbers were included to guide users to those resources.

Development details. The recency of information and usefulness of contact information define this criterion. Knowing that the phone numbers, locations, hours, availability, and access were accurate was essential to creating a resource that could actually serve others. Right before we placed an order to print the materials, we called each location to confirm the address and hours.

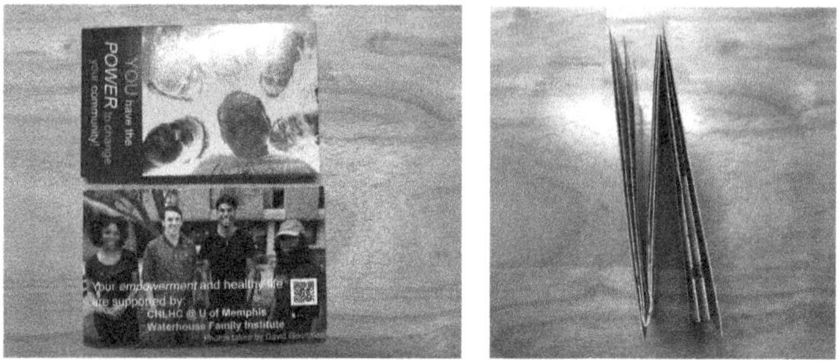

Front and back of the visual aid

Side view

Figure 11.7 Product design of the visual aid.

Evaluation and strength of evidence. Monitoring the process of resource development, the usefulness of the content, and then finally assessing the resource are addressed in this final criterion. We were fortunate to have a large team to advise us in constructing the elements in the piece. All of us were working from various perspectives but were unified by the SNS approach to the project. A communication researcher, Community Health Worker, statistician, two research assistants, and close colleagues reviewed more than ten drafts of the content and examined it for plain language, visual/meaning clarity, usefulness, alignment of purpose, access of design, and accuracy. Assessment of the outcomes of its use is detailed in the upcoming sections.

Incorporating the Visual Aid Resource into the Intervention

To examine the utility of the tailored visual aid, student-interventionists were divided into two groups and given an additional training session: (1) a control group, in which students delivered HIV intervention with the general materials (e.g., pamphlets and condoms); the student-interventionists in the control group chose what to feature in the conversations with their peers, and (2) a VHL group, in which student-interventionists were given the visual aid that had numbered contents that could guide their conversation with their peers. Regardless of the group they joined, all student-interventionists received materials, including pamphlets (e.g., "what is HIV?" "What is PrEP?" "What is an STD?") and male and female condoms as conversational facilitators. Student-interventionists reviewed the materials and were quizzed to ensure accuracy in training content.

Students had two face-to-face meetings with their network associates (peers/community members). In the first meeting, student-interventionists obtained informed consent from their network associates after thoroughly explaining the study's nature and its procedures. Student-interventionists reported that they took approximately 15 minutes on the first meeting. In the second meeting, student-interventionists in each group (control and VHL) delivered the HIV intervention to peers in the ways they were trained. The student-interventionists reported that they spent approximately 30 minutes on the second meeting, but some of the meetings exceeded an hour because peers asked questions and talked about their concerns.

The network associates completed baseline measures (Time 0: T0) following the first meeting and the second survey (Time 1: T1) after the second meeting. After a two-week interval, these peers/community members participated in the third survey (Time 2: T2). All surveys were administrated with Qualtrics online survey system to emphasize confidentiality. The appropriate university's institutional review board approved this study.

Participants

Student-interventionists identified their network associates, which included their friends, family members, classmates, roommates, and other individuals who could benefit from the HIV intervention. Student-interventionists adopted the following inclusion criteria: individuals who were (1) 18 years or older, (2) able to have two face-to-face meetings, (3) able to read and speak English, (4) able to receive and answer phone calls for verification purpose, (5) not previously recruited, and (6) able to provide informed consent.

> Students spent significant class time throughout the semester asking questions and exchanging their own strategies to deliver the PrEP/HIV communication intervention. Some students managed their peers' (possible) resistance to listen to HIV intervention by using an opening prompt like, "Hey, do you know how many people in Memphis are positive for HIV?" Others used male and female condoms as a conversational starter. "Can you guess what I got in my class today?" Recruiting participants and delivering the intervention was not easy for everyone. The students were not isolated interventionists. Guided by Donna and our class experience, they were a team.

Data Analysis

To examine the visual aid's effectiveness, we conducted a series of repeated-measures one-way analysis of variance (ANOVAs) to compare variables across three surveys/times.

Results

Of a total of 206 community members examined in the second semester of the study in which the visual aid resource was used, 142 completed all three surveys in the study. After the verification phase (phone calls to each participant), we retained 129 cases (62.4%) for analysis. Sampled participants described their gender as 65.1% female, and the majority of them described themselves as heterosexual/straight (92.2%). The mean age was 23.47 (*SD* = 6.31). Participants, as a whole, identified themselves as African American (52.7%), Caucasian (31.8%), Asian (3.1%), Hispanic (1.6%), and multiple race (10.9%). In the control group, participants identified as 38.0% African American, 49.3% Caucasian, 4.2% Asian, 1.4% Hispanic, and 7.0% multiple race. In the VHL group, participants identified themselves as 70.7% African American, 10.3% Caucasian, 1.7% Asian, 1.7% Hispanic, and 15.5% multiple race.

Participants as a whole described their relationship with student-interventionists as family (22.5%), work-related (1.6%), school-related (1.6%), friend (64.3%), and other (4.7%). Despite our efforts to randomize participants, the ratio of these relationships between the control group and the VHL group is slightly different. In the control group ($n = 71$), participants described their relationship as family (26.8%), work-related (2.8%), school-related (4.2%), friend (60.6%), and other (5.6%). On the other hand, the VHL group described their relationships with student-interventionists as family (17.2%), school-related (8.6%), friend (69%), and other (3.4%). See Table 11.1 for the demographic characteristics.

Overall, the participants received our HIV intervention quite positively (*mean* = 4.5, *SD* = 0.54). There is no statistically significant difference on their reaction based on the intervention groups: $t(127) = -0.459$, $p = 0.647$; their sexual orientation: $F(1,127) = 0.817$, $p = 0.368$; race: $F(1,10) = 0.091$, $p = 0.770$; employment status: $F(8,120) = 0.985$, $p = 0.451$; and relationships with student-interventionists: $F(4,123) = 0.308$, $p = 0.872$.

HIV Knowledge

When we combined knowledge items into one continuous variable, the repeated-measure ANOVA test revealed that participants across the two groups increased their knowledge significantly across three surveys: Wilk's $\lambda = .533$, $F(1.838, 233.443) = 72.02$, $p < .001$, $\eta^2 = .467$, but no statistically significant differences between groups were observed along with the changes: Wilk's $\lambda = .985$, $F(1.838, 233.443) = 1.020$, $p = .357$, $\eta^2 = .008$.

To examine the group differences on specific knowledge items, we conducted series of repeated-measure ANOVAs and found that the visual aid appeared to be effective or less effective on certain knowledge items. The knowledge score of the VHL group on the item "I believe HIV/AIDS is a deadly disease" increased more significantly throughout three surveys compared with the control group: Wilk's $\lambda = .954$, $F(1.796, 228.123) = 4.042$, $p = .023$, $\eta^2 = .031$. The knowledge score of the control group on the item "if a pregnant woman tests positive for HIV, she can receive treatment that will prevent her baby from becoming infected with HIV" increased more significantly throughout three surveys compared with the VHL group: Wilk's $\lambda = .610$, $F(1.643, 208.723) = 3.807$, $p = .032$, $\eta^2 = .029$. The knowledge score of the control group on the item "HIV medicine is so expensive, only rich people can afford it" increased more significantly throughout three surveys compared with the VHL group: Wilk's $\lambda = .865$, $F(1.902, 241.527) = 4.284$, $p = .016$, $\eta^2 = .033$. See Table 11.2 for complete knowledge scores.

Table 11.1 Network Associates' demographic characteristics

	Total (N = 129)	*Control group (n = 71)*	*VHL group (n = 58)*
Age	*23.47 (SD = 6.31)*	*24.28 (SD = 6.70)*	*22.65 (SD = 5.82)*
Sex assigned at birth	81 (62.8%)	47 (66.2%)	24 (41.4%)
Female	48 (37.2%)	24 (33.8%)	34 (58.6%)
Male	2 (1.6%)	2 (2.81%)	0 (0%)
Sexual orientation	7 (5.4%)	7 (9.9%)	0 (0%)
Homosexual/Gay	120 (93.0%)	62 (87.3%)	58 (100%)
Bisexual			
Heterosexual			
Race	68 (52.7%)	27 (38.0%)	41 (70.7%)
African American	41 (31.8%)	35 (49.3%)	6 (10.3%)
Caucasian	2 (1.6%)	1 (1.4%)	1 (1.7%)
Hispanic	4 (3.1%)	3 (4.2%)	1 (1.7%)
Asian	10.9%)	5 (7.0%)	9 (15.5%)
Multi race			
Occupation	48 (37.3%)	35 (49.3%)	13 (22.4%)
Employed more than 32 h/w	20 (15.5%)	8 (11.3%)	12 (20.7%)
Employed less than 32h/w	3 (2.3%)	2 (2.8%)	1 (1.7%)
Unemployed	25 (19.4%)	11 (15.5%)	14 (24.1%)
Student (not employed)	3 (2.4%)	2 (2.8%)	1 (1.7%)
Homemaker	5 (3.9%)	1 (1.4%)	4 (6.9%)
Student + employed more than 32 h/w	25 (19.4%)	12 (16.9%)	13 (22.4%)
Student + employed less than 32 h/w			

SD, Standard deviation.

Table 11.2 Changes in knowledge scores

	Control group (n = 71)			*VHL group (n = 58)*		
	T0 M (SD)	*T1 M (SD)*	*T2 M (SD)*	*T0 M (SD)*	*T1 M (SD)*	*T2 M (SD)*
Total	3.64 (.383)	4.10 (.346)	4.02 (.359)	3.66 (.367)	4.02 (.451)	3.99 (.437)
Item 1	3.32 (1.22)	3.65 (1.20)	3.41 (1.27)	3.45 (1.30)	3.24 (1.28)	3.12 (1.38)
Item 2	2.00 (.97)	2.34 (1.25)	2.45 (1.22)	2.26 (1.13)	3.28 (1.36)	3.24 (1.36)
Item 3	3.93 (1.23)	4.23 (1.14)	4.13 (1.04)	4.02 (1.13)	4.24 (.98)	4.24 (.87)
Item 4	4.73 (.51)	4.86 (.39)	4.79 (.41)	4.71 (.56)	4.74 (.48)	4.59 (.70)
Item 5	3.08 (.91)	3.87 (1.22)	3.76 (1.05)	3.14 (.85)	3.97 (.97)	3.91 (.78)
Item 6	3.34 (.86)	4.32 (.69)	4.20 (.71)	3.50 (.86)	4.03 (.88)	4.10 (.89)
Item 7	4.00 (.63)	4.41 (.62)	4.34 (70)	3.74 (.72)	4.26 (.61)	4.21 (.61)
Item 8	3.92 (.87)	4.42 (.81)	4.25 (.81)	3.84 (.86)	4.24 (.63)	4.28 (.70)
Item 9	4.59 (.62)	4.76 (.49)	4.73 (.48)	4.47 (.68)	4.56 (.66)	4.61 (.62)
Item 10	3.46 (.86)	4.17 (.81)	4.13 (.83)	3.43 (1.13)	3.59 (1.14)	3.62 (1.04)

M, mean; *SD*, standard deviation; knowledge items.

(*Continued*)

	Control group (n = 71)			VHL group (n = 58)		
	T0 M (SD)	T1 M (SD)	T2 M (SD)	T0 M (SD)	T1 M (SD)	T2 M (SD)
Item 1	I believe HIV/AIDS is an incurable disease.					
Item 2	I believe HIV/AIDS is a deadly disease.					
Item 3	People become infected with HIV only because of unprotect sex with unknown individuals.					
Item 4	Only white homosexual men get infected with HIV.					
Item 5	A person's HIV status can be determined in 10 minutes with a simple gum swab.					
Item 6	If a pregnant woman tests positive for HIV, she can receive treatment that will prevent her baby from becoming infected with HIV.					
Item 7	HIV test results are usually unreliable.					
Item 8	People can be tested for HIV at no charge.					
Item 9	You can always tell if someone has HIV by how they look.					
Item 10	HIV medicine is so expensive, only rich people can afford it.					

Vested Interest (VI)

The VI subscales were summed to examine overall vested interest. The repeated-measure ANOVA test revealed that overall vested interest increased through T0 to T2: Wilk's λ = .317, $F(1.943, 246.721) = 152.403$, $p < .001$, $\eta^2 = .545$. There was no difference on the overall VI score between two groups: Wilk's λ = .975, $F(1.943, 246.721) = 1.362$, $p = .016$, $\eta^2 = .011$. Among the changes on each of six VI variables throughout three surveys, we found that the score on *severity* among the VHL group reduced more significantly than that of the control group: Wilk's λ = .9525, $F(1.923, 244.253) = 3.188$, $p = .045$, $\eta^2 = .024$. The changes on other VI variables over three surveys did not show any group differences. See Table 11.3 for the overall VI scores.

Outcomes

Of 129 participants, 31 (24.0%) took an HIV test after receiving an HIV intervention from a student-interventionist; 10 participants (7.8%) contacted the

Table 11.3 Vested interest scores

	Control group (n = 71)			VHL group (n = 58)		
	T0 M (SD)	T1 M (SD)	T2 M (SD)	T0 M (SD)	T1 M (SD)	T2 M (SD)
Total	2.21 (.366)	2.74 (.47)	2.69 (.42)	2.20 (.33)	2.65 (.31)	2.70 (.28)
certainty	1.97 (.61)	2.33 (.75)	2.23 (.70)	1.98 (.56)	2.14 (.64)	2.23 (.57)
immediacy	1.59 (.56)	1.86 (.63)	1.87 (.63)	1.57 (.53)	1.77 (.57)	1.92 (.58)
salience	1.99 (.88)	2.12 (.80)	2.18(.90)	2.01 (.77)	2.20 (.80)	2.29 (.78)
self-efficacy	2.46 (.60)	3.01 (.58)	2.90 (.56)	2.44 (.65)	2.97 (.56)	2.95 (.52)
response-efficacy		4.41 (.64)	4.25 (.71)		4.35 (.57)	4.14 (.51)
severity	3.35 (.38)	3.34 (.40)	3.32 (.42)	3.28 (.44)	3.05 (.48)	3.12 (.59)

M, Mean; *SD*, standard deviation.

PrEP coordinator after receiving an HIV intervention; 5 participants (3.9%) are currently taking PrEP; 88 participants (68.2%) talked about HIV intervention with at least one person who is important to them; and 93 participants (72.1%) know their HIV status. The Chi-square test revealed that there are no group differences on these outcome variables.

What Does It Mean?

Overall, the intervention was successful in increasing network associates' knowledge about HIV and PrEP and vested interest to elicit recommended behaviors. To our surprise, the use of our visual aid did not bring significant difference to network associates' knowledge, vested interest, and their behaviors as a whole. However, there were slight differences observed on the subscale items. The use of our visual aid was particularly powerful in emphasizing useful, effective treatments for HIV. That is, after the intervention, network associates in the VHL group recognized HIV as a non-deadly disease. Their score on decreased severity also supports this change. The control group was more effective in emphasizing the benefits for pregnant women to protect their children and help them envision the costs associated with HIV treatment.

There is another possible explanation for the differences between two groups. Despite our efforts to randomize participants, the control group possessed more family relationships compared with the VHL group. Conversations about pregnancy and finance may have been more easily and openly discussed within family relationships compared to other types of relationships (e.g., work, school, and friends). With similar logic, relationships pertaining to work and friends may be an effective channel to deliver general, overall benefits of HIV intervention. This underscores the importance and power of existing relationships held between the message senders and recipients of the intervention when determining what resources and strategies should be featured and emphasized in the intervention.

> Donna reported that many students contacted her to ask questions and to refer their peers for testing. Throughout the semesters, our students took part in post-AIDS conversations because they understood the nature of HIV, the associated stigma, and the importance of reasonable access to resources. In the post-intervention survey, students reported that engaging in conversations about HIV intervention was at first not easy, but they were stunned to observe the positive impacts they made on their own communities. In two semesters, 97% of student-interventionists noted that they would continue to share the HIV information they learned from this project because they know it can empower others.
>
> In this journey, not so unlike other health communication intervention journeys, we see the through-line of resistance to the many steps we took along the way. Except this resistance unfortunately reified the stigma of silence we sought to weaken, not among our students but among our institutional stakeholders. We noticed deeply rooted stigma and silence surrounding HIV; colleagues had doubts about the recommendations made

in the visual resource, suspected that we were protected in our claims about transmission and safety. HIV researchers in other silos on campus were quickly uninterested in an intervention driven by visual communication and relationships. Administrators in our own piece of the academic world were critical of the course design that led students directly into the path of engaged research about HIV. There were many barriers that seemed to embody the stigma of silence that we sought to ameliorate. We stand amazed at the resilience and openness of our students to not only teach and lead others to better health literacy, but to find it for themselves over the course of this project.

***

I told my class about Ms. Barbo and her son, Timothy. I gave them the book title. It's still up for sale. She was brave – in that insular white community in central Kansas – to come out and talk about an illness that was scrubbed out of any conversations or media. I wanted to impart to my students what it was like to be witness to the massive shift in knowledge, treatment, and care of HIV between 1986 and 2020. Ms. Barbo is my indexing event, the voice I heard when going with friends to be tested, when getting my own HIV tests, and when deciding to walk into new research territory as a novice in this subject matter. Ms. Barbo's experience and willingness to share had immense significance for me. And so a student asked me, after I shared the story, "Did you ever get in touch with her and tell her?" And I hadn't. I had thought of her, remembered her, told my classes about her over the years, but had never reached out to her to let her know the lasting impact of her story and her son's life. That night, after my student inquired if I had gotten in touch, I looked up Beverly Barbo.

This study was funded by *The Waterhouse Family Institute for the Study of Communication and Society* at Villanova University, College of Arts and Sciences.

References

Baker, D. W. (2006). The meaning and the measure of health literacy. *Journal of General Internal Medicine, 21*, 878–883. https://doi.org/10.1111/j.1525-1497.2006.00540.x

Baker, D. W., Wolf, M. S., Feinglass, J., Thompson, J. A., Gazmararian, J. A., & Huang, J. (2007). Health literacy and mortality among elderly persons. *Archives of Internal Medicine, 167*(14), 1503–1509.

Berkman, N. D., Sheridan, S. L., Donahue, K. E., Halpern, D. J., & Crotty, K. (2011). Low health literacy and health outcomes: An updated systematic review. *Annals of Internal Medicine, 155*(2), 97–107. https://doi.org/10.7326/0003-4819-155-2-201107190-00005

Center for Disease Control and Prevention. (2005). Use of social networks to identify persons with undiagnosed HIV infection --- seven U.S. cities, October 2003--September 2004. *Morbidity and Mortality Weekly Report.* Retreieved from https://www.cdc.gov/mmwr/preview/mmwrhtml/mm5424a3.htm

Centers for Disease Control and Prevention. (2016). *HIV testing in the United States.* Retrieved from https://www.cdc.gov/nchhstp/newsroom/docs/factsheets/hiv-testing-us-508.pdf

Center for Disease Control and Prevention. (2017a). *HIV in the United State: At a glance.* Retrieved from https://www.cdc.gov/hiv/statistics/overview/ataglance.html

Center for Disease Control and Prevention. (2017b). *HIV surveillance report, 2016.* Retrieved from http://www.cdc.gov/hiv/library/reports/hiv-surveillance.html.

Center for Disease Control and Prevention. (2017c). *Learn about health literacy.* Retrieved from https://www.cdc.gov/healthliteracy/learn/

Collier, K. L., Colarossi, L. G., & Sanders, K. (2017). Raising awareness of pre-exposure prophylaxis (PrEP) among women in New York City: Community and provider perspectives. *Journal of Health Communication, 22*(3), 183–189.

Dawson-Rose, C., Cuca, Y. P., Webel, A. R., Solís Báez, S. S., Holzemer, W. L., Rivero-Méndez, M., … Lindgren, T. (2016). Building trust and relationships between patients and providers: An essential complement to health literacy in HIV Care. *Journal of the Association of Nurses in AIDS Care, 27*(5), 574–584. https://doi.org/https://doi.org/10.1016/j.jana.2016.03.001

Denning, P., & DiNenno, E. (2017). *Communities in crisis: Is there a generalized HIV pidemic in lmpoverished urban areas of the United States?* Retrieved from https://www.cdc.gov/hiv/group/poverty.html

Dixon, L., Salinas, M., & Marques, L. (2016). Advances and challenges in conducting research with diverse and vulnerable populations in a healthcare setting: Reducing stigma and increasing cultural sensitivity. In R. Parekh & E. W. Childs (Eds.), *Stigma and prejudice: Touchstones in understanding diversity in healthcare* (pp. 303–324). Humana Press. https://doi.org/10.1007/978-3-319-27580-2_17

Doak, C. C., Doak, L. G., & Root, J. H. (1996). *Teaching patients with low literacy skills* (2nd ed.). Philadelphia, PA: J. B. Lippincott Company.

Ergene, T., Çok, F., Tümer, A., & Ünal, S. (2005). A controlled-study of preventive effects of peer education and single-session lectures on HIV/AIDS knowledge and attitudes among university students in Turkey. *AIDS Education & Prevention, 17*(3), 268–278.

Friedman, A. L., Kachur, R. E., Noar, S. M., & McFarlane, M. (2016). Health communication and social marketing campaigns for sexually transmitted disease prevention and control: What is the evidence of their effectiveness? *Sexually Transmitted Diseases, 43*(2S), S83-S101. https://doi.org/https://doi.org/10.1097/olq.0000000000000286

Girault, P., Green, K., Clement, N. F., Rahman, Y. A. A., Adams, B., & Wambugu, S. (2015). Piloting a social networks strategy to increase HIV testing and counseling among men who have sex with men in greater Accra and Ashanti region, Ghana. *AIDS and Behavior, 19*(11), 1990–2000. https://doi.org/10.1007/s10461-015-1069-z

Gwadz, M., Cleland, C. M., Perlman, D. C., Hagan, H., Jenness, S. M., Leonard, N. R., … Kutnick, A. (2017). Public health benefit of peer-referral strategies for detecting undiagnosed HIV infection among high-risk heterosexuals in New York City. *Journal of Acquired Immune Deficiency Syndromes, 74*(5), 499–507. https://doi.org/10.1097/QAI.0000000000001257

Hersh, L., Salzman, B., & Snyderman, D. (2015). Health literacy in primary care practice. *American Family Physician, 92*(2), 118–124.

Hicks, G., Barragan, M., Franco-Paredes, C., Williams, M. V., & del Rio, C. (2006). Health literacy is a predictor of HIV/AIDS knowledge. *Health Services Research, 38*(10), 717–723.

HIV.gov. (2016). *Federal efforts to scale up PrEP and reduce new HIV infections.* Retrieved from https://www.hiv.gov/federal-response/policies-issues/prep-framework

HIV.gov. (2017). *Fast facts.* Retrieved from from https://www.hiv.gov/hiv-basics/overview/data-and-trends/statistics

Hood, J. E., & Friedman, A. L. (2011). Unveiling the hidden epidemic: A review of stigma associated with sexually transmissible infections. *Sexual Health, 8*(2), 159–170.

Kalichman, S. C., Benotsch, E., Suarez, T., Catz, S., Miller, J., & Rompa, D. (2000). Health literacy and health-related knowledge among persons living with HIV/AIDS. *American Journal of Preventive Medicine, 18*(4), 325–331. https://doi.org/https://doi.org/10.1016/S0749-3797(00)00121-5

Kaphingst, K. A., Kreuter, M. W., Casey, C., Leme, L., Thompson, T., Cheng, M. R., ... Filler, C. (2012). Health literacy INDEX: Development, reliability, and validity of a new tool for evaluating the health literacy demands of health information materials. *Journal of Health Communication, 17*(sup3), 203–221.

Kimbrough, L. W., Fisher, H. E., Jones, K. T., Johnson, W., Thadiparthi, S., & Dooley, S. (2009). Accessing social networks with high rates of undiagnosed HIV infection: The social networks demonstration project. *American Journal of Public Health, 99*(6), 1093–1099. https://doi.org/10.2105/AJPH.2008.139329

Lightfoot, M. A., Campbell, C. K., Moss, N., Treves-Kagan, S., Agnew, E., Dufour, M. S. K., ... Lippman, S. A. (2018). Using a social network strategy to distribute HIV self-test kits to African American and Latino MSM. *JAIDS: Journal of Acquired Immune Deficiency Syndromes, 79*(1), 38–45.

Linley, L., An, Q., Song, R., Valverde, E., Oster, A. M., Qian, X., & Hernandez, A. L. (2016). HIV testing experience before HIV diagnosis among men who have sex with men -21 jurisdictions, United States, 2007–2013. *Morbidity and Mortality Weekly Report.* Retrieved from https://www.cdc.gov/mmwr/volumes/65/wr/mm6537a3.htm

Mahajan, A. P., Sayles, J. N., Patel, V. A., Remien, R. H., Ortiz, D., Szekeres, G., & Coates, T. J. (2008). Stigma in the HIV/AIDS epidemic: A review of the literature and recommendations for the way forward. *AIDS, 22*, S67-S79. https://doi.org/10.1097/01.aids.0000327438.13291.62

Miller, C. H., & Adame, B. J. (2016). Scales for measuring the dimensions of vested interest. In D. K. Kim & J. Dearing (Eds.), *Health communication measures* (pp. 265–278). New York: Peter Lang.

Osborn, C. Y., Paasche-Orlow, M. K., Davis, T. C., & Wolf, M. S. (2007). Health literacy: An overlooked factor in understanding HIV health disparities. *American Journal of Preventive Medicine, 33*(5), 374–378. https://doi.org/10.1016/j.amepre.2007.07.022

Parnell, T. A. (2015). *Health literacy in nursing: Providing person-centered care.* Springer Publishing Company.

Petrocelli, J. V., Tormala, Z. L., & Rucker, D. D. (2007). Unpacking attitude certainty: Attitude clarity and attitude correctness. *Journal of Personality and Social Psychology, 92*(1), 30.

Sani, A. S., Abraham, C., Denford, S., & Ball, S. (2016). School-based sexual health education interventions to prevent STI/HIV in sub-Saharan Africa: A systematic review and meta-analysis. *BMC Public Health, 16*(1), 1069. https://doi.org/10.1186/s12889-016-3715-4

Schulz, P. J., & Nakamoto, K. (2013). Health literacy and patient empowerment in health communication: The importance of separating conjoined twins. *Patient Education and Counseling, 90*(1), 4–11. https://doi.org/http://dx.doi.org/10.1016/j.pec.2012.09.006

Siegler, A., Mouhanna, F., Giler, R. M., McCallister, S., Yeung, H., Jones, J., ... Sullivan, P. S. (2018, March). *Distribution of active PrEP prescriptions and the PrEP-to-need ratio, US, Q2 2017.* Paper presented at the Conference on Retroviruses and Opportunistic Infections, Boston, MA.

Smith, R. A. (2007). Language of the lost: An explication of stigma communication. *Communication Theory, 17*(4), 462–485. https://doi.org/doi:10.1111/j.1468-2885.2007.00307.x

Terui, S., Goldsmith, J. V., Daugherty, C. D., & Briscoe, J. R. (2019). A student-driven HIV/PrEP communication intervention using a modified social network strategy. *Journal of American College Health*, 1–5. https://doi.org/10.1080/07448481.2019.1664554

Terui, S., Huang, J., Goldsmith, J. V., Blackard, D., Yang, Y., & Miller, C. H. (2020). Promoting transformative community change for equitable health: Peer education and intervention for pre-exposure HIV prophylaxis. *Journal of Health Communication.* https://doi.org/https://doi.org/10.1080/10810730.2020.1730526

Tique, J. A., Howard, L. M., Gaveta, S., Sidat, M., Rothman, R. L., Vermund, S. H., & Ciampa, P. J. (2017). Measuring health literacy among adults with HIV infection in Mozambique: Development and validation of the HIV literacy test. *AIDS and Behavior, 21*(3), 822–832.

Witte, K., Meyer, G., & Martell, D. (2001). *Effective health risk messages: A step-by-step guide.* Thousand Oaks, CA: SAGE.

Wolf, M. S., Gazmararian, J. A., & Baker, D. W. (2005). Health literacy and functional health status among older adults. *Archives of Internal Medicine, 165*(17), 1946–1952.

Woodring, J. V., Kruszon-Moran, D., Oster, A. M., & McQuillan, G. M. (2014). Did CDC's 2006 revised HIV testing recommendations make a difference? Evaluation of HIV testing in the US household population, 2003–2010. *JAIDS Journal of Acquired Immune Deficiency Syndromes, 67*(3), 331–340.

Yuen, E. Y., Dodson, S., Batterham, R. W., Knight, T., Chirgwin, J., & Livingston, P. M. (2015). Development of a conceptual model of cancer caregiver health literacy. *European Journal of Cancer Care.* https://doi.org/10.1111/ecc.12284

Afterword

On Localocentricity and "Post-AIDS"

Ambar Basu

I start with the proposition that the dominant language of "post-AIDS" currently in circulation inflicts violence — structural violence — and necessitates a counter-call, towards *localocentricity*. As I attempt to explain why, I offer my thoughts on the dominant language of "post-AIDS," on structural violence, and the idea of localocentricity.

In her influential essay in the *Journal of Medical Humanities*, Walker (2020) rightfully argues that there is no "post" to HIV and AIDS. In other words, HIV and AIDS is a "present" phenomenon that is likely to continue to be so unless the multiple spokes of the HIV and AIDS wheel, so to speak, are adequately addressed in every part of the globe, particularly in Global South, which has historically borne and bears the inequitable burden of the disease. It is no news that health, illness, well-being, etc., are consistently imagined in technologized biomedical vocabulary. Even as researchers have emphasized and re-emphasized a focus on the social, cultural, geopolitical, and economic drivers of health, the mainstream languages on health and its corollaries derive legitimation via the myriad technocratic advances of biomedicine. While such advancements are crucial, equally – if not more – crucial are efforts to make health more equitable, and that would mean addressing the socio-cultural necessities of health, particularly for those individuals and communities at the margins of our global "civil societies."

The prevailing discourse on "post-AIDS" fantasizes a world that is free of HIV and AIDS, a world in which humans and their agents are in control of the prevention and spread of the disease; and that the condition of such a "post-AIDS" world is achievable through an undisputed harnessing of the powers of technologies such as HAART and PrEP. As Walker notes, the prevailing discourse on "post-AIDS" is made possible by biomedical innovations. Yet, it is problematic to embrace the prevailing logic of "post-AIDS" because of the (over)simplicity it accords to complex and layered phenomena like HIV and AIDS. I argue that such an embrace is not just problematic, it is tantamount to obfuscating the possibilities of structural violence embedded in "post-AIDS" logics.

Farmer (2005) has worked with the concept of structural violence for some time now. He explains that structural violence is suffering or violence that is "'structured' by historically given (and often economically driven) processes and

DOI: 10.4324/9781003000945-15

forces that conspire –– whether through routine, ritual, or, as is more commonly the case, the hard surfaces of life –– to constrain agency (p. 40)." Farmer adds that structural violence mostly occurs when locally rational choices that human agents can or are willing to make are curtailed by structures[1] such as "racism, sexism, political violence, and grinding poverty" (Farmer, 2005, p. 40). In other words, violence inflicted on human beings by structures – whereby human agents are harmed by existing structures or suffer because of an utter lack of or an inequitable access to structures necessary for a dignified and healthy life – amounts to structural violence.

Structural violence is insidious insofar as it is not easily observable; it "all too often defeats those who describe it" (Farmer, 2005, p. 40). The magnitude of suffering is so deep that it is often too difficult to render visible, represent, or narrate. I'd like to believe that to understand and document structural violence, it is imperative to make evident the erasures – of lives, voices, dignities – it creates. For example, through my research with a community of women sex workers in Kolkata, India, I have come to understand that structures of modernity create conditions for the historiographic erasure of members of this community. By that, I mean their marginalization – geographic, economic, legal, discursive, etc. – from mainstream civil society platforms such as education, employment, and democratic decision-making apparatii precludes or absents them from history; their narratives and their selves are erased from space and collective conscience – existence, in other words – now and in the future.

In an analogical rationality, "post-AIDS" conceives similar erasures – discursively and materially, for those living with HIV and AIDS (which in itself marks margins) and particularly for those at the margins of HIV and AIDS, such as (most) commercial sex workers across the globe. The authors in our book clearly reason how these violences materialize. For one, the discourse absents the fact that millions of vulnerable individuals and communities do not have access to HAART and/or PrEP. A substantial section of this population who know about these medical technologies but are not able to access them only adds to violations they face for living with HIV and/or AIDS in the first place. The dominant "post-AIDS" discourse, as a structure here, inflicts material structural violations by shifting the focus away from the need to make adequate health services available for everyone. Poverty and erratic housing, for instance, present particular challenges to prioritizing clinical care over other needs. Further, the discourse that "all will be well" IF one abides by the medical technologies of diagnosis and prevention absents the myriad of material and discursive structural violence, most profoundly, the stigma that comes with HIV and AIDS and the subsequent denial of fundamental human rights for being vulnerable to HIV and AIDS. The most vulnerable to HIV and AIDS across the globe are women and minorities, discerningly those who are historically marginalized in terms of race, gender, occupation, sexuality –– sex workers, queer individuals, and minority women, to name a few. Not to forget the "uncertainty, anxiety, ongoing negotiation (emotional, social, economic) and the many daily challenges of living with an illness without a cure" (Walker, 2020, p. 9434). In short, the prevailing "post-AIDS" rhetoric, espoused by agents who (seek to) control the global dynamics of population health as a site for aggressive profiteering (Dutta & Pal, 2020), is geared towards sustaining social, cultural, economic, and political structures that hide scars and gaping sores that living with HIV and AIDS entails in a world of increasing health (and other democratic) inequities.

My research with sex workers in India and with transgender women in sex work in the U.S. points to the deficiencies inherent in the preponderant "post-AIDS" rationality. Sex workers across the world mostly continue to live at the margins of society and at the intersectionality of various forms of discrimination. Members of the sex worker community in Kolkata, India, I interpret (in my research with the community) point to structural configurations that deny them and their children the right to even dream about a future they envisage. HIV testing, for one, is more of a marker of further discrimination and a likely loss of their ability to provide for their family. Access to HAART, much less PrEP, is more of a mirage that causes more consternation than confidence (Basu, 2011, 2017). For several transgender women in sex work who participated in my research project, their association with HIV and AIDS technologies that are at the center of the prevailing "post-AIDS" lexis, is at best layered. Some participants explained that the availability of HAART made living with HIV a manageable condition; a good number of others spoke not only of the vulnerability of HIV and AIDS as an occupational hazard, but they also emphasized the framing of their health and vulnerability to HIV and AIDS in terms of the violences they face, such as a near-complete lack of mental health services, stigma, abandonment by family and relatives, lack of social standing, lack of employment, little or very expensive access to health insurance, and medical professionals unwilling to engage with their unique health needs. I have come to understand, repeatedly, that the dominant "post-AIDS" discourse, in its quest to serve biomedical interests, is characterized by its abject expurgation of the embodied lived struggles – what I call localocentric articulations (see Basu, 2010; Basu, Ketheeswaran, & Cusanno, 2020; Dillon & Basu, 2014) – of those acutely vulnerable to HIV and AIDS.

As a counter to the prevalent "post-AIDS" discourse then, I offer a politics of localocentricity, one that is situated in an "ongoing project of recognizing the agentic capacities of peoples, communities, societies" in the "extractive spaces of the (Global) South" (Dutta & Pal, 2020, p. 349). Localocentricity refers to the idea of foregrounding those local scapes/spaces/sites within and of which the local makes its world their own. This idea offers possibilities for larger phenomena and singularity of lives to collide in slippery relationships between individual plots and collective sense-making (see Das, 2007) as individuals and communities navigate the local-global to narrativize lives in ways that often do not matter to the mainstream. Being centered on this local enables a microscopic interrogation of how macro–meso–microstructures cause violence to the margins and the simultaneous storying–repulsion–negotiation–transformation of this violence. Localocentricity invites an inversion; it embraces a call to center how the bricks of hegemonic violence are re-laid to dislocate the hegemony.

Here, the local becomes celebrated in opposition to the oppressive politics of the mainstream and the resulting erasures of the margins from discourses and materiality that are made to matter by those in control of the mainstream. This local, both messy and discrete, authenticates vocalizations of dispossession, resistance, and survival. It is intimately connected to the politics of voice in the everyday, and it becomes even more and acutely political when related to the everyday of the margins.

In the Introduction to this book, we made it clear that this collection of essays is a deliberate political effort to communicatively upend the "post-AIDS" myth and, more importantly, blow the proverbial whistle on the staggering violence it propagates. To that end, localocentricity advances a politics that denies the (euphoric) logics of an AIDS-free world marketed by agencies in the Global North that have historically monopolized the discourses and resources relevant to HIV and AIDS.

Note

1 Structures broadly refer to institutions and forms of social organizing that facilitate or limit human agents' access to resources (Basu, Ketheeswaran, & Cusanno, 2020). Structures define and limit the possibilities that are available to individuals and communities as they navigate their lived exigencies. Examples of structures are medical services, modes of transportation, legal systems, education, food, clean spaces, shelter, policies, civil society organizations, media platforms, national and international political actors, national and global health organizations, global trade and arms treaties, etc. Structures at these multiple levels work intersectionally to influence life outcomes of human agents who create and reify such structures as well as engage with them to transform them. Structures are embedded in material reality as well as in communicative practices, with one influencing the other.

References

Basu, A. (2010). Communicating health as an impossibility: Sex work, HIV/AIDS, and the dance of hope and hopelessness. *Southern Communication Journal, 75*(4), 413–432. https://doi.org/10.1080/1041794x.2010.504452.

Basu, A. (2011). HIV/AIDS and subaltern autonomous rationality: A call to re-center health communication in marginalized sex worker spaces. *Communication Monographs, 78*(3), 391–408. doi: 10.1080/03637751.2011.589457.

Basu, A. (2017). Reba and her insurgent prose: Sex work, HIV/AIDS and subaltern narratives. *Qualitative Health Research, 27*(10), 1507–1517. doi: 10.1177/1049732316675589.

Basu, A., Ketheeswaran, N., & Cusanno, B. R. (2020). Localocentricity, mental health and medical poverty in communication about sex work, HIV and AIDS among trans women engaged in sex work. *Culture, Health & Sexuality*, Advance online publication. https://doi.org/10.1080/13691058.2020.1817562.

Das, V. (2007). *Life and words: Violence and the descent into the ordinary.* Berkeley: University of California Press.

Dillon, P. J., & Basu, A. (2014). HIV/AIDS and minority men who have sex with men: A meta-ethnographic synthesis of qualitative research. *Health Communication, 29*, 182–192. https://doi.org/10.1080/10410236.2012.732911.

Dutta, M.J., & Pal, M. (2020). Theorizing from the Global South: Dismantling, resisting, and transforming communication theory. *Communication Theory, 30*(4), 349–369. doi: 10.1093/ct/qtaa010.

Farmer, P. (2005). *Pathologies of power: Health, human rights, and the new war on the poor.* Berkeley: University of California Press.

Walker, L. (2020). Problematizing the discourse of "Post-AIDS." *Journal of Medical Humanities, 41*(2), 95–105. https://doi.org/10.1007/s10912-017-9433-9.

Index

Note: **Bold** page numbers refer to tables; *italic* page numbers refer to figures and page numbers followed by "n" denote endnotes.